Diagnosis and Therapy of Tattoo Complications

Current Problems in Dermatology

Vol. 52

Series Editors

Peter Itin Basel

Gregor B.E. Jemec Roskilde

Diagnosis and Therapy of Tattoo Complications

With Atlas of Illustrative Cases

Volume Editors

Jørgen Serup Copenhagen
Wolfgang Bäumler Regensburg

242 figures, 239 in color, and 8 tables, 2017

KARGER

Basel · Freiburg · Paris · London · New York · Chennai · New Delhi · Bangkok · Beijing · Shanghai · Tokyo · Kuala Lumpur · Singapore · Sydney

Current Problems in Dermatology

Prof. Jørgen Serup
Bispebjerg University Hospital
Department of Dermatology D
Copenhagen (Denmark)

Prof. Wolfgang Bäumler
Department of Dermatology
University of Regensburg
Regensburg (Germany)

Library of Congress Cataloging-in-Publication Data

Names: Serup, Jørgen, editor. | Bäumler, Wolfgang, 1959- editor.
Title: Diagnosis and therapy of tattoo complications : with atlas of illustrative cases / volume editors, Jørgen Serup, Wolfgang Bäumler.
Other titles: Complemented by (work): Tattooed skin and health. | Current problems in dermatology ; v. 52. 1421-5721
Description: Basel ; New York : Karger, 2017. | Series: Current problems in dermatology, ISSN 1421-5721 ; vol. 52 | Complemented by Tattooed skin and health / volume editors, Jørgen Serup, Nicolas Kluger, Wolfgang Bäumler.
Basel ; New York : Karger, 2015. | Includes bibliographical references and indexes. | Includes bibliographical references and index.
Identifiers: LCCN 2016059608 (print) | LCCN 2016059920 (ebook) | ISBN 9783318059779 (hard cover : alk. paper) | ISBN 9783318059786 (e-ISBN) | ISBN 9783318059786 (e-book)
Subjects: | MESH: Tattooing--adverse effects | Laser Therapy--methods | Tattooing--methods | Skin Diseases--diagnosis | Skin Diseases--therapy
Classification: LCC GT2345 (print) | LCC GT2345 (ebook) | NLM WR 140 | DDC 391.6/5--dc23
LC record available at https://lccn.loc.gov/2016059608

Bibliographic Indices. This publication is listed in bibliographic services, including Current Contents® and Index Medicus.

Disclaimer. The statements, opinions and data contained in this publication are solely those of the individual authors and contributors and not of the publisher and the editor(s). The appearance of advertisements in the book is not a warranty, endorsement, or approval of the products or services advertised or of their effectiveness, quality or safety. The publisher and the editor(s) disclaim responsibility for any injury to persons or property resulting from any ideas, methods, instructions or products referred to in the content or advertisements.

Drug Dosage. The authors and the publisher have exerted every effort to ensure that drug selection and dosage set forth in this text are in accord with current recommendations and practice at the time of publication. However, in view of ongoing research, changes in government regulations, and the constant flow of information relating to drug therapy and drug reactions, the reader is urged to check the package insert for each drug for any change in indications and dosage and for added warnings and precautions. This is particularly important when the recommended agent is a new and/or infrequently employed drug.

www.karger.com
Printed on acid-free and non-aging paper (ISO 9706)
ISSN 1421–5721
e-ISSN 1662–2944
ISBN 978–3–318–05977–9
e-ISBN 978–3–318–05978–6

Contents

Preface

This book is prepared as a small textbook for fellow clinicians, who in the future will face patients suffering from tattoo complications. Tattoo complications is a new subspecialty in medicine; however, this new field has not yet been integrated in medical education. In view of the high number of tattooed individuals, clinicians will consistently see patients with health problems in tattooed skin. However, clinicians often have doubts about how to diagnose and treat these complications.

It is important to recognize that patients with tattoo complications truly are patients since their disease burden is comparable to other cumbersome skin diseases. Patients with tattoos have to some degree been neglected in the past. There are many patients with tattoo complications but they are scattered over many specialties.

The topic of this book deserves special attention because tattooing, which is minor surgery, is an unauthorized injection of significant amounts of pigment particles and myriads of chemicals of tattoo inks into the human body with a broad spectrum of possible risks. These are displayed in the clinical setting where the treating doctor encounters the clinical manifestations on a face-to-face basis so to speak. The field of tattoo complications is refined and not easy. Fortunately, many tattooed individuals do not suffer complications and just enjoy having their tattoo.

Refined diagnosis and disease classification are the requisites to rational therapy. Laser removal of tattoos is covered in four chapters including novel treatment. Surgical treatment of complications is covered in a separate chapter with dermatome shaving as a prioritized method along with a review of medical treatment options. A summary chapter presents a guide to treatment of tattoo complications and tattoo removal.

Last but not least, an extensive material of cases illustrating the different types and classes of tattoo complications is displayed in the format of an atlas including selected clinical photos and brief case summaries with comments and educational notes. The clinician can use this atlas for pattern recognition and as a visual guide to diagnosis of new cases. The atlas follows the new diagnosis classification system described in the book and submitted to the WHO International Classification of Diseases 11th revision (ICD-11).

This book on the diagnosis and therapy of tattoo complications is printed in the series Current Problems in Dermatology by Karger Publishers, Switzerland, as volume 52 – a follow-up of the recently published book *Tattooed Skin and Health*, volume 48, 2015, of the same series. Volume 48 describes basics, cultures, practices, as well as general health aspects and regulations of tattooing including the many safety issues related to tattoo inks. The two books are complementary, and one book is indispensable relative to the other if deep insight in all aspects of the topic is sought. Karger Publishers has taken a further initiative to support research and education in the field of tattoo complications by including the new section Tattoo and Body Art in their classical and fully indexed journal *Dermatology*, originally started in 1893. With this triplet, Karger Publishers has been established as the world leader in scientific publication in the field of tattooing.

The European Society of Tattoo and Pigment Research (ESTP) inaugurated in 2013 in Copenhagen, Denmark, stands behind the mentioned publications. The ESTP organizes biannual international congresses: Copenhagen 2013, Bruges 2015, and Regensburg 2017.

This book was only possible thanks to generous contributions of the esteemed faculties of the chapter authors. Karger Publishers also did a marvelous job with this book, and it was a privilege to work with the Karger team.

Jørgen Serup, MD, DMSc,
Professor of
Dermatology and Chairman of ESTP
The 'Tattoo Clinic', Bispebjerg University
Hospital, Copenhagen, Denmark

Wolfgang Bäumler, MSc, PhD
Professor and Treasurer of ESTP
University of Regensburg, Department of
Dermatology, Regensburg, Germany

Serup J, Bäumler W (eds): Diagnosis and Therapy of Tattoo Complications. With Atlas of Illustrative Cases.
Curr Probl Dermatol. Basel, Karger, 2017, vol 52, pp 1–17 (DOI: 10.1159/000450773)

From Technique of Tattooing to Biokinetics and Toxicology of Injected Tattoo Ink Particles and Chemicals

Jørgen Serup

The 'Tattoo Clinic', Department of Dermatology, Bispebjerg University Hospital, Copenhagen, Denmark

Abstract

Tattoo colourants are colourful nano- and microparticles, which are practically insoluble and thus permanent once installed in the dermis by the tattooist. Tattoo ink also has soluble ingredients and contaminants. Pigments can distribute via the lymph and possibly also directly to the blood, and a minute fraction may over time undergo metabolic breakdown and as hapten(s) induce allergic reactions of red tattoos. Carbon black of black tattoos has a tendency to agglomerate and form larger bodies that can elicit foreign body reactions in black tattoos and even granuloma formation with overlap to sarcoidosis in the clinic. Very little is known about the biokinetics and safety profile of the many tattoo pigments in use, and no specific pigment-related chemical of tattoo ink causing identified adverse reactions in humans has been depicted. Inks have many ingredients and contaminants. Insoluble and soluble ingredients of inks supposedly have very different characteristics of absorption, distribution, metabolism, and excretion, with pigments being extremely slowly excreted, contrasting soluble ingredients with fast elimination. Tattoos are a single-dose exposure. Controlling the safety of tattoo inks by banning potentially critical chemicals hitherto has been unsuccessful due to lacking documentation of clinical and epidemiological relevance and because the tattoo industry is already internationally established, free, and in the ownership of the people. Doctors treating patients with tattoo complications consequently have a key role in identifying risk situations and local outbreaks, which needs clarification, therapy, and the intervention of authorities. In the treatment of complications, as seen in general practice and in other specialties, basic insight into the fate of tattoo pigments in the body is necessary. Tattoo complications are complicated and facetted with many entities and disease mechanisms; they are a new subspecialty in medicine and dermatology.

Tattooing – the permanent decoration of the skin after installation or injection of physical colourants in the dermis – is old and dates millennia back [1, 2]. Tattoos made a historical move from the original use by tribes in the pacific region, the orient, Africa, South and North America, Greenland, and the arctic zone to sailors, who introduced tattoos in the harbour cities of Europe and made them popular among lower-class people. A

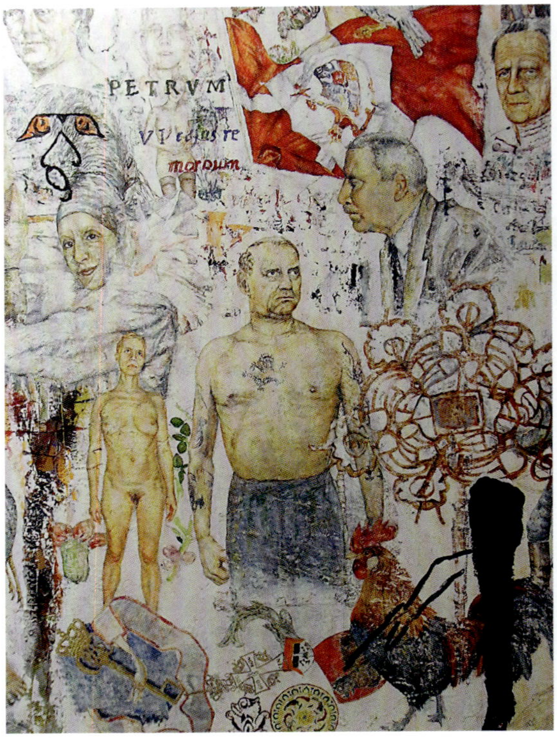

Fig. 1. Frederik IX, King of Denmark from 1947 to 1972. The tattooed king is displayed in a large fresco-style painting in the foyer of a ministerial building in Copenhagen, made by H.C. Rylander from 1990 to 2002. The painting illustrates the history of Denmark and includes points of recent changes of civil and national life. The king's more formal portrait is painted in small size in the upper right corner. The painting was made from an authentic photo of the king, which was displayed in the window of 'Tato-Jacks' tattoo parlour in Nyhavn 17, Copenhagen, the world's oldest tattoo parlour still in business. The police had the portrait removed the day after the photo was put on display in the window, but English and Swedish newspapers nevertheless published it as a shocking photo.

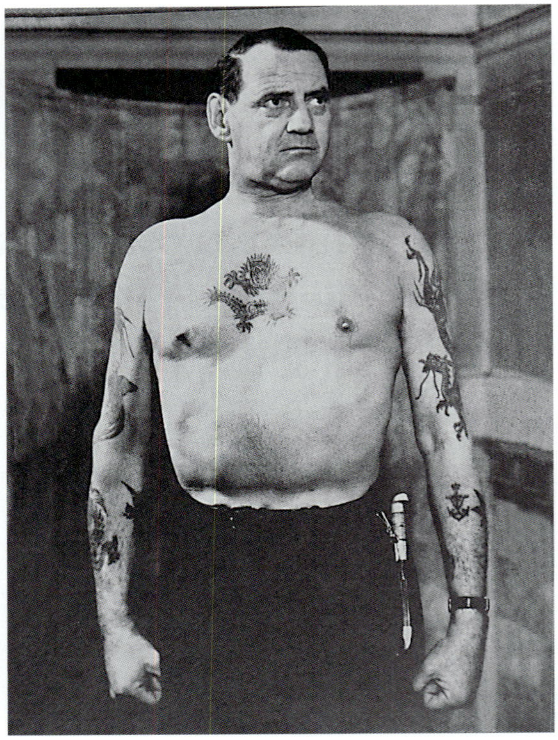

Fig. 2. The original photo of Frederik IX on display in the tattoo parlour Nyhavn 17, Copenhagen. In the photograph, the king spontaneously positioned himself as laymen proud of their large tattoos typically do: breast high, firm look to one side, pronated arms, and handgrip.

more recent move was from the use among criminals and prostitutes in the beginning of the 20th century to the present situation with a broad acceptance of tattoos widely independent of social class, with tattoos even being used by kings (fig. 1). Nevertheless, many people today still consider tattoos to be a negative social stigma closing opportunities in life, and there is an ever-ongoing conflict with the natural skin ideal.

Today some 15% of the population of industrialised countries are tattooed, with a double prevalence in youngsters; recently with females and males being tattooed equally frequent [2]. From prevalence measured in a number of countries, nearly 100 million Europeans and about 500 million global citizens can be estimated to be tattooed. Among various subgroups with a special affection to tattoos, there is a group of people, who develop an addiction to tattoos and become extensively tattooed all over the skin (fig. 2). Being heavily exposed, they represent a special risk group of toxicological interest.

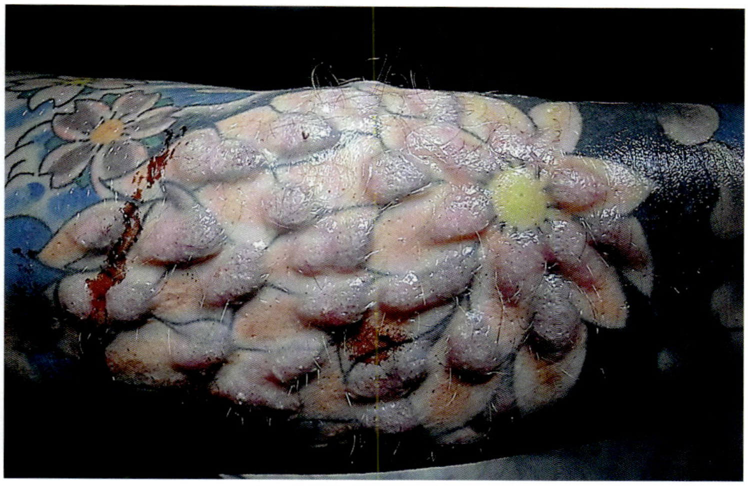

Fig. 3. Allergic tattoo reaction in the colour red with excessive hyperkeratosis on the forearm of a man.

Tattooing spontaneously grew to magnum size over the last century, in particular in the recent two decades. Now it is established as a huge industry with many commercial stakeholders; nevertheless, it is still wild and in the ownership of the people. Tattooing grew big before modern societies developed strict regulations of other fields of chemical exposure of the human body to risk elements such as drugs as well as industrial and environmental chemicals including carcinogens and pollutants in contact with skin. Today the tattoo business with tattooists and manufacturers of tattoo inks, needles, and other utilities, such as tattoo machines, is remarkably little regulated and a free bird working smoothly across national borders, helped by Internet trades. This situation contrasts the sophisticated, influential national and international regulation of drugs, cosmetics as well as nutritional and other products. The tattoo industry has different strata, some who are responsible, others not.

Compared to other exposures of the skin and the human body, tattooing of today is probably the largest ongoing global experiment on exposure of humans to rather unknown chemicals and particles introduced into the body by direct injection of the skin. Fortunately, major hazards with many victims apparently have not happened, and the empiric and not protocolled experiment of tattooing has until now not provoked a situation in which regulators were forced to limit the business. However, the risk of the tattooed is surely not nil, and an increasing number of complications associated with tattooing, as exemplified by infections and allergies, grew up parallel to its popularity. Today tattoo complications are a challenge to the health system. Doctors in general practice and in various specialties shall be prepared to diagnose and treat tattoo complications in the future. Complications are presently treated by different specialties, but it is a new subspecialty in dermatology (fig. 3).

The European Union has very recently defined tattoo inks as consumer products and established expert groups, who have published extensive reports on standards for measurement of ingredients of inks and the state of play, with a final report on tattoo safety including a review of the clinical panorama of complications and known hazards [3–5]. The Council of Europe published resolutions on critical substances in tattoo inks back in 2003, with an update in 2008 called ResAp(2008)1 [6]. Despite major limitations of this

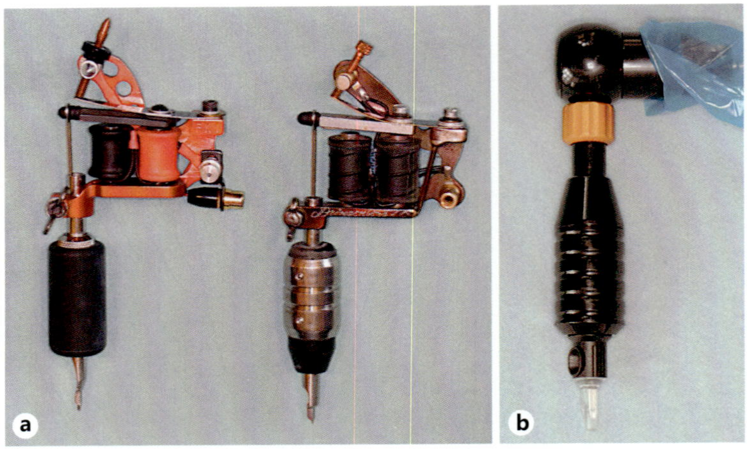

Fig. 4. a Examples of electric coil machines, the dominating type of machine for the last century. Needles and handgrip are separate units, which can be autoclaved by the tattooist or bought as single-use or integrated units. **b** Rotor machine only working with single-use integrated needle and handpiece. The motor is in a closed compartment.

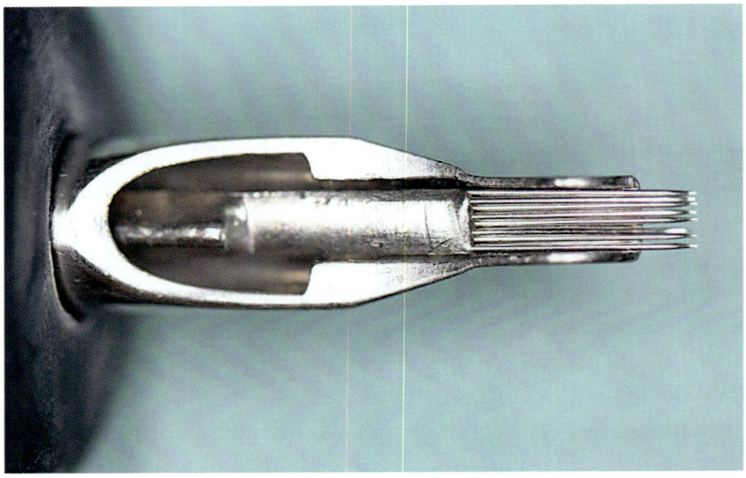

Fig. 5. Modern needle of the type 'shader' with a number of stylus needles amalgamated into a brush.

guide as to clinical and epidemiological significance, some countries nevertheless introduced national regulations with 'negative lists' copied from the resolution but included no 'positive list' directing towards safer tattooing in future practice. Relevant literature also include the book *Dermatologic Complications with Body Art*, the book *Tattooed Skin and Health* (Karger Publishers), the comprehensive report 'Tattoos – Health, Risks and Culture' published by the Danish Council on Health and Disease Prevention, and a detailed toxicological review in *The Lancet* by Laux et al. [2, 7–9].

Tattooing: Techniques and Practices

The basic technique of tattooing has remained the same since the beginning, namely penetration of the epidermal barrier with several needle pricks allowing the colourant to find its way via the needle track to a permanent position in the outer part of the dermis. Originally, tattooing was made by hand using a primitive sharp instrument shaped like a pen. The colourants were crude materials such as soot or natural minerals found in nature. Since about the year 1900, electric machines based on electromagnetism and with a coil engine have be-

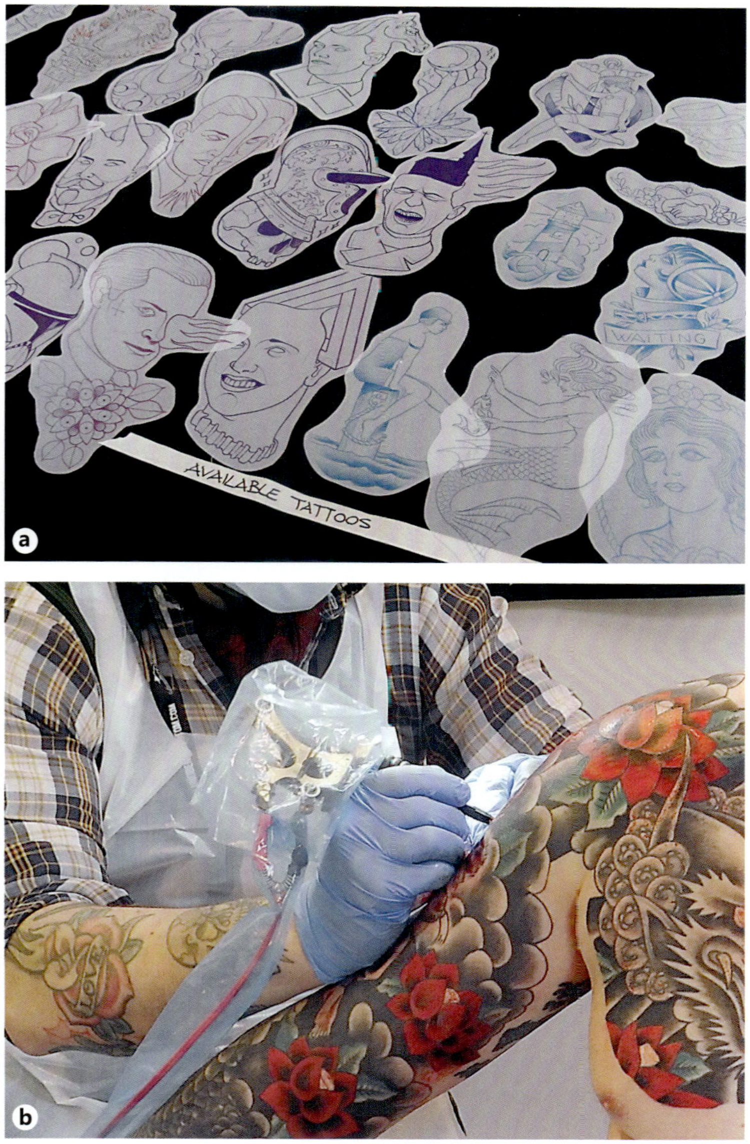

Fig. 6. a Tattooists' display of a selection of tattoo motifs available to the customer. A motif is copied onto the skin and then tattooed. **b** A tattooist during operation. The tattooist dips the tip of the needle from time to time in a small cup with the ink, which is similar to handwriting with a steel pen in the old days. Inks can be mixed or diluted with water.

come extensively used and finally came to dominate the tattoo industry all over the world, blooming with the increasing popularity of tattoos among people (fig. 4a, b). Very recently, motor-driven rotor machines of the type 'Hawk Cheyenne' have become commonly used. Rotor machines are easier to keep clean and they work with a single-use and sterilised hand piece with an integrated needle (fig. 5).

Tattooists, who may be more or less experienced, mostly perform tattoos. It is an art and craftsmanship that shall be learned over a period of time and under supervision. Tattoos can be based on samples from a catalogue copied on the skin or individualised depending on the customer's wish (fig. 6a, b). As mentioned, tattooists use electric coil machines and rotor machines. The

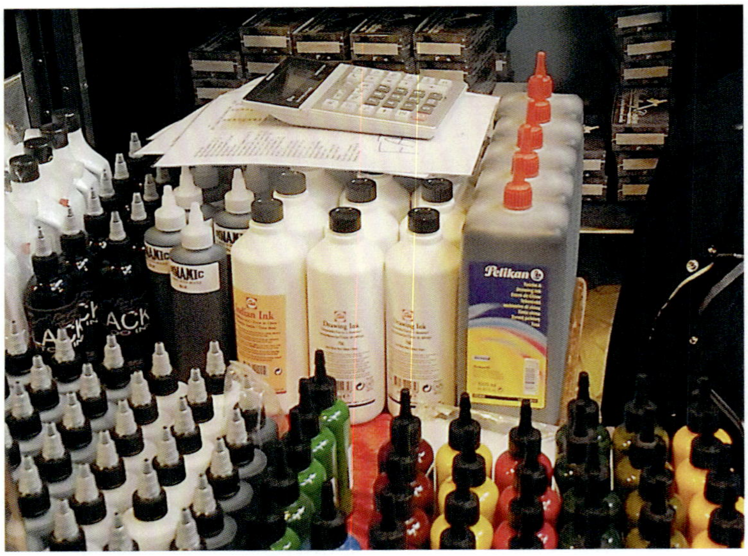

Fig. 7. Tattoo inks for sale at a tattoo convention in Copenhagen. Hundreds of products are offered, including Indian and Pelikan ink used by architects, artists, and others for writings and drawings on paper. The producer of Pelikan ink directly states on the product label that the product is not for tattooing.

basic needle is a simple and solid metal stylus, which is different from a hollow medical injection needle with a channel inside. Tattoo needles are divided into 'liners' and 'shaders'. A 'liner' is used for the initial drawing of the contour of the tattoo from a template. It is typically made with three individual stylus needles amalgamated in one final needle with the profile of a triangle. The needle is dipped into a small cup with ink. The tattoo ink held between the three needles then makes its way into the skin by the oscillating manoeuvre of the needle driven by the engine and dose the ink as the needle repeatedly penetrates the epidermal barrier. A tattoo machine performs some 3,000 needle oscillations per minute. The tattooist controls the depth of the injection, the number of passes, the total amount of ink on the needle, and by constantly wiping the skin under supervision of the operation also directly the amount of ink being injected, making up the tattoo with the desired intensity of colour. 'Shaders' are composed of 4–16 needles or more amalgamated in 1 broad needle working like a brush. There are several types and profiles. 'Shaders' are used for filling out the motive between the linings and they dose the colourant in the skin in a horizontally even distribution. The dose of tattoo ink injected in the body is primarily dependent on the area of the tattoo, the tattoo instrument, the type of needle used, and the tattooist. There is no fixed or standardised dose. Obviously, the dose of tattoo ink per surface area and the total exposure of the body to a specific ink must show huge variation. Tattooing is, as a fundamental fact, single-dose exposure and not chronic or accumulative dosing. It is one shot of many different bullets.

Tattoo needles vary a lot in technical quality, which can be easily checked under a magnifying lens or a surface microscope. Some needles may be falsely marked with the European quality stamp CE. Some contain nickel. Needles of poor quality are more traumatic to the skin and may have hooks that traumatise and make cuts. The dose and absorption of tattoo ink are obviously higher if the needle having or not having a hook traumatises the skin, if the tattooist is an amateur, and if the tattooists deliberately inject too much ink ambitious to produce a densely coloured tattoo as the customer may wish or even insist on. Some tattoos are performed by amateurs at home

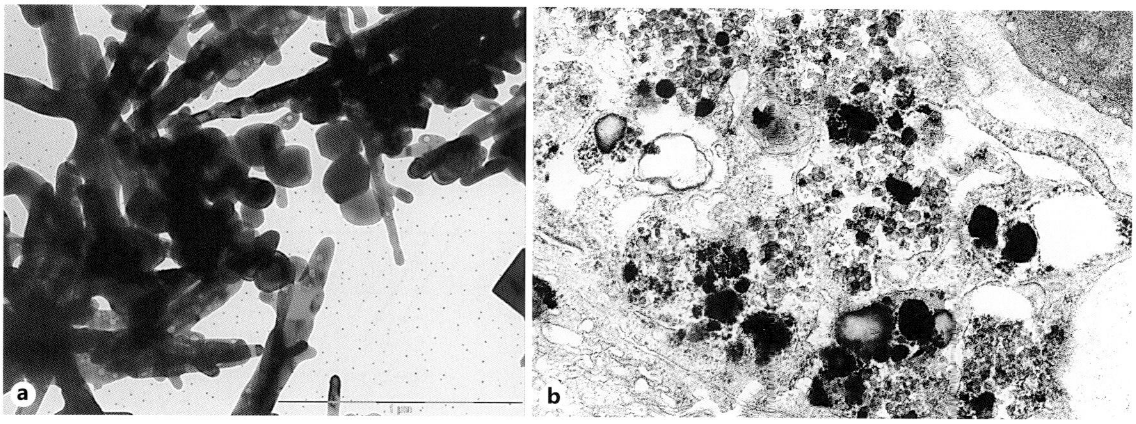

Fig. 8. a Scanning electron microscopy of tattoo pigment in a commercial tattoo ink stock product with primary particles sized <100 nm, i.e. nanoparticles. Particles tend to agglomerate already in the ink bottle. Courtesy of Panum Institute, Copenhagen. **b** Transmission electron microscopy of tattooed human skin. Detail of a mast cell with irregular pigment elements in the cytoplasm indicating the physical breakdown of particles. Courtesy of Dr. T. Kobayasi, Bispebjerg University Hospital, Copenhagen.

and under primitive conditions, others in outdoor markets and at parties. The vast majority of tattoos are made by professional tattooists in their parlours.

Cosmetic tattoos, also called permanent make-up, are mostly performed by cosmetologists. Their instruments are essentially identical to the instruments used by tattooists and work according to the same principle, albeit they are often more refined and of higher quality. Pencil-shaped and elegant rotor machines with a single-use integrated hand piece and needle dominated the permanent make-up business for years. In the USA, the term 'micropigmentation' was introduced in 1986 [10]. According to European standard, it is synonymous to cosmetic tattooing and permanent make-up. Instruments and inks commonly used in this business represent no special technique or principle, neither regarding instrument nor regarding specific pigments or inks used, albeit colour libraries differ, with some inks claimed to be 'semipermanent'. There are a countless number of different tattoo needles and machines.

Tattoo Colourants and Inks

Tattoos are made to mark the skin permanently with colour from a tattoo ink stock product (fig. 7). Black and red are the most popular colours, but a broad range of other colours and nuances is used. The colourant is not a soluble chemical but a pigment particle, i.e. a physical particle sized from about 30 to 6–800 nm depending on the type of pigment (fig. 8a, b) [11]. Black pigment, carbon black, is smaller and in the nanoparticle range, i.e. sized less than 100 nm. Pigment particles are of extremely low solubility in hydrophilic and lipophilic solvents. The low solubility of pigments is the key prerequisite behind their robustness and permanent stay in the dermis. Robustness also implicates that pigments are highly resistant to enzymatic and other modes of breakdown in the tissues including digestion by macrophages. Pigments often are chemically coated to make them stable without too much aggregation and agglomeration happening during production, storage, and use [12]. Pigment particles have an electric load on the surface. Some are physiochemically active, in particular carbon black. Carbon black

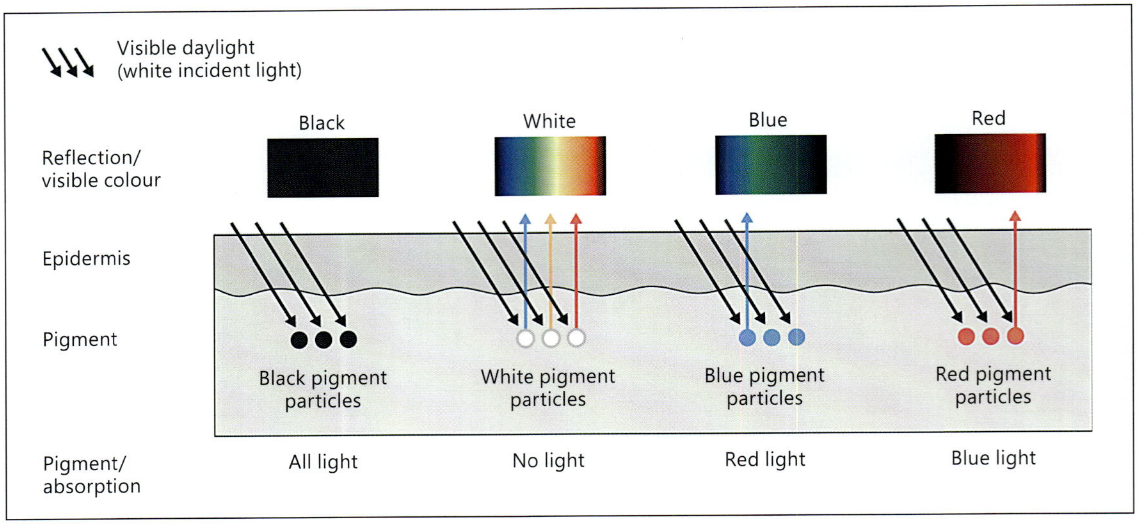

Fig. 9. Illustration of the interaction between incident white daylight (indicated with black arrows) and the reflected light of different colours, depending on the pigment inside the skin in differently coloured tattoos. The incident daylight penetrates the epidermis and contains all primary colours in full spectrum. Black pigment absorbs all light, in contrast to white pigment, which reflects every part of the spectrum. Coloured pigments absorb the complementary colour to the reflected light, which appears as the tattoo's colour. For example, the red pigment absorbs the blue-green part of the light, but not the red part, which then can be reflected and creates the tattoo's visible colour as seen from outside, red. Reproduced with permission from the Council on Health and Disease Prevention [2].

may over time and in situ in the dermis agglomerate and form large clusters sized several microns. The host organism may perceive such large agglomerates as foreign bodies, resulting in an inflammatory response causing symptoms [13]. The foreign bodies sometimes result in classical granuloma formation in the tattoo and even trigger sarcoidosis in other organs, supposedly by an autoimmune mechanism [14, 15].

Pigments of today are industrial materials produced as raw materials in enormous amounts for several purposes other than tattoo inks [16]. The chemical purity can be as low as 80%, thus with many contaminants and unknown chemicals. Azo pigments with the azo group –N=N– and phthalocyanines with a polycyclic molecular structure and copper are commonly used as red and green/blue pigments. Tattoo ink stock products are dispersions of pigments in water with a number of other ingredients added such as tensides, whiteners, and fillers including silica and barium sulphate. Witch hazel extract and shellac may be added to make the ink have a desired viscosity. A number of inks contain preservatives such as parabens. Some established manufacturers label the main ingredients, but many do not. The Colour Index (CI) number indicates the chemical class of the main pigment. The Chemical Abstract Service (CAS) registry number indicates the precise chemical name and structure of the pigment chemical.

The colour of a tattoo as perceived by the eye is the result of daylight absorbed by the tattoo pigment in the dermis and the light reflected back to the surroundings of wavelengths not being absorbed by the pigment particles (fig. 9). Thus, pigments are automatically photoactive with absorption of light in a special range of the light spectrum, determining the colour we visually see. Absorption may result in photochemical process-

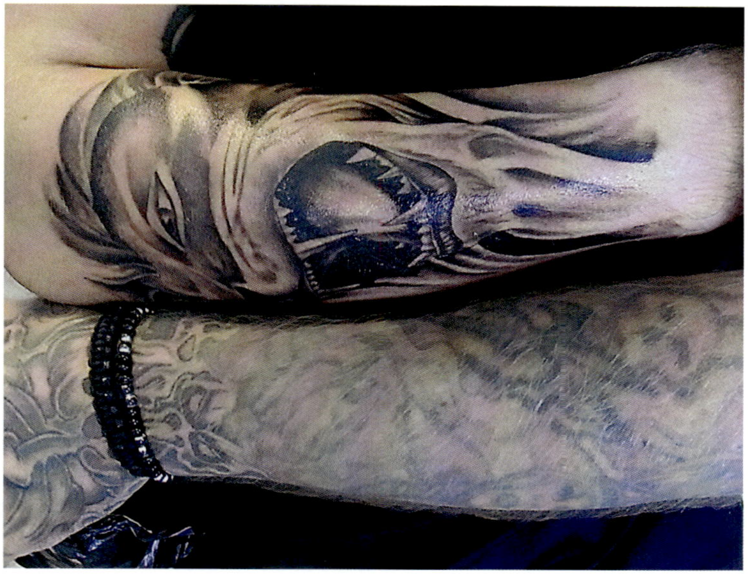

Fig. 10. Newly tattooed skin of the forearm (top) compared to skin of the opposite side tattooed only a few years before (bottom).

es with some active breakdown of pigment to a range of chemical split products in particular if the pigment absorbs light in the blue end of the spectrum (the tattoo colour then visible is red) or directly in the UV band. The closer the absorbance is to UV, the stronger the photochemical energy. Red pigment is, for the reason of basic physics, more prone to photochemical breakdown and, therefore more easily undergoes bleaching over time. Thus, the tattoo colour itself together with exposure to sun and daylight over time influence the chemical breakdown of pigments into metabolites, with the risk that toxic, sensitising, or otherwise dangerous chemicals are formed, with the red end of the spectrum among all colourful pigments being of higher potential risk of unforeseeable events.

Injected Dose of Tattoo Ink and Local Distribution in the Skin

It is known that new tattoos are brighter in colour than older tattoos, and sometimes the tattoo may completely lose the original colour (fig. 10). Thus, over decades, some change of the pigment may occur, with visible disappearance of pigment from the tattoo. However, the chemical breakdown with pigment replaced by metabolites that can be colourless does not automatically mean that the pigment chemicals were completely washed out of the skin. Other processes such as epidermal changes, redistribution of pigment in the skin, and dermal fibrosis may also blur the visual impression and make the tattoo look bleached. Nevertheless, it is likely that in most tattoos, at least some slow elimination of pigment takes place over years. Moreover, regarding the formulation and particularly regarding the pigment, tattoo ink shall be seen as an extremely slow-release formulation.

When making a tattoo, an amount of tattoo ink is injected in the dermis (fig. 11a, b). Already during tattooing, some pigment flows back via needle tracts to become wiped off by the tattooist as part or normal routine. During early healing, a significant amount of the ink originally deposited in the dermis escapes backwards to the skin surface and the bandage, where pigment may be observed in the debris from the tattoo wound. If in-

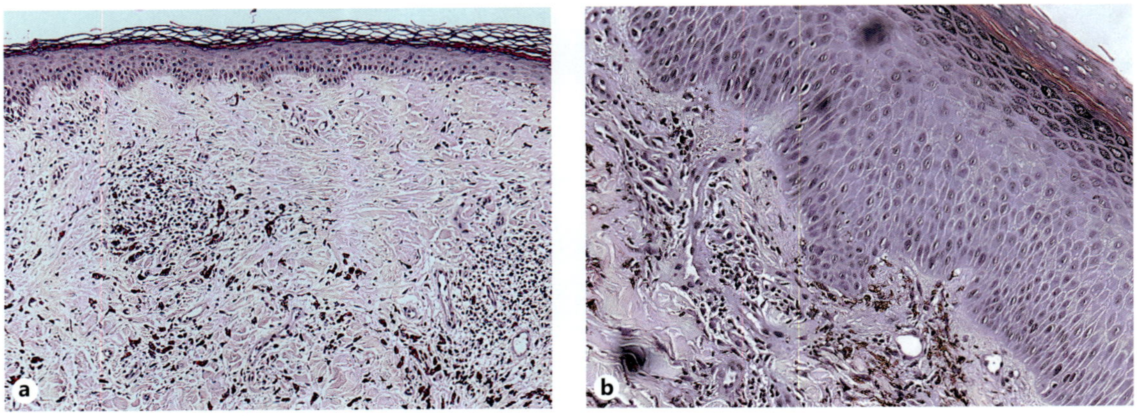

Fig. 11. a Skin biopsy from tattooed skin with an allergy to red pigment. HE stain. Clusters of pigment and lymphocytic infiltration accumulate around blood vessels and under the epidermis. Clusters represent large agglomerates. Primary particles are under the resolution of light microscopy, as are breakdown chemicals released from particles and the hapten responsible for the allergic reaction. **b** Detail from the outer dermis and epidermis with subepidermal pigment, cellular infiltration, and a discrete agglomerate of pigment, which has escaped over the basement membrane on its way out of the skin.

fection occurs, large amounts of pigment may escape to the surface, leaving colourless dots or general weakening of colour of the tattoo after healing. Escape of pigment to the surface ends when the basement membrane between epidermis and dermis is healed, which happens after 1–2 weeks. Pigments normally cannot pass this barrier and thus are trapped in the dermis despite their spontaneous tendency to drift out of the skin. Pigments of the dermis originally installed in the vertical needle tracks down to mid-dermal level shortly after installation relocate and move towards the surface, as described above, but also with a move following the interstitial flow directed the way of lymphatic drainage of that tattooed skin site as well as the blood vessels. Shortly after tattooing, pigments may appear in the regional lymph nodes and cause tenderness and swelling. Lymph nodes are quite efficient in stopping tattoo pigment. Nodes store pigments for years. Thus, the regional lymph nodes are tattooed invisibly along with the skin. The perivascular tissue with collagen envelopes is a relative barrier to particles, which tend to concentrate and accumulate in the perivascular tissue. According to a study on gold particles in mice and rats, some unknown fraction of small-sized particles pass directly to the blood, become circulated, and reach a variety of distant organs [17–19]. Soluble ingredients of inks have different biokinetics and are distributed directly to the blood.

The precise dose of tattoo pigment injected in human skin by tattooing cannot be determined with acceptable precision and thus remains unknown. The percentage of pigment in tattoo ink by w/v typically is in the range of 10–30%. Rodents' skin is thin and, when it comes to tattooing, not suitable as a conclusive experimental surrogate of human skin. Nevertheless, elegant studies in mice on selected pigments can when extrapolated to human skin maybe illustrate some theoretical magnitude of order of pigment in the dermis [20, 21]. Studies demonstrate large amounts of tattoo chemicals and their breakdown products being deposited in tattooed mice skin, with accumulation of chemicals in sentinel nodes. These studies were followed by one study on pigskin and one on human cadaver skin [22, 23]. Experimental studies clearly indicate that red and yellow azo pigments are sensitive to photochemical breakdown, and over time, a significant amount of pigment disappears out of the skin [24, 25]. However, there remains a huge knowledge gap regarding the very many aspects of tattoo pigments, chemicals and human skin including the influence of sun, daylight and laser light. Obviously, experiments with one class of pigment or a few model pigments, such as the azo pigment named pigment red 22, cannot be uncritically extrapolated to every pigment in general use. Carbon black, titanium dioxide, and iron oxide pigments are expected to have other characteristics than azo pigments. Many variables determine the local dose. These are anatomical site, skin thickness, elasticity and other features of the skin, the tattoo consisting of one or several colours, the area of tattooed skin, the desired colour intensity of the tattoo, the percentage of pigment in the ink and ink viscosity, the instruments used for tattooing, in particular the needle, and the professional performance of the tattooist. The tattooist can be a professional tattooist, a cosmetician, or an amateur.

From the toxicological point of view, the precise dose and absorption of specific colourants as well as the specific ingredients and contaminants of inks are of pivotal interest, since every ingredient and every contaminant among dozens of such components of inks have their own biokinetic profiles and specific safety issues. With so many inks on the market mostly of unknown composition and considering the variability of dosing, the precise dose and exposure of the human body by tattooing to chemicals and particles are truly unknown and impossible to put on one simple formula.

Absorption, Distribution, Metabolism, and Excretion of Tattoo Ink Ingredients

Tattoo inks are, as mentioned, composed of practically insoluble pigment and a number of ingredients and contaminants of variable solubility with water as the vehicle [16]. Alcohols may be added to the vehicle to help solubility of lipophilic substances. Alcohols are not added in concentrations, which are efficient as preservative. Industrial preservatives may be added without being labelled on the product. Nickel is a very common contaminant, and a study found nickel in small amounts in every ink out of 58 inks studied and exceptionally also in higher concentrations [26]. Chrome may now and then also be present.

After injection of tattoo ink in the skin, as mentioned, absorption of soluble ingredients and relocation of pigment in the skin takes place along with local metabolism depending on the ingredient (fig. 12). Absorption of soluble substances by the blood may peak within minutes, hours, and days followed by metabolism and excretion in the liver and the kidney. Pigments have a very different and certainly a much more delayed absorption. The bulk of pigment remains embedded locally in the dermis between collagen fibres producing the permanently colourful tattoo as desired. As mentioned, pigments are primarily distributed to the lymphatics and then stored permanently in the regional nodes. However, a minor fraction of pigments, especially small-sized particles, may reach the blood circulation directly and become distributed to several organs, in particular the liver, where Kupffer cells have the normal function to depict and inactivate circulating bodies. The Kupffer cells in the liver and mast cells in tissues and lymph nodes are active in clearing tissues for particles by phagocytosis.

After tattooing, the major part of absorption of pigment from the skin with distribution to the lymph, blood, and other systems has probably occurred after about 6 months. Pigments are assumed to be equally robust to metabolism and biologic breakdown in the skin and in other organs to which the pigment becomes distributed. Because pigments are persistent for several years and even lifelong, it is the general opinion that the

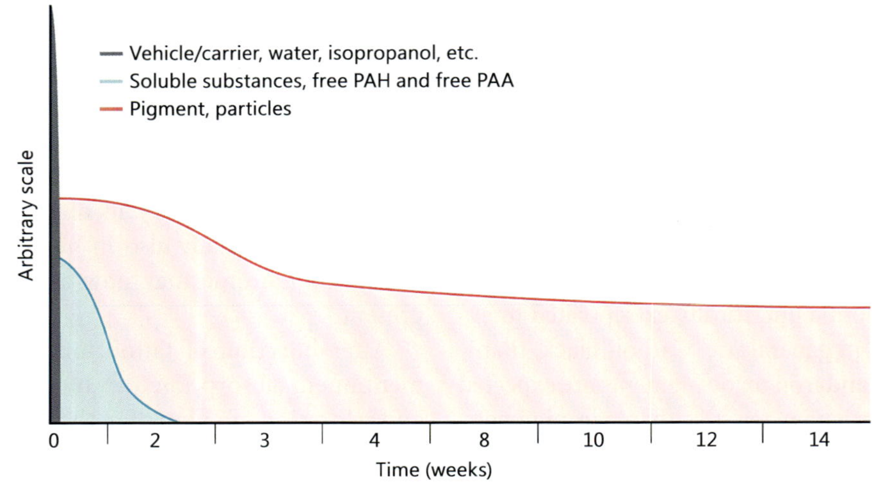

Fig. 12. Hypothetical illustration of the distribution and elimination of tattoo ink after injection into the skin. Inert carriers (water and isopropyl alcohol) are eliminated from the skin in the course of minutes or a few hours, and free chemical substances in the course of hours or a few days. Pigment particles are redistributed in the tissue and are distributed to the lymph nodes, among other places, in the course of days or a few weeks, but most of the pigment particles are permanently deposited in the dermis for years with very little elimination. This provides permanent colouring of the skin and determines the tattoo's visible colour. Reproduced with permission from the Council on Health and Disease Prevention [2].

breakdown of pigment and the formation of chemical breakdown products occur in a very slow rate, depending on the specific pigment, exposure to sun, etc. Slow-rate degradation and elimination of tattoo pigment over decades is expected to result in daily dose exposures of the body, which is under detection limits of any analytical method applied to critical substances, such as the chemicals on the negative list of the ResAp(2008)1 of the Council of Europe resolution [6].

In the discussion of the biokinetics and toxicology of tattoo ink, it is fundamental to recognise the simple fact that *tattooing is a single-dose exposure* of particles and chemicals and not a chronic or accumulative exposure.

Risk Assessment, Safety Strategy, and the Role of Doctors and Clinics

The 'Tattoo Clinic' of Bispebjerg University Hospital, Copenhagen, Denmark, has published a material of 493 patients with clinical tattoo complications collected from 2008 to 2015. As described in this publication, the clinical spectrum of tattoo complications of today is dominated by bacterial infections, allergies in red tattoos and sometimes in tattoos of other colours, and papulonodular reactions of black tattoos. Moreover, there is a large group of special events, such as urticaria, neurosensory disorder, ulceronecrotic reaction, traumatic sequels of tattooing, and sequels of tattoo removal by caustics and lasers [27]. A new classification of chronic inflammatory tattoo reactions is introduced. There is a large group of people who experience psychosocial complications and wish to have the tattoo removed if possible. In the literature, a few hundred case reports were published over a century, described in extensive reviews [28–32]. A review by Wendt et al. [33] from 2013 summarised more recent case reports of tattoo complications that occurred after modern organic pigments had taken over.

In the Bispebjerg University Hospital study, red tattoos with allergic reactions and black tattoos with papulonodular reactions have been identified as part of today's groups of major problems, in addition to bacterial infections and psychosocial problems [27]. Papulonodular reactions of black tattoos are predisposed to develop sarcoid granulomas and be associated with or trigger sarcoidosis that also affects internal organs [13–15].

Making safe inks is an important ambition, and finding culprit chemicals in tattoo inks causing reactions and omitting them is a logical approach. However, in clinical and basic research there are presently only two conclusive cases in which ingredients of inks can be linked directly to common tattoo complications observed in the clinic. One case is azo pigments as a chemical class of colourants associated with allergic reactions with an unknown chemical breakdown supposed to contribute to a hapten formed over time in the skin as responsible for allergic sensitisation and reactions in the red tattoo [27, 34]. The other case is nonallergic reactions in black tattoos of the papulonodular type, where black pigment particles agglomerate in the skin and form foreign bodies of a size that causes an inflammatory reaction and, with special predisposition of the individual, even sarcoid granuloma and sarcoidosis [14, 15, 27]. However, there is no identified specific chemical(s) that can explain allergic reactions of tattoos as seen in red tattoos, and the problem in black tattoos is primarily a physical problem related to particle properties with agglomeration happening in the skin over time. Phototoxicity reactions, another major group mainly causing mild complaints, has no specified chemical cause even if pigments absorbing light in the blue end of the spectrum, i.e. tattoos of red, black, and dark colour, are more prone to photochemical breakdown.

Safety assessment according to concepts of traditional toxicology involves in vitro studies, animal studies, and clinical observations mentioned in increasing order of evidence. Safety assessment of tattoo inks in the past primarily addressed pigments and pigment breakdown products with an emphasis on carcinogenic, mutagenic, and reproduction-toxic substances in new inks or being formed as metabolic breakdown products. This field only represents a narrow field of potential safety issues in play, as seen from the clinical perspective. Attempts have been made to establish derived safety assessment of tattoo inks based on toxicological models already used in school toxicology, i.e. calculation of 'derived dose of no effect level' (DNEL), 'derived dose of minimal effect' (DMEL), and 'margin of safety' (MOS), with effect understood as a specified toxic effect. However, these risk estimates require as a prerequisite the kind of unsafe substances to be characterised with knowledge about the precise risk organ(s), and there must be some linearity between dose and risk. The substance shall be bioavailable, i.e. of some reasonable solubility, which pigments are not. Calculations also include information about dose of exposure and biokinetics as well as washout of the substance, information that is not easily available. Robust pigment particles fall outside the scope of meaningful derived risk assessment. Thus, these risk models often used in toxicology are not applicable to risk assessment of pigments of tattoo inks.

Carbon black pigment often contains a number of polycyclic aromatic hydrocarbons (PAH), and red azo pigments may contain or be degraded to primary aromatic amines (PAA). In in vitro and in some animal studies, both classes of chemicals were associated with mutagenic events and risk of cancer, with PAH being relevant as a carcinogen on airway exposure. However, when extrapolated to tattooing, it is a major limitation that such studies are based on chronic and repeated exposure over extended periods. It has not been shown that cancers in humans can be induced by single-dose exposure to PAH or PAA. Thus, with tattooing as a single-dose exposure, it is not possible to draw any positive conclusion about a cancer risk of PAH and PAA in tattoo inks, when humans are tattooed. Indeed, an extensive review of the medical literature only traced exceptional skin cancers in tattooed people, and there was no reported case with two skin cancers in the same tattoo [35]. Since light-induced skin cancer is already very common, the conclusion was that reported cancers observed in tattoos occurred merely by coincidence. A recent study of photocarcinogenicity in mice showed that the incidence of light-induced cancer in skin tattooed black with an ink banned due to a high content of a potential carcinogen actually was *reduced*, explained by absorbance of UVB by pigment in the dermis resulting in reduced backscattered UV light toward the epidermis [36]. The only type of skin tumour associated with tattoos is keratoacanthoma, which is clinically innocent and benign despite convergent histopathology mimicking squamous cell carcinoma, which was recently documented in a large material of patients [37]. There have been no convincing reports of internal cancer induced by tattooing or of reproduction-toxic events. Nevertheless, due to the potential mutagenic effect of PAH and PAA and since even a single dose given on a critical day of foetal growth might be reproduction toxic, there is *international consensus that pregnant women and women who could be pregnant shall not be tattooed.* Doctors asked the question if tattoos can cause cancer accordant with consensus among specialists in the field and in accordance with the medical literature, and a recent report by the European Union responded that on the background that millions of people are tattooed, *the state of the art opinion is that tattoos are not associated with cancers* [5].

The European Council very recently evaluated a possible toxicological standard test program that might be applied to new inks and cover other aspects and mechanism of relevance, i.e. aspects beyond carcinogenic, mutagenic and reproduction-toxic effects [38]. The expert group concluded that, with pigments being particles of extremely low solubility, the vast majority of standard tests used in other fields such as drug evaluation and testing of cosmetic ingredients are not applicable to tattoo inks, because such use of established test methods is not validated in relation to physical pigments and tattoo inks. Important fields exemplified by sensitisation to red pigments by a hapten developed after a long time cannot be assessed with methods such as the guinea pig maximisation test and the lymph node assays. The agglomeration phenomenon of black pigment is not covered by a known standard test. A major field not covered with validated tests is photosensitivity reactions and photochemical breakdown of pigment.

Metal in inks is also a challenge. Tattoo inks of today are generally free of mercury and cadmium, which in the past caused allergy of tattoos made with cinnabar and cadmium sulphate used for decades as inorganic pigments. Metals such as barium, aluminium, and occasionally lead might raise safety concerns; however, clinical cases of tattoo complications caused by these metals have not been reported except for a case suggested to be a reaction to aluminium [39]. Metals of primary concern as sensitizers are nickel and chromium VI. Nickel supposed to be metallic is common in tattoo inks as a contaminant originating from production units with stainless steel vessels and is thus unlikely to be sensitising [26]. Analytical methods determine metals as total concentrations and not as ionic nickel or chromium VI, which are the active allergens [40]. There is no recognised standard for measurement of the two metallic sensitizers as the European Union also stated in a report on analytical methods for tattoo inks [5, 40]. There remains a relevant concern that metallic sensitizers may now and then be a significant part of pigment raw materials in particular found in iron oxide pigments as contaminants of the original pigment source material used in pigment production. Nickel even is a registered carcinogen, which is not considered relevant in relation to tattooing.

Allergy of red tattoos associated with azo pigment is one of the commonest tattoo complications. Azo pigments causing allergy of red tattoos are known to act as haptens, i.e. indirect and composite allergens with an epitope and tissue protein complex making up the active allergen [34]. Azo pigment cannot be tested by standard patch testing, which is negative even if the person is patch tested directly with the red culprit ink [34]. The allergen is not available in the ink bottle. Physical particles as such are not allergens but chemical substances released from particles that might act as sensitizer. Sensitisation is not elicited by simple PAA breakdown products of the azo pigment even if PAA now and then may be present in tattoo ink products. Sensitisation can take months or years to develop. Thus, despite clinical allergy of red tattoos also with cross-sensitivity reaction of older tattoos being one of the commonest tattoo complications, there is no in vitro, animal, or human test, which can depict azo pigments with allergenic potential and thus help the development of allergy-safe inks free of sensitising chemical. The specific chemical of potential risk and serving as epitope remains unidentified.

Pigment micro- and nanoparticles is another field of safety concern. As mentioned, pigments, in particular carbon black, may aggregate and agglomerate in situ and form foreign bodies causing tissue reaction including granuloma formation and sarcoidosis [14, 15]. Pigment particles accumulated and agglomerated in lymph nodes may also cause swelling and inflammation of the node. Carbon black nanoparticles and other pigment particles may reach the blood stream and distant organs, in particular the liver; however, there have not been clinical reports indicating distant organ events related to pigments and tattooing, except for inflammatory reactions of regional lymph nodes, which typically are transient.

With present knowledge, the ResAp(2008)1 resolution of the Council of Europe has, despite enthusiasm among regulators, become positioned in research as hypothetical, hampered by lack of documented clinical and epidemiological relevance. It was not implemented efficiently, and it is unlikely that tattooing realistically can become safer by strict adherence to the resolution. Established tattoo ink manufacturers already have self-discipline and avoid problematic ingredients such as salts of mercury, cadmium, and, as much as production allows, nickel and chromium. The main concern is tattoo inks made by overseas manufacturers, who cannot be identified. There are several examples of imported inks from such sources, with fake labelling, dubious ingredients, and not to mention contamination with bacteria despite false claim of sterility printed on the label. Some even copy bottles of known brands.

Tattooed individuals who are addicted to tattooing and carry tattoos covering major parts of their skin are a group of special toxicological interest, a group of voluntary 'guinea pigs' exposed to exorbitant doses of pigment. There have been no reports of survival rates of such persons or special acute hazards, or long-term events of skin and other organs observed in this high-exposure group.

Because of practically no regulation of the tattoo field and for a number of other reasons, the doctor holds a key position in pragmatic tattoo safety handling. The lack of risk assessment applicable to tattoo inks, the lack of valid test systems, models, and analytical standards, and the reality of tattooing being huge in the society highlight the importance of doctors and clinics, who actually are confronted with the patients and thus shall diagnose and treat tattoo complications up to best performance. This includes duly reporting of severe and accumulated cases to relevant authorities to help their surveillance and control of local outbreaks. The Food and Drug Administration in the USA, the European Union (RAPEX notification by national competent authority), and France have established active vigilance systems inviting doctors' reporting of cases of tattoo complications, but these systems are very little used. The vast majority of countries have no vigilance system in place, but authorities are generally interested in being notified about severe cases of tattoo complications. Tattoo complications as well as their diagnosis and interpretation leading to proper therapy are difficult and a matter of being familiar with this very special field. There is limited support from standard textbooks. Tattoo complications itch and influence quality of life, and the patients often contact their doctor [41]. Prevention of tattoo complications in the large-scale population has a pragmatic approach and strategy described as 'seamless prevention of tattoo complications' with realistic actions to reduce the problem where other undertakings have hitherto failed [2, 42].

Purely by fortune and thanks to critical care and antibiotic treatment provided by hospitals and clinics, the very severe and life-threatening complications of tattooing causing death, in particular sepsis, have not been reported in the medical literature for decennia, contrasting the fatalities reported in the old literature.

References

1 Laumann A: History and epidemiology of tattoos and piercings. Legislation in the United States; in de Cuyper C, Pérez-Cotapos M-L (eds): Dermatologic Complications with Body Art. Heidelberg, Springer, 2010, pp 1–11.

2 Tattooing – Health, Risks and Culture. The Council on Health and Disease Prevention, Copenhagen, 2015, pp 1–165. www.vidensraad.dk.

3 European Commission: JRC Technical Reports. Safety of tattoos and permanent make-up, compilation of information on legislative framework and analytical methods. Report of work package 1. Administrative arrangement N. 2014-33617 conducted on behalf of DG JUST, 2015.EUR 27528 EN; ISBN 978–92–79–50394–8 (PDF); DOI 10.27788/542617.

4 European Commission: JRC Technical Reports. Safety of tattoos and permanent make-up. State of play and trends in tattoo practices. Report of work package 2. Administrative arrangement N. 2014-33617 conducted on behalf of DG JUST, 2015. EUR 27394 EN; ISBN 978–92–79–52789–0 (PDF); DOI 10.2788/924128.

5 European Commission: JRC Technical Reports. Safety of tattoos and permanent make-up. Final report of work package 3. Administrative arrangement N. 2014-33617 conducted on behalf of DG JUST, 2016. EUR 27247 EN; ISBN 978–92–79–58783–2 (PDF); DOI 10.2788/011817.

6 Council of Europe: Resolution Res-ap(2008)1 on Requirements and Criteria for the Safety of Tattoos and Permanent Make-Up. Strasbourg, 2008.

7 de Cuyper C, Pérez-Cotapos M-L (eds): Dermatologic Complications with Body Art. Heidelberg, Springer, 2010.

8 Serup J, Kluger N, Bäumler W (eds): Tattooed Skin and Health. Curr Probl Dermatol. Basel, Karger, 2015, vol 48.

9 Laux P, et al: A medical-toxicological view of tattooing. Lancet 2016;387:395–402.

10 Zwerling CS, Dixon LH, Christensen FF, Goldstein NF (eds): Micropigmentation Millennium. Alfaretta, Apex Book Manufacturing, 2010, ISBN 978–0–615–48414–3.

11 Høgsberg T, Loeschner K, Löf D, Serup J: Tattoo inks in general use contain nanoparticles. Br J Dermatol 2011;165: 1210–1218.

12 Dirks M: Making innovative tattoo ink products with improved safety: possible and impossible ingredients in practical usage; in Serup J, Kluger N, Bäumler W (eds): Tattooed Skin and Health. Curr Probl Dermatol. Basel, Karger, 2015, vol 48, pp 118–127.

13 Høgsberg T, Jacobsen NR, Clausen P, Serup J: Black tattoo inks induce reactive oxygen species production correlating with aggregation of pigment nanoparticles but not with polycyclic aromatic hydrocarbon content. Exp Dermatol 2013;22:464–469.

14 Kluger N: Sarcoidosis on tattoos: a review of the literature from 1939–2011. Sarcoidosis Vasc Diffuse Lung Dis 2013; 30:86–102.

15 Sepehri M, Carlsen K, Serup J: Papulo-nodular reactions in black tattos as markers of sarcoidosis. Study of 92 tattoo reactions from a hospital material. Dermatology 2017, in press. DOI 10.1159/000453315.

16 de Cuyper C, D'Hollander D: Materials used in body art; in de Cuyper C, Pérez-Cotapos M-L (eds): Dermatologic Complications with Body Art. Heidelberg, Springer, 2010, pp 13–28.

17 Gopee NV, Roberts DW, Webb P, Cozart CR, Siitonen PH, Warbritton AR, Yu WW, Colvin VL, Walker NJ, Howard PC: Migration of intradermally injected quantum dots to sentinel organs in mice. Toxicol Sci 2007;98:249–257.
18 Sadauskas E, Jacobsen NR, Danscher G, Stoltenberg M, Vogel U, Larsen A, Kreyling W, Wallin H: Biodistribution of gold nanoparticles in mouse lung following intrathecal installation. Chem Cent J 2009;3:1–7.
19 Tang J, Xiong L, Wang S, Wang J, Liu L, Li J, Yuan F, Xi T: Distribution, translocation and accumulation of silver nanoparticles in rats. J Nanosci Nanotechnol 2009;9:4924–4932.
20 Gopee NV, Cui Y, Olson G, Warbritton AR, Miller BJ, Couch LH, Warner WG, Howard PC: Response of mouse skin to tattooing: use of SKH-1 mice as a surrogate model for human tattooing. Toxicol Appl Pharmacol 2005;209:145–158.
21 Engel E, Vasolid R, Santarelli F, Maisch T, Gopee NV, Howard PC, Landthaler M, Bäumler W: Tattooing of skin results in transportation and light-induced decomposition of tattoo pigments – a first quantification in vivo using a mouse model. Exp Dermatol 2009;19:54–60.
22 Engel E, Santarelli F, Vasolid R, Maisch T, Ulrich H, Prantl L, König B, Landthaler M, Bäumler W: Modern tattoos cause high concentration of hazardous pigments in skin. Contact Dermatitis 2008; 58:228–233.
23 Engel E, Spannberger A, Vasolid R, König B, Landthaler M: Photochemical cleavage of a tattoo pigment by UVB radiation or natural sunlight. J Dtsch Dermatol Ges 2007;5:583–589.
24 Cui Y, Spann AP, Couch LH, Gopee NV, Evans FE, Churchwell MI, Williams LD, Doerge DR, Howard PC: Photodecomposition of pigment yellow 74, a pigment used in tattoo inks. Photochem Photobiol 2004;80:175–184.
25 Lehner K, Santarelli F, Penning R, Vasolid R, Engel E, Maisch T, Gastl K, König B, Landthaler M, Bäumler W: The decrease of pigment concentration in red tattooed skin years after tattooing. J Eur Acad Dermatol Venereol 2011;25: 1340–1345.
26 Jacobsen E, Tønning K, Pedersen E, Bernth N, Serup J, Høgsberg T, Nielsen E: The Danish Environmental Protection Agency. Report on Chemical Substances in Tattoo Ink, 2012, report 216 (English version). ISBN 978–87–92779–87–8. www.mst.dk/publications/English.
27 Serup J, Sepehri M, Hutton Carlsen K: Classification of tattoo complications in a hospital material of 493 adverse events. Dermatology 2017, in press. DOI 10.1159/000452148.
28 Goldstein N: Complications from tattoos. J Dermatol Surg Oncol 1979;5: 869–878.
29 Jacob CJ: Tattoo-associated dermatoses: a case report and review of the literature. Dermatol Surg 2002;28:962–965.
30 Kazandjieva J, Tsankov N: Tattoos: dermatological complications. Clin Dermatol 2007;25:375–382.
31 Kluger N: Cutaneous complications related to permanent decorative tattooing. Expert Rev Clin Immunol 2010;6:363–371.
32 Kluger N: Acute complications of tattooing presenting in the ED. Am J Emerg Med 2012;30:2055–2063.
33 Wenzel SM, Rittmann I, Landthaler M, et al: Adverse reactions after tattooing: review of the literature and comparison to results of a study. Dermatology 2013; 226:138–147.
34 Serup J, Hutton Carlsen K: Patch test study of 90 patients with tattoo reactions: negative outcome of allergy patch test to baseline batteries and culprit inks suggests allergen(s) are generated in the skin through haptenization. Contact Dermatitis 2014;71:255–263.
35 Kluger N, Koljonen V: Tattoos, inks and cancer. Lancet Oncol 2012;13:e161–e168.
36 Lerche C, Sepehri M, Serup J, Poulsen T, Wulf HC: Black tattoos protect against UVR-induced skin cancer in mice. Photodermatol Photoimmunol Photomed 2015;31:261–268.
37 Takai T, Misago N, Murata Y: Natural course of keratoacanthoma and related lesions after partial biopsy: clinical analysis of 66 lesions. J Dermatol 2015;42: 353–362.
38 Safer tattooing – overview of current knowledge and challenges of toxicological assessment. Council of Europe, the European Directorate for the Quality of Medicines and Health Care (EDQM). Report, 2016 (unpublished).
39 Pontén A: Lichenoid reaction in a red tattoo and contact allergy to aluminium (abstract). 1st Eur Congress Tattoo Pigment Res, Copenhagen, November 2013.
40 Prior G: Tattoo Inks, Analysis, Pigments, Legislation. Berlin, Epubli GmbH, 2014. ISBN 978–3–8442–8611–3.
41 Hutton Carlsen K, Serup J: Patients with tattoo reactions have reduced quality of life and suffer from itch: Dermatology Life Quality Index and Itch Severity Score measurements. Skin Res Technol 2015;21:101–107.
42 Serup J: Seamless prevention of adverse events from tattooing: integrated strategy emphasizing the customer-tattooist interaction; in Serup J, Kluger N, Bäumler W (eds): Tattooed Skin and Health. Curr Probl Dermatol. Basel, Karger, 2015, vol 48, pp 236–247

Prof. Jørgen Serup, DMSc
Department of Dermatology D41, Bispebjerg University Hospital
Bispebjerg Bakke 23
DK–2400 Copenhagen NV (Denmark)
E-Mail joergen.vedelskov.serup@regionh.dk

Serup J, Bäumler W (eds): Diagnosis and Therapy of Tattoo Complications. With Atlas of Illustrative Cases.
Curr Probl Dermatol. Basel, Karger, 2017, vol 52, pp 18–29 (DOI: 10.1159/000450775)

Individual Risk and Prevention of Complications: Doctors' Advice to Persons Wishing a New Tattoo

Jørgen Serup

The 'Tattoo Clinic', Department of Dermatology, Bispebjerg University Hospital, Copenhagen, Denmark

Abstract

Doctors who are consulted about health and tattoo risks have an important role in the prevention of an individual's tattoo complications. Tattooing is a tremendous exposure of the human body to needle operation, particles, and chemicals. The risk is related to a person's health condition, level of insight, decision-making, and to the operation of tattooing, tattoo inks and utensils, tattoo parlour, and the aftercare. Tattooing is painful minor surgery performed without anesthesia. It can be associated with syncope. It is major needle trauma with histamine release and wheal and flare in the operation field. The skin barrier is broken. Bacterial infections come early. Chronically intermittent and mild complaints affect 4/10 of all the tattooed, and 2/10 have sensitivity to sun. Chronic complications with allergy in red tattoos and nodules due to pigment agglomeration and foreign body formation in black tattoos are less common but certainly at the level of cumbersome skin disease. Reactions to black tattoos are strongly associated with sarcoidosis. There are many other distinct entities of tattoo complications. A campaign called 'Tattoo – know your risk' is presented with detailed fact sheets about tattoos, tattoo problems, how to reduce risk, and a checklist for the tattoo customer before decision-making. The sheets with keynote information are useful aids for doctors giving advice to persons curious about acquiring a tattoo.

The risk of tattoo complications may be potential and general, as exemplified by the reproduction-toxic risk of the population when females are exposed large scale to brands, ingredients, and contaminants of tattoo ink stock products on market. The risk may also be individual, with a focus on the specific risk to the individual being in a certain health condition and in the process of selecting the precise tattoo design, the tattoo parlour, and the tattooist. The situation and scene determine what can be done regarding advice and prevention of tattoo complications and hazards.

The primary aim of this chapter is to describe individual tattoo-associated risk factors, which doctors realistically can consider when a person wishing a new tattoo asks for their advice. Deciding on a new tattoo, which can be the very first a person acquires in a process moving from naïve and healthy skin towards tattoo addiction with multiple tattoos all over the skin, is a milestone decision for life.

Obviously, advice at a personal level cannot be strictly limited to the individual risk related to the specific health condition of the person. Risk assessment and advice also shall address the full sequence of risky events and risk exposures associated with the completed course of acquiring a new tattoo, namely

- Predictors of risk according to health limitations of the person wishing a new tattoo.
- Risks of making a wrong decision due to an inferior state of information, with the person having a lack of knowledge about the pros and cons of tattooing, seen as a decision for life taken without any informed consent.
- The risk associated with the tattoo operation, which is a form of minor surgery made with no anesthesia, mostly under primitive conditions and by persons who in most countries are not formally authorized and educated to perform the refined operation of tattooing despite the need of craftsmanship and other skills. It is not directly transparent that the tattooist is truly a professional.
- The risk associated with the tattoo parlour and the utensils, i.e. tattoo inks, needles, machines, etc.
- The risk of infection and the risk associated with aftercare.
- Chronic complaints and complications related to tattoos, with tattoo inks baring potential risks.

Events associated with risk and specific risk factors may in practice be isolated or shared. Bacterial infection is an example of a shared risk, with the causative bacteria being an isolated risk and a conditio sine qua non. The pathogen may originate from the person being tattooed, the tattooist, the parlour, the needle, or the ink, and clinical infection may depend on the spontaneous resistance of the tattooed, the amount of inoculum, the bacterial strand, the degree of traumatization of the skin, and the quality of care, disinfection, sterility, and aftercare.

Being tattooed always carries a potential risk, and risk prediction is about rating the degree of risk on behalf of the individual and respectful to the person's free right to make their final decision to become tattooed or not. If this decision is positive, the aim of a doctor's advice is restricted to influencing the circumstances of tattooing with the ambition to limit risks and prevent hazards.

This chapter provides a brief introduction to the theme. Detailed information on tattoo complications can be found in a number of recent reviews and reports [1–7]. The European Union has recently summarized the present knowledge on tattoos and clinical risks in extensive reports [8–10]. In-depth information, especially on how to diagnose tattoo complications, is provided in the chapter by Serup [this vol., pp. 58–73].

State of Play of Tattoos and Tattooing

Having a tattoo has always had a sunny side and a dark side. Many are just happy with their tattoo with no regrets, no complaints, and no medical complications. This is the main reason why tattooing has grown from a history of magic tattoos used by tribes into a popular fashion of modern societies all over the world with hundreds of millions of people being tattooed. The widespread use of tattoos and their new position as acceptable by many people, thus no more seen as an automatic marker of subculture and low social class, create a situation in which tattoo complaints and complications – the dark side – are significantly manifested. With so many people tattooed, even rare occurrences become many by number. Disease due to tattoo complications shall of course be diagnosed and treated following quality standards generally used in the health system. However, the incidence and prevalence of tattoo complications in today's society are quite little known and may depend on country, segments of the population, gender, and other variables.

The tattoo industry, with far more tattooists than dermatologists, thousands of parlours, and hundreds of manufacturers of inks and utensils, has grown into a billion-dollar industry, working across national borders and with no efficient control. Tattooing is a cultural phenomenon of age and in the people's ownership, and it is settled in a position of splendid consolidation. A complete ban of tattooing is out of reach. The industry cannot be controlled anymore because of knowledge gaps in science and lacking transparency and international consensus on how to make progress in prevention. In this situation, doctors' interest and active role with advice to individual persons wishing a new tattoo become of importance for the prevention of tattoo complications in practice. Tattoo complication is disease. Facing the failure of implementing an international regulation of the tattoo business, a realistic approach to prevention, a strategy building on classical methods of prevention named 'Seamless prevention of adverse events from tattooing', has been introduced [6, 11].

The European Union recently published a detailed report on the state of play of tattooing and the tattoo industry in Europe [9].

Tattoo Complaints and Complications by Definition

It is important to distinguish chronic complaints, which are mild and often clinically insignificant, from chronic complications, which are more severe and often require medical treatment.

Tattoo complications are defined as more serious adverse reactions or events after tattooing and healing of the tattoo, which manifest as objective abnormalities or pathologies associated with clinical and subjective symptoms of a severity considered disease or disablement. The sufferers, in general, request medical advice and treatment.

Tattoo complaints only show mild subjective or objective abnormal experiences or observations acquired along with and caused by the tattoo. Persons with chronic and intermittent complaints generally do not seek medical advice or treatment. Tattoo complaints are far more common in the tattooed population than genuine medical complications are.

There is a broad overlapping spectrum ranging from minor and intermittent complaints commonly seen to significant medical complications eventually leading to invalidation and death, the latter being very uncommon or exceptional today. This is illustrated in the pyramid of tattoo adverse effects shown in figure 1.

The Clinical Spectrum of Tattoo Complaints and Complications

Tattoo complaints and complications mostly are limited to one 'problematic tattoo' and thus manifested in the skin. However, various organs can be involved. The tattoo ink is injected into the skin across the spontaneously rather tough epidermal barrier to chemicals coming from outside. Inks are watery formulations with dispersed and insoluble pigment particles and a number of more or less soluble ingredients and contaminants [12]. Pigments, for the major part, remain permanently in situ in the dermis at the injection site, while soluble substances within the first days after tattooing will reach the blood stream and become distributed to several organs, metabolized, and excreted by the liver and the kidneys [6, 7]. Depending on the type, pigments may undergo some slow degradation over years, and the colour may bleach under the influence of sunlight.

Complaints and complications, consequently, may be *acute or subacute* caused by the physical injury of the tattoo procedure, caused by microorganisms introduced with the tattoo needle and due to soluble ink ingredients, or *chronic or chronically intermittent* caused by pigment par-

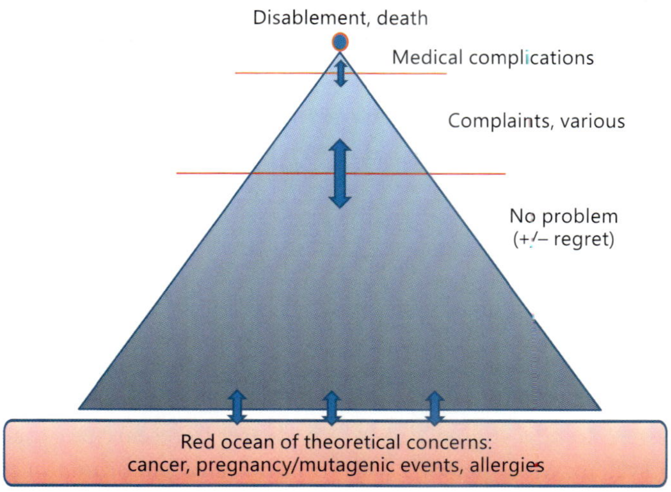

Fig. 1. The tattoo risk pyramid. The pyramid illustrates magnitudes of order of tattoos not causing a problem (except for regret), tattoos with intermittent complaints, tattoos complicated with diseases, and on the top the few cases with very serious complications and hazards with disablement and death. On the bottom there is a 'red ocean' of theoretical risk factors and concerns, which despite millions of persons being tattooed, have resulted in no measurable problem to the tattooed. This is either because there is no real problem or because a problem is rare, clinically insignificant, overseen, or falls under detection limits of methods of observation. Important complications in the clinic, namely allergic reactions of red tattoos, pigment aggregation with nodules in black tattoos, and photosensitivity, have found no precise causation related to tattoos or the ink. With the precise causation of the mentioned reactions being unknown, it is not possible to eliminate risks, and pragmatic approaches to prevention need to be used. This contrasts infectious tattoo complications, where rational strategies emphasizing hygiene and sterility can be practiced and make tattooing safer.

ticles or their local metabolites, diseases and abnormal reactions of the person including allergy, and external factors such as the sun. Additionally, *psychosocial* problems and eventually social invalidation may develop and make the tattooed person regret the tattoo and want it removed.

Two recent studies from Copenhagen, Denmark, have addressed *complaints in tattooed persons* [13, 14]. One study included persons attending an STD clinic for a checkup. In the other study, persons enjoyed sunbathing on the beach and were thereby spontaneously exposing their uncovered skin to the researcher. The studies agreed that chronic and intermittent complaints are very common (table 1). Studies found chronic and intermittent complaints in as many as 4/10 of all tattooed persons, and increased sensitivity to sun in 2/10. The main symptoms were intermittent itch and pain, swelling, and redness. The swelling was often papular. Dark-coloured tattoos, especially black tattoos but also red and blue tattoos, more often caused complaints. Sufferers often accepted their complaints and just applied a sun blocker or covered the tattoo with some textile if the problem was sensitivity to sun. Tattooed persons in general said they were reluctant to seek the advice of a doctor partly because they may feel ashamed and partly because they may feel the

Table 1. Prevalence of chronically intermittent tattoo complaints: summary of two studies [13, 14]

	STD clinic study [13]	'Beach' study [14]	Pooled/total
Total number studied	154	144	298
Complaining	65/154 (42%)	60/144 (42%)	125/298 (42%)
Photosensitivity among those with complaints	24/65 (37%)	31/60 (52%)	55/125 (44%)

In total, 4/10 have complaints and 2/10 have photosensitivity, which is 44% of all complaints.

doctor is unlikely to be qualified enough or motivated to help them with this self-inflicted problem. Many felt their tattoo to be a stigma also in relation to the health system. Most persons will first ask their tattooist for advice. During the process of tattooing, tattooed persons develop a level of confidence with the tattooist to a degree, which can be compared to a patient-doctor relationship [15].

Medical *complications in tattooed persons* are reported as case reports collected over a century and described in review articles [2–4]. Some reports are obsolete since the type of pigment is no longer used, as exemplified by red cinnabar pigment composed of mercury sulfide. A recent publication from the 'Tattoo Clinic', Bispebjerg University Hospital, on a large series of 493 complications showed allergy in red tattoos, papulonodular reactions in black tattoos, bacterial infections, and psychosocial complications to be the commonest complications, but the spectrum of medical tattoo problems is broad and includes a broad range with many specific entities each with their characteristic disease mechanism [16]. A new entity, which has been common but obscured for years, was identified, namely inflammatory reactions of black tattoos due to pigment agglomeration with foreign body formation and sometimes granuloma formation, associated with a high risk of sarcoidosis. The study and the spectrum of tattoo complications are discussed in detail in the chapter by Serup [this vol., pp. 58–73].

The distinction between tattoo complaints and complications nevertheless has overlaps and is clearer to researchers than it is to laymen. The *multifaceted panorama of problems of tattoos* as felt and uncritically reported via the Internet by the tattooed themselves was studied in a questionnaire study in German-speaking countries by Klügl et al. [17]. In total 3,411 questionnaires were available for the analysis. Persistent problems in the tattoo were reported by 6%, i.e. intermittent edema, itching, elevated skin, acne, skin papules, and numbness. Moreover, 3% stated other health problems such as psychic problems and light sensitivity. However, due to its design, the study has an inbuilt limitation, because respondents will respond on the background of their personal threshold of seeing a problem and actively respond to an Internet invitation. The study contributes to the mapping of the type of problems perceived by tattooed persons and may illustrate the magnitude of order, but it cannot document the epidemiological incidence and prevalence of events. The study indicates that many tattooed people accept their chronic complaints, since only few consulted their doctor and received prescriptions. Tattooed persons may already from early on, after having experienced major pain and discomfort associated with acquiring the tattoo in the tattoo parlour, have learned that tattooing and tattoos are bound to skin problems, which are to overcome. With a changed mind-set, they might be prepared to ac-

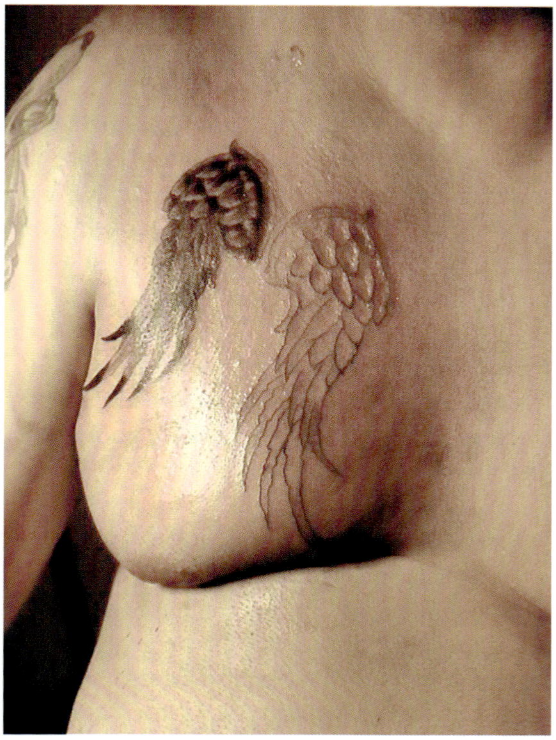

Fig. 2. Newly made tattoo with obligatory wheal and flare reaction due to massive needle trauma causing histamine release in the traumatized skin. The itchy and cumbersome reaction is expected and normal; it fades after a few hours.

cept intermittent discomfort of their tattoo and not see it as abnormal. Moreover, the study reported that during tattooing as well as in the first days and weeks after tattooing, 67.5% suffered skin problems and 6.6% systemic reactions. Systemic reactions directly after tattooing were dizziness, headache, nausea, or fever. The study, thus, strongly indicated that problems are much more frequent during tattooing and during the wound-healing phase than they are after months and years. People learn to live with problems that cannot be eradicated. However, even mild tattoo problems, despite being acceptable, are limitations the individuals did not suffer from before they were tattooed.

The Obligatory Trauma of Tattooing and Health Problems Associated with the Process of Being Tattooed

Acute tattoo trauma is obligatory (fig. 2). During tattooing the person inevitably suffers acute pain, itch, and acute inflammation with swelling and redness in the tattooed skin depending on the technique of tattooing and the individual predisposition, with persons with urticaria factitia being at special risk of severe reaction. The acute reaction is a needle trauma driven by the traumatic release of histamine provoked by the thousands of needle pricks performed down to the mid-dermal level [18, 19]. Such *urticarial needle trauma* locally in the tattooed skin with wheal and flare extending to the surrounding skin normally fades within hours or a day. Urticarial reactions are more advanced if the needle is of poor quality or damaged. In addition, amateur tattooists overworking the skin with major physical traumatization leaving a traumatic wound may with such an inferior technique provoke advanced acute reactions with severe inflammation followed by wound-healing problems and scarring, which ultimately leads to pigment defects in the tattoo due to escape of pigment during the prolonged phase of healing. Traumatization can also result in profuse bleeding and blur the operation field during tattooing. Persons with deficient coagulation and on special medications such as anticoagulants and nonsteroidal anti-inflammatory drugs, pain killers, have an increased risk of bleeding. During tattooing some persons may show *systemic adverse reactions* and faint due to the pain of tattooing or if they are dehydrated or hungry. Tattooing is always painful, but for some people it can be very painful. Fainting or syncope during tattooing can also have a medical background, i.e. cardiac disease with hypotension and arrhythmia, thromboembolism, epilepsy, diabetes with hypoglycemia, etc. Tattoo parlours and tattooists are not equipped and not educated to prevent and treat life-threatening hazards during tattooing. Fainting is rather common, while death during tattooing, luckily, is exceptional.

Healing of the tattoo wound after tattooing typically will take 1–3 weeks. The tattooed skin becomes inflamed with dense cellular infiltration. A crust of necrotic epidermis is formed on the surface of the skin. The crust holds tattoo pigment, which flew back through needle tracks and out to the surface. The skin manages to reject as much pigment as it can until the basement membrane zone has recovered after a few days, holding the pigment back in the dermis, where it was injected by the tattooist. During healing and some weeks thereafter, the pigments, which were installed in the dermis primarily in the needle tracts, reposition and move towards the outer dermis. Pigments also move towards the vasculature targeting the lymph and the general circulation. Tattoo healing, obviously, is associated with symptoms and discomfort, which normally fade parallel to the healing of the tattoo. Tattooing breaks the microbial barrier of the skin and represents a high-risk situation with respect to invasion of bacteria and other microbial contaminants from various sources, i.e. the person being tattooed, the ink, the instruments, in particular the tattoo needle, the parlour, and the tattooist. Consequently, *bacterial infections peak the first day(s) after tattooing*. The earlier the infection occurs, the higher the risk that it may become invasive and cause sepsis. Tattoo infections are discussed in the chapter by Serup [this vol., pp. 30–41]. The risk of infection not only depends on the practice of tattooing but also on the aftercare. There is no standard of aftercare, and the range of practices is overwhelming depending on the opinion and experience of the individual tattooist. It is common to wrap the tattoo wound with a plastic film as a 'moist' wound-healing treatment, which is after a few days followed by a cream or an ointment, which can have panthenol as an empirical ingredient. There appears to be no documentation of rationale of different wound care practices. Aftercare itself implicates a risk that human pathogens causing infection are introduced.

Risks from commercial tattoo ink stock products, pigments, and ingredients as well as their absorption, distribution, metabolism, and excretion are discussed in the chapter by Serup [this vol., pp. 1–17].

Tattoo-Related Health Problems from the 'Think before You Ink' Perspective and Doctors' Advice to Persons Asking about Their Individual Risk

Potential risks, especially carcinogenicity as well as mutagenic and reproduction-toxic side effects, of tattoo inks related to the content of polycyclic aromatic hydrocarbons and primary aromatic amines remain a theoretical concern; however, neither cancer of the skin nor of internal organs has been confirmed to be a problem in the clinic [6, 7, 10, 20]. Reproduction-toxic events are critical and difficult to detect, and pregnancy and tattooing remains a recognized relevant safety concern. *Thus, when being asked, the doctor can respond that the state of the art opinion is that being tattooed carries no increased risk of cancer, but women who are pregnant and women who could possibly be pregnant are recommended to refrain from tattooing.* This opinion finds confirmation in a recent expert report of the European Union [10].

Individual predisposition to complaints and complications are manifold, and a panorama of risk factors shall be considered and applied to the particular case asking for advice. The 'Tattoo Clinic' of Bispebjerg University Hospital, Copenhagen, Denmark, developed a number of fact sheets with precautions and advices. It is part of a campaign directed towards persons being in the process of deciding on a new tattoo. Sheets condense the many medicals facts about tattoos and tattooing, and the material is also useful as convenient information for doctors and others. The English version of the campaign with the title 'Tattoo – know your risk' is available on the web page of the European Society of Tattoo and Pigment Research (ESTP), www.ESTPresearch.org. The original Scandinavian version, 'Tatovering – tænk før du tør' is available on the web page of Bispebjerg Hospital, www.bispebjerghospital/campaigns. Both versions have direct access on Google by searching the name of the campaign. Patients asking for advice can be given the links. Other campaigns are also available on the Internet under the label 'Think before you ink'.

The fact sheets of the campaign of Bispebjerg University Hospital are shown below. They represent a sequence of information with sheets 1 and 2 prepared for the person with initial curiosity about having a tattoo, and sheets 3 and 4 for the person who may have decided to have a tattoo but wishes advice on how to have the tattoo made the safest way. The escape and safer run is to refrain from being tattooed. The sheets have some overlap of information, and the language is prepared to be hopefully easily understood by nonprofessionals.

Fact Sheets

1. Do You Know These Fundamental Facts about Tattooing?

- About 15% of the general population is tattooed; the young generation about 30% and in the elderly fewer.
- Increasingly women and very young people are getting tattoos – this is the trend.
- Many tattoo businesses of variable standard have opened, and in addition a large number of amateur operators are active.
- In reality, there is no 'control' or effective regulation of tattooing and tattoo ink.
- *Getting a tattoo is your responsibility. There is, practically, no room for regret. It is a decision for life, and nobody can guarantee your safety.*
- About four-in-ten of all people with a tattoo have some chronic or intermittent problems with the tattoo with periodic itching and swelling. About 1-in-5 do not tolerate sun on their tattoo.
- More serious problems that require medical treatment are quite rare. However, they can be severe and incapacitating.
- Allergy to red colour and shades of red are, together with infections, the most common complications. Also nodules in black tattoos can create problem and be associated with the disease sarcoidosis.
- In spite of a theoretical possibility of cancer in tattooed skin, this has not been seen to be a problem, but neither have cancers in skin and other organs been excluded.
- Pregnancy and tattooing is a NO GO because of potential risk to the fetus in early pregnancy related to chemicals in tattoo inks.
- *No tattoo ink is perfectly safe* with regard to the chemicals it contains which can cause allergy or other harm. Inks are industrial products with known and unknown ingredients. Nearly all inks contain nickel contaminant. The ink manufacturer does not assume any liability and often is unknown. Inks from established suppliers are supposed to be safest. No authority can 'sort' inks into harmful and safe inks, thus ensuring your safety. There exists no EU approval or CE quality stamp of tattoo inks even if it is claimed or sold like that. The ink is pricked into your skin, but only if you dare!
- 10% of new stocks of ink contain bacteria from the manufacturer – bacteria such as Staphylococci, Streptococci and Coli, which can give you serious infections. The bacteria may be there even if the ink bottle is labelled 'Sterile'. International infections can be spread in the ink. Low cost inks, so-called 'china inks' bought on the internet and produced in countries with high prevalence of bacteria resistant to antibiotics (MRSA) carries special risk.

Original inks from well-established manufacturers carry less risk.

- Many people with tattoos change their ideas as they get older, and may have problems in their work and private lives because of the tattoo, its position or the motif chosen.
- It is not true that tattoos can be easily removed using laser treatment. It is also very expensive.
- Magnetic resonance scanning (MR) can make tattoos sting, burn, and swell in connection with some investigation later in life. This is because the tattoo pigment in the skin can be magnetic. Cosmetic tattoos are more prone to MR burn.

2. Problems with Tattoos

- Bacterial infections and problems with healing in fresh tattoos. The infections can spread, become deep and cause abscesses. You can get blood poisoning with high fever, also called sepsis or septicaemia. The condition is life threatening and acute treatment in hospital is needed.
- Allergies in red tattoos and shades of red with chronic itching and swelling that affects your quality of life. This is like getting a skin disorder that is as severe as other chronic itching skin disorders. Corticoid cream does not work. Best treatment is removal of the pigment by surgery. Laser removal can boost the allergy and make it worse.
- Small tender nodules in black tattoos that are not an allergy. Seen in particular when too much pigment is pricked into the skin. Sun makes it worse. Nodules in black tattoos can be manifestation of the disease sarcoidosis, which can affect different organs including the lung. A black tattoo can trigger the development of sarcoidosis. Consult a Doctor.
- Episodes of stinging nettle-like swelling in the tattoo lasting from a few days to weeks.
- Abnormal skin growth where the skin bulges and becomes extremely scaly, coarse and hard.
- Abnormal scar formation, possibly as a so-called hypertrophic scar or keloid depending on individual predisposition.
- Seepage of pigment into the surrounding skin called 'pigment fan' with unwanted colouration and migration of pigment into the lymphatic system, exceptionally with chronic swelling of the skin and the subcutaneous layer (lymphedema). The pigment follows the lymph and is often found in the lymph nodes far from the tattoo. You cannot see it and will not know it is there. It is normal that lymph nodes are tattooed invisibly along with the skin. Ink ingredients go into your body.
- Sensitivity to light with stinging, itching, pain and swelling in the sun.
- Chronic pain without any visible change in the tattoo, can be severe and invalidating, a 'pain syndrome'.
- Transfer of infectious liver diseases (hepatitis B and C) and HIV occurs rarely today with tattoos because tattooists nowadays normally wear gloves. Other virus infections can cause problem. Warts can spread and become sown into a tattoo. A cosmetic tattoo can trigger facial herpes.

3. Your Personal 'Checklist' before You Make a Decision to Get a Tattoo

- Are you completely healthy, or are you temporarily under the weather after a cold for example; do you have a chronic condition (there are many types of chronic disorders); or are you receiving immune system suppressant therapy with a biological medicine, cancer medicine or other potent medicine that affects your entire body and changes how it reacts and how a new tattoo may heal?
- Do you have a chronic infection such as HIV, viral liver inflammation (hepatitis) or another chronic infection?
- Do you have a more widespread skin condition such as eczema and psoriasis?

- Are you a carrier of harmful bacteria such as penicillin-resistant staphylococci (MRSA) or other resistant bacteria (ESBL)?
- Do you have a tendency to form ugly scars, particularly the 'keloid' type?
- Do you or did you suffer from the disease *sarcoidosis*, which primarily attacks the lungs? If so, consider that you have an over 500-fold increased risk that a new tattoo, in particular a black tattoo, can trigger a fresh outbreak of sarcoidosis or a relapse of your disease, which also may become manifested in the new tattoo, in other parts of the skin (scar sarcoidosis, erythema nodosum), and in internal organs.
- Do you have a blood clotting disorder or are you receiving anti-coagulation treatment?
- Do you suffer from a disease with sudden seizures, epilepsy, disturbances in heart rhythm, etc.?
- Do you have a rubber allergy with latex hypersensitivity? In that case, a tattoo can be life-threatening if the tattooist uses rubber gloves.
- Do you have a severe nickel allergy or perhaps chromate allergy? Inks contain traces of nickel; a few inks have higher concentrations and may induce a widespread allergic reaction in your entire skin. Allergy to preservatives also can be a problem.
- Are you a blood donor? As a blood donor, your health is suspect for about six months (depending on country) after getting a tattoo. You cannot give blood again until you have been shown to be free of HIV and viral liver infections.
- *Are you a woman and pregnant, are trying to get pregnant, or perhaps could be pregnant without realising it?* In that case you should consider the fact that tattoo ink can contain chemicals that affect cell division and could potentially harm a baby, particularly in the early stages of pregnancy. No ink is safe if you are pregnant.
- Are you emotionally unstable, in a stressed situation or have problems with the tattooing process? In that case, don't do it – tattooing always adds a risk you didn't had before.
- Have you given serious consideration to the tattoo motif? Choose your motif with care and avoid extreme pictures or pictures you probably will regret (examples from real life: a cat eating a cheese sandwich, an erect penis, both seen as large tattoos on the legs of young girls).
- Have you considered your future work situation? Be perfectly clear that visible tattoos will exclude you from companies that do not accept visible tattoos, or could lower your prospects in a company. Many people value tattoos negatively.
- Will you still like the tattoo in 10, 20 and 30 years? Trends come and go!
- Do not get a tattoo if you are younger than 18, and never encourage minors to get one.

4. How to Reduce the Risk when You Get a Tattoo

- *Red tattoo inks more than any other colour may cause severe allergy.* Avoid red colours and red shades such as orange, pink, violet, burgundy, etc. These shades often contain red pigment combined with other pigments.
- Have a tattoo that is as small as possible in tattooed area (the larger the tattoo, the more pigment in the skin, the greater the risk) and always on a place that can be covered by clothes. NEVER on the face, neck and hands, in many countries illegal because of the high risk of unforeseeable social disablement later in life. If possible, avoid the lower half of the arms and legs – if you regret the tattoo, summers will be rather hot wearing long sleeves or trousers! Or at least find a compromise if you really insist having a tattoo that will be visible and on display.
- Avoid tattoos on the wrists and ankles. These cause more problems due to the function of the joints necessitating stretching the skin at joint motions.

- Avoid those parts of the skin ('up sides') that are particularly exposed to the sun because sun-triggered problems are very common. Sunlight also breaks down the pigment to new chemical compounds which can cause allergy and problems. The sun over time make coloured tattoos bleach and even can change the colour from blue to dirty green, or white to black, for example.
- Do not let the tattooist tattoo over brown moles because these can develop into melanoma, a highly malignant skin cancer. Melanoma may not be detected early enough if the tattoo pigment covers the mole. Delay in diagnosing melanoma can easily be fatal.
- Demand that the tattooist uses only the amount of ink necessary, and not use excessive amounts of ink in the skin. Intensely coloured tattoos cause more problems.
- Think twice about impulse tattoos including 'party tattoos' and tattoos made under peers' pressure. Say 'No Thanks' and take time to consider. It is your skin, your life, your risk and your decision.
- Choose your tattooist carefully. Make sure you know his right name; that hygiene is good; and that needles and gloves are only used once. The tattooist should be experienced and not an amateur – tattooing is a skilled craft that must be learnt. Never get a tattoo from a travelling tattooist including those who work at festivals. Avoid getting a tattoo abroad and particularly in countries where the incidence of penicillin-resistant staphylococci (MRSA) is high.
- Ensure by yourself and insist that the ink bottles used for your tattoo are completely new and clean and from a generally recognised manufacturer. As a minimum, the manufacturer's name and full identity should be printed on the bottle which also shall have some form of declaration of ingredients especially a CI number, i.e. colour index number telling the chemical code of the pigment, which is then identified. Do not be tattooed with low-price ink, so-called 'china ink', or copies of brand-name tattoo ink.
- Sterile water should always be used for diluting ink and tattooing shadows – you can yourself buy sterile water at the pharmacy and take it with you. Distilled water is not necessarily sterile. Do never use water from the taps.
- *Always ask the tattooist for a slip stating the name, type and manufacture of the inks used on you, including the CI number.* This is important if you develop a complication and need to consult a doctor because of a tattoo problem. The tattooist does not keep personal records of customers – you must do this yourself by getting a slip. Store the slip safely somewhere. You can even take an I-phone photo of the ink bottle and the label. It is your assurance if an ink on the market is shown to have catastrophic effects and must be suddenly recalled from the market due to medical hazards coming up. Contaminated ink has been the cause of regional outbreaks. If anybody has had dangerous inks applied to their skin they need to report to a hospital to get early treatment in particular if high fever and symptoms of blood poisoning.

References

1 De Cuyper C, Pérez-Cotapos M-L: Dermatologic Complications with Body Art. Tattoos, Piercings and Permanent Make-Up. Berlin, Springer, 2010.

2 Kluger N: Cutaneous complications related to permanent decorative tattooing. Expert Rev Clin Immunol 2010;6:363–371.

3 Wenzel SM, Rittmann I, Landthaler M, et al: Adverse reactions after tattooing: review of the literature and comparison to results of a study. Dermatology 2013;226:138–147.

4 Simunovic C, Shinohara MM: Complications of decorative tattoos: recognition and management. Am J Clin Dermatol 2014;15:526–536.

5 Serup J, Kluger N, Bäumler W (eds): Tattooed Skin and Health. Curr Probl Dermatol. Basel, Karger, 2015, vol 48.

6 Serup J, Harrit N, Linnet JT, Møhl B, Olsen O, Westh H: Tattoos – Health, Risks and Culture (report). Copenhagen, The Council on Health and Disease Prevention (Vidensråd for forebyggelse), 2015, pp 1–178. www.vidensraad.dk.

7 Laux P, Tralau T, Tentschert J, Blume A, Al Dahouk S, Bäumler W, Bernstein E, Bocca B, Alimonti A, Colebrook H, de Cuyper C, Dähne L, Hauri U, Howard PC, Janssen P, Katz L, Klitzman B, Kluger N, Krutak L, Platzek T, Scott-Lang V, Serup J, Teubner W, Schreiver I, Wilkniss E, Luch A: A medical-toxicological view of tattooing. Lancet 2016; 387:395–402.

8 European Commission: JRC Technical Reports. Safety of tattoos and permanent make-up. Compilation of information on legislative framework and analytical methods. Report of work package 1. Administrative arrangement N. 2014-33617 conducted on behalf of DG JUST, 2015.EUR 27528 EN; ISBN 978–92–79–50394–8 (PDF); DOI 10.27788/542617.

9 European Commission: JRC Technical Reports. Safety of tattoos and permanent make-up. State of play and trends in tattoo practices. Report of work package 2. Administrative arrangement N. 2014-33617 conducted on behalf of DG JUST, 2015. EUR 27394 EN; ISBN 978–92–79–52789–0 (PDF); DOI 10.2788/924128.

10 European Commission: JRC Technical Reports. Safety of tattoos and permanent make-up. Final report of work package 3. Administrative arrangement N. 2014-33617 conducted on behalf of DG JUST, 2016. EUR 27247 EN; ISBN 978–92–79–58783–2 (PDF); DOI 10.2788/011817.

11 Serup J: Seamless prevention of adverse events from tattooing: integrated strategy emphasizing the customer-tattooist interaction; in Serup J, Kluger N, Bäumler W (eds): Tattooed Skin and Health. Curr Probl Dermatol. Basel, Karger, 2015, vol 48, pp 45–47.

12 Jacobsen E, Tønning K, Pedersen E, Bernth N, Serup J, Høgsberg T, Nielsen E: The Danish Environmental Protection Agency. Report on Chemical Substances in Tattoo Ink, 2012, report 216 (English version), ISBN 978–87–92779–87–8. www.mst.dk/publications/English.

13 Høgsberg T, Carlsen KH, Serup J: High prevalence of tattoo complaints among a young population tattooed with recent organic pigments. J Eur Acad Dermatol 2013;27:846–852.

14 Carlsen KH, Serup J: Photosensitivity and photodynamic events in black, red and blue tattoos are common. A 'beach study'. J Eur Acad Dermatol 2014;28: 231–237.

15 Kristensen MW: Tattooist-customer relationships in a diversified environment of professional tattooists and 'scratchers'; in Serup J, Kluger N, Bäumler W (eds): Tattooed Skin and Health. Curr Probl Dermatol. Basel, Karger, 2015, vol 48, pp 45–47.

16 Serup J, Sepehri M, Hutton Carlsen K: Classification of tattoo complications in a hospital material of 493 adverse events. Dermatology 2017, in press. DOI 10.1159/000452148.

17 Klügl I, Hiller K-A, Landthaler M, Bäumler W: Incidence of health problems associated with tattooed skin: a nation-wide survey in German-speaking countries. Dermatology 2010;221:43–50.

18 Groth L, Serup J: Cutaneous microdialysis in man: effects of needle insertion trauma and anesthesia on skin perfusion, erythema and skin thickness. Acta Derm Venereol 1998;78:5–9.

19 Groth L, Jørgensen A, Serup J: Cutaneous microdialysis in the rat: insertion trauma and effect of anesthesia studied by laser Doppler perfusion imaging and histamine release. Skin Pharmacol Appl Skin Physiol 1998;11:125–132.

20 Kluger N, Koljonen V: Tattoos, inks and cancer. Lancet Oncol 2012;13:e161–e168.

Prof. Jørgen Serup, DMSc
Department of Dermatology D41, Bispebjerg University Hospital
Bispebjerg Bakke 23
DK–2400 Copenhagen NV (Denmark)
E-Mail joergen.vedelskov.serup@regionh.dk

Serup J, Bäumler W (eds): Diagnosis and Therapy of Tattoo Complications. With Atlas of Illustrative Cases.
Curr Probl Dermatol. Basel, Karger, 2017, vol 52, pp 30–41 (DOI: 10.1159/000450777)

Tattoo Infections, Personal Resistance, and Contagious Exposure through Tattooing

Jørgen Serup

The 'Tattoo Clinic', Department of Dermatology, Bispebjerg University Hospital, Copenhagen, Denmark

Abstract

Bacterial infection of tattoos remains a common complication. Pyogenic bacteria can cause infections shortly after the tattoo is made. Severity of infection varies from minor to major, ultimately with life-threatening septicemia. Viral infections may be introduced, i.e. HVB, HVC, and HIV. The risk of infection depends on the following triad: microbial pathogen and its aggressiveness, individual resistance of the tattooed, and inoculation and exposures by the tattoo needle and in the tattoo parlor. Some infectious risks can be controlled. Persons with weaknesses can refrain from tattooing. Tattoo parlors and tattooing can be hygienic and clean albeit not sterile; much has improved helped by hygiene guidelines of professional tattooists' organizations and through control instituted by local and national authorities. Tattoo inks remain a potential source of infection difficult to control in a low-priced competitive market operating over the Internet and across national borders. Ten percent of new inks are contaminated with bacteria pathogenic to humans, independent of a claim of 'sterility'. Known brands and established manufacturers are considered safer. Work is in progress aiming at common European standards for tattoo hygiene. Doctors have a role not only in treating tattoo infections but also in reporting cases to the competent authority in their country to support the monitoring of tattoo infections at any time, as an instrument for the authority to detect local outbreaks of tattoo infections early and prevent that new tattoo customers become infected. It is a potential risk of the future that new and very aggressive bacteria not seen in the past may unexpectedly show up in the tattoo scene.

A main function of the skin integument is to be a barrier to microorganisms invading the body and causing infection. With thousands of needle penetrations of the epidermal barrier performed under conditions that are never sterile, tattooing represents a potentially major risk of infection of the skin and the body. Performed in accredited hospitals and clinics, tattooing would be considered minor surgery and require a sterile setting and utensils. However, tattooing has its own historical background behind practices of today.

Tattoo infections are common, relative to the range of tattoo complications; nevertheless, they are far more rare than expected considering tattooing procedures and practices as well as the many professional levels of operators including amateurs. This may have two reasons. Most tat-

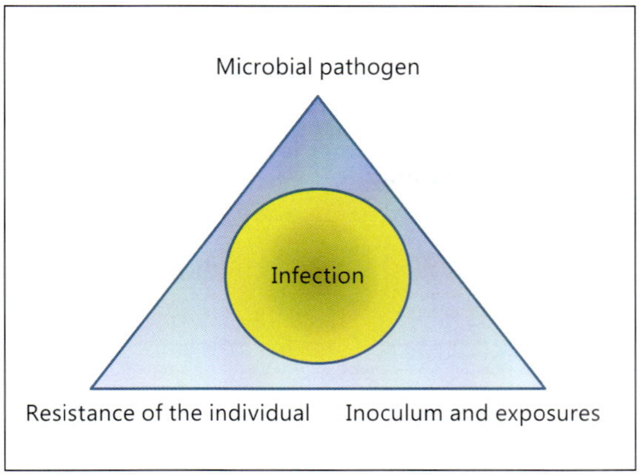

Fig. 1. The principal vectors determining a clinically manifested tattoo infection.

tooed people are young and healthy. Most tattooists are responsible and aware about the risks of infection and thus already take precautions to limit the risks. In some countries, authorities control tattoo parlors to make sure the practice is up to requirement. The Netherlands have been in the forefront with regulation and control of tattooing, known as the Amsterdam model [1–3].

The risk of infection has three important vectors, namely the microbial pathogen, the resistance of the individual to infection, and the inoculum and exposure represented by the tattooing operation having a sequence of different exposures and risks (fig. 1). The literature on rare cases and the spectrum of more typical tattoo infections are extensive [4–10].

Microbial Pathogens Causing Tattoo Infections

Tattoo infection is in a privileged situation in which the etiologies and associated clinical manifestations have been known for many years. Microbiology is highly developed, as is antibiotic therapy. However, exposure to pathogens depends on geography, country, culture, and standard of tattoo parlors. Detailed information on how, where, and when a tattoo was acquired is needed in patient care as basic information. Tattoo infections acquired in places with a high prevalence of bacterial strains resistant to antibiotics require a careful approach. However, independent of country, particularly *pyogenic bacteria* are the main cause of tattoo complications albeit local and endemic microbial pathogens always shall be considered. The recent literature includes cases of tattoo infections with environmental mycobacteria, but such type of infection is very rare compared with pyogenic infection, and the interest in the literature is disproportionate relative to reality [11, 12]. Typical tattoo infections are illustrated in figures 2a, b, 3a–d, and 4a–d.

The following is a brief summary of the literature on different classes of microbial pathogens and their manifestations. Most of the infections mentioned as uncommon are rare, endemic, or historical.

Common Bacterial Infectants and Infections

These are caused by *Staphylococcus aureus*, *Streptococcus pyogenes*, and occasionally *Pseudomonas aeruginosa*. Other bacteria such as *Escherichia coli* may also cause infection. Pyogenic bacteria reaching the blood may cause life-threatening septicemia and endocarditis.

The clinical picture is as follows:

- Minor or minute infection of a tattoo or parts of a tattoo with folliculitis or pimples. Infection is often innocent and self-limiting.
- Superficial tattoo infection and impetigo associated with or followed by abscess in the tattooed skin. Source: the person being tattooed (may be a chronic carrier of pathogenic bacteria), the tattoo ink, or the tattoo parlor having an inadequate hygienic standard. Infection may be mild or moderate but may progress if untreated.
- Regional tattoo infection with horizontal spread in the surrounding skin and tissue with

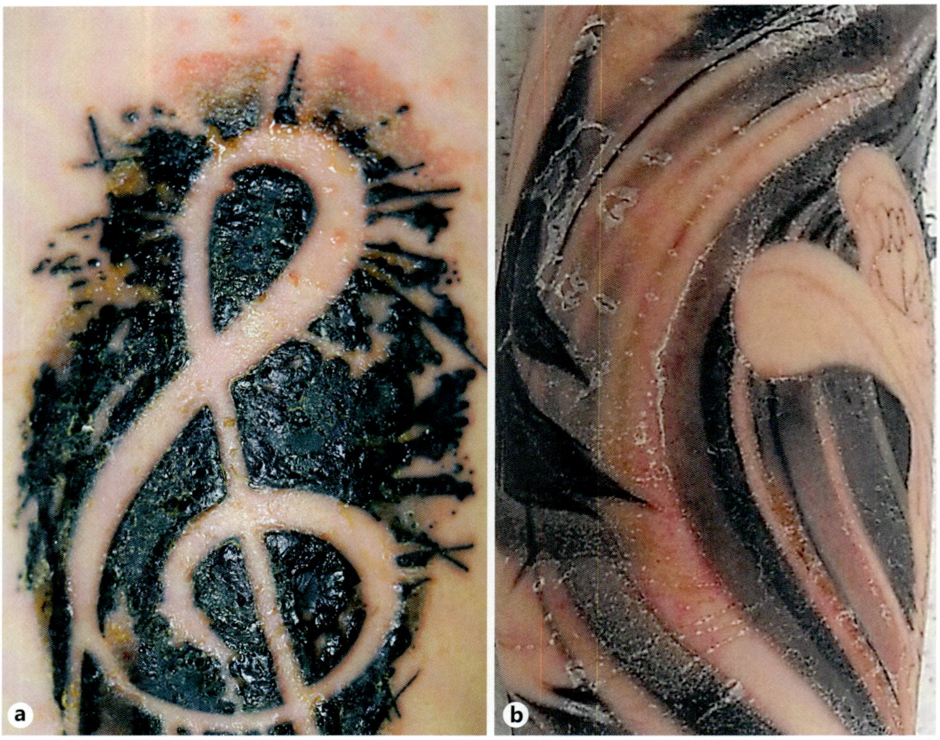

Fig. 2. Pyogenic bacterial infections in tattoos. **a** Superficial infection, impetigo. Epidermal changes dominate. **b** Profound nonulcerating infection, cellulite. Epidermal signs of infection are minor and secondary. The general condition may be affected. Further information and illustrations are shown in the atlas, pp. 145–148.

erysipelas. Source: see 'Superficial tattoo infection'. Infection requires antibiotic treatment and may be severe.

- Progressive infection affecting deep structures with cellulitis or necrotizing fasciitis [13]. Source: see 'Superficial tattoo infection'. Infection is acute, severe, and potentially life threatening. Acute surgery can be necessary.
- Systemic infection with septicemia, sepsis and possibly complicated with endocarditis and distant organ abscess. Source: see 'Superficial tattoo infection'. Infection is acute and life threatening. Acute treatment in hospital and especially early treatment are needed to prevent septic shock.

Uncommon or Endemic Bacterial Infectants and Infections

- Tuberculosis *(Mycobacterium tuberculosis)* by inoculation with local infection of the tattoo, and potentially widespread infection. Source: infected materials or persons in the tattoo parlor or in the environment.
- Atypical mycobacteria (environmental contaminants) by inoculation with local infection of the tattoo. Source: tattoo ink or contaminated tap water used for dilution of ink.
- Leprosy *(M. leprae)* by inoculation with local infection and potentially disseminated lepromatous disease. Source: tattoo instruments and tattooist or environment.

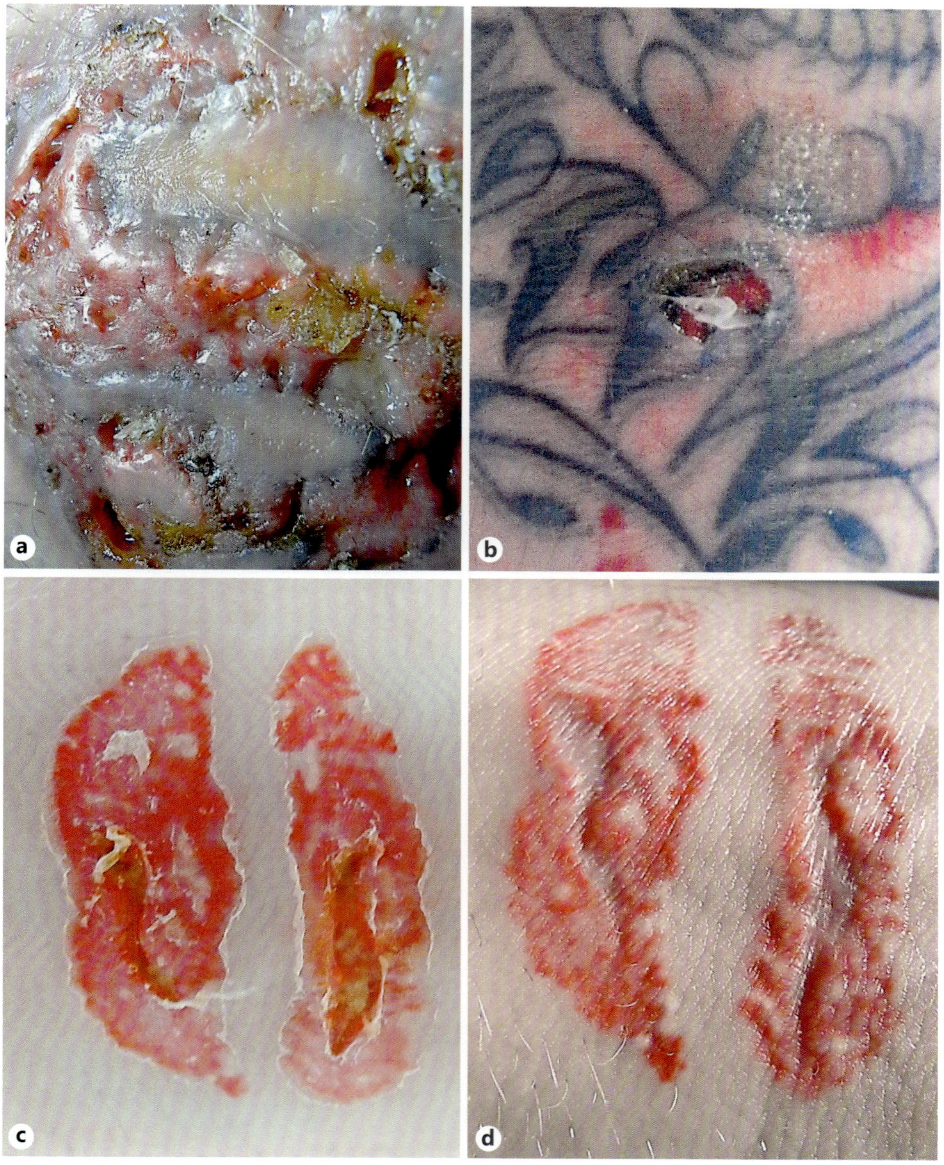

Fig. 3. Pyogenic tattoo infections with ulceration. **a** Allergic tattoo reaction of a red tattoo with secondary bacterial infection. **b** Bacterial infection with deep ulceration. **c** Primary bacterial infection of a red tattoo, superficial ulceration. **d** Same tattoo as pictured in **c** during healing with loss of pigment in infected sites.

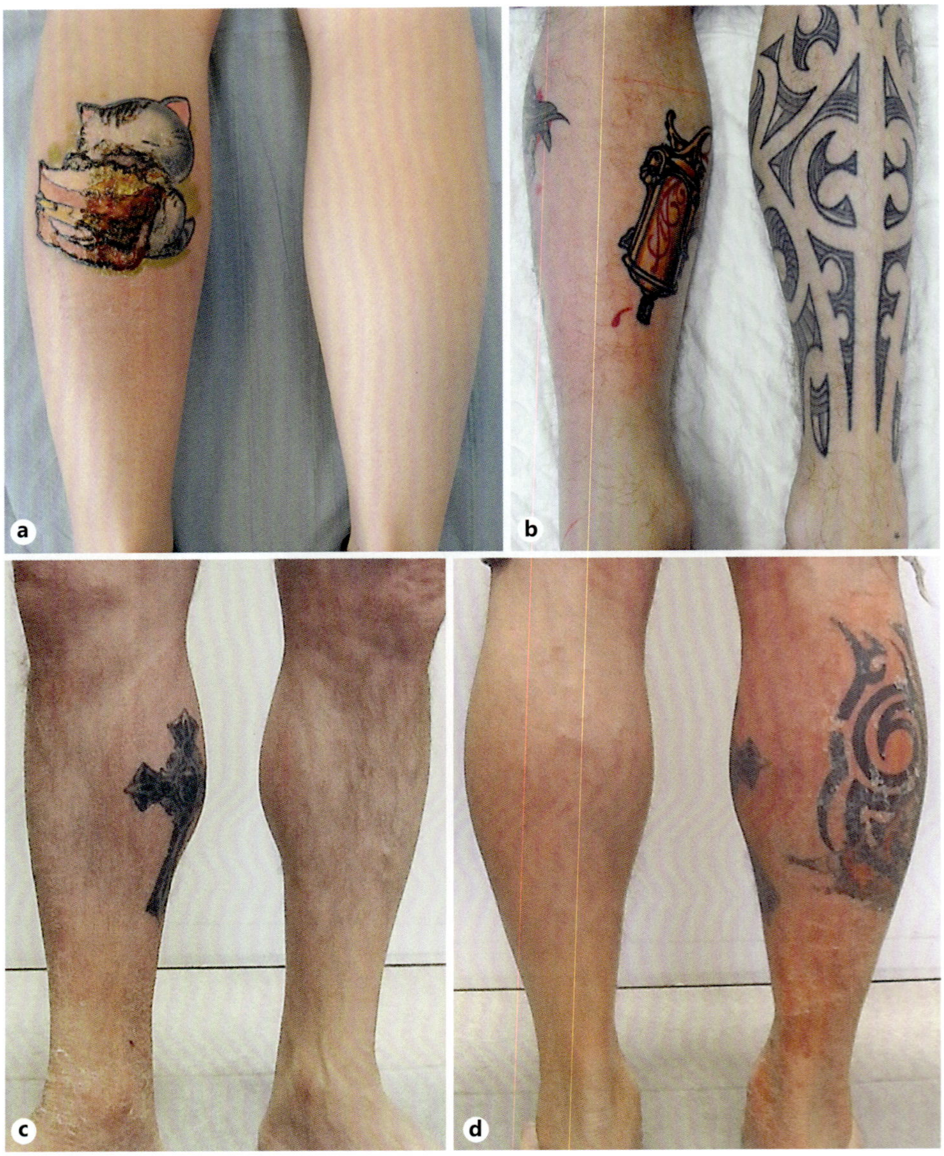

Fig. 4. Pyogenic tattoo infection of the legs. **a** Local tattoo infection with impetigo. **b** Tattoo infection with cellulite, redness, and swelling of the leg. **c** Tattoo infection with swelling and signs of erysipelas, with demarcation line of redness. **d** Posterior aspect of the tattoo pictured in **c**.

- Syphilis *(Treponema pallidum)* by inoculation with ulcus durum in the tattoo, regional lymph node swelling, or unnoticed with debut as second-stage syphilis. Source: a personal contact or the tattooist (historical case from Philadelphia, where the tattooist used sputum to disperse pigment).
- Chancroid (*Haemophilus ducreyi*, a Gram-negative *Streptobacillus*) by inoculation with ulcus molle in the tattoo and regional lymph gland swelling. Source: the person being tattooed, a contact, or the tattooist. This bacterium easily infects by inoculation (classical venereology, the 'autoinoculation test').
- Tetanus *(Clostridium tetani)* by inoculation, manifested as classical tetanus with muscle spasms; life-threatening in persons not vaccinated against this bacterium. No efficient antibiotic is available.

Viral Infectants and Infections

- Common warts, verruca vulgaris *(Papillomaviruses)* with viral warts primarily in the tattoo or in the skin surrounding the tattoo. Source: often the person being tattooed.
- Water warts, *Molluscum contaginosum* (DNA poxvirus) in the tattoo with local spread primarily in the surrounding skin. Source: often the person being tattooed, their relatives, or their children.
- Herpes simplex *(herpes simplex virus)* manifested as a primary herpes simplex attack in the tattooed skin or as a flare-up of herpes already hosted by the person, with lips, perioral skin, and genitals as anatomical sites of risk.
- Vaccinia with widespread herpes simplex infection all over the skin in predisposed individuals such as persons with atopic dermatitis; serious infection that may require treatment in hospital.
- Hepatitis B and C *(hepatitis virus B and C)* manifested as general malaise followed by hepatitis, but often the infection is subclinical [14]. There are no local signs of infection of the tattoo. It may ultimately and over years progress into fibrotic liver disease and hepatic failure with death. Source: another person or reuse of needles, which carries a high risk of transfer.
- HIV infection (*human immunodeficiency virus*, a retrovirus) manifested as general malaise followed by multi-organ manifestations and severe immunodeficiency. In the tattoo, there is no sign of local infection. Source: another person or transfer by reuse of needles as practiced in certain environments [15].

Fungal and Other Uncommon Infectants and Infections

- Fungal infections *(dermatophytes and other fungi pathogenic to humans)* may be inoculated in the tattoo and cause local infection. Source: the tattoo parlor, instruments, contacts, or persons. Manifested as 'ringworm' or atypical long-lasting and eczematous reaction of the tattooed skin progressing into the surrounding skin. Infection with the *Acremonium* species with mycetoma has been described.
- Exceptional inoculations associated with tattooing are leishmaniasis caused by protozoan parasites genus *Leishmania*, zygomycosis caused by mold fungi of the Zygomycota phylum, and blastomycosis caused by the dimorphic microfungus *Blastomyces dermatitidis* of the family Ajellomycetaceae. Infections may be cutaneous, mucocutaneous, visceral, and even pulmonary depending on the infective agents.

Treatment of infections depends on the case and the pathogen causing infection and shall be decided by the responsible doctor in cooperation with local microbiologists, guided by the sensitivity of the pathogen to antibiotics or other treatment. During treatment, it is important to report to the local authority, since outbreaks of infection among customers of a particular tattoo parlor is always an issue. Sometimes culture of bacteria from the tattoo ink bottle is possible. Tattooists are mostly, but not always, eager to have the case concluded and the risk eliminated from their parlor. There may also be other routines of the parlor needing a revisit.

Individual Resistance of the Person Being Tattooed

Healthy young individuals normally have high spontaneous resistance to pyogenic bacteria in contact with skin, but development of clinical infection also depends on the strain of bacteria, the exposure, and the inoculum. With some viral infections, hepatitis B and C as well as HIV, there is no efficient spontaneous resistance, and anyone can become infected. With hepatitis B and C, only a small inoculum is required. Viruses live in biologic material, and therefore direct transfer of a virus from one person to another sharing a tattoo needle carries a special risk.

Persons with reduced spontaneous resistance have an increased risk of being infected while having a tattoo. Conditions of inferior resistance are malnourishment, drug addiction, alcoholism, immune deficiency and ongoing immunosuppressive therapies, severe chronic disease, diabetes, etc. However, there are also situations when resistance is only temporarily reduced, i.e. in persons who are tired, burdened by problems and stress, mentally out of balance, or suffering from a psychiatric disorder.

Hospital infections – new infections acquired by patients during their stay in hospital – are in most countries in the range of 8–10%, despite prevention to reduce the problem, including sterile conditions of surgery. This illustrates the influence of weakened health on susceptibility to infection [16].

Carriers of methicillin-resistant *S. aureus* (MRSA) and persons with a history of recurrent bacterial infections carry a higher risk of also getting an infection in a new tattoo, and added to that, a risk that the infection cannot be treated successfully.

Persons with low resistance to infections shall not be tattooed. It is the shared responsibility of the person being tattooed and the tattooist that spontaneous resistance is good at the time of getting a tattoo. General practitioners can advise their patients with relevant chronic health problem against tattooing.

Inoculum and Exposure to Pathogens in the Tattoo Parlor

The inoculum with the pathogen causing clinical infection may originate from the following sources:

- The tattooed person
- The tattooist and other persons in the room
- Tattoo ink
- Needles, machines and other utensils, and tattoo trauma facilitating infection
- The tattoo parlor
- Aftercare being incorrect
- The environment of the tattooed during the tattoo healing phase

The tattooed person, the tattooist, and other persons in the tattoo parlor may infect the tattooed by direct or indirect contact. Disinfection of the skin subject to tattooing is rational as prevention, but bacteria may be hosted in other parts of the skin, such as in the nostrils and in the anogenital region. If hand hygiene is not good, indirect transfer of bacteria to the area of the tattoo operation may happen. Reuse of tattoo needles practiced by some amateurs and in environments such as prisons, obviously, carries a high risk of transfer of infectious material, especially hepatitis viruses and HIV [15, 17].

Tattoo ink contaminated with bacteria represents an important risk of bacterial infections by inoculation [18–20]. *Ten percent of newly bought tattoo inks stock products were found to be contaminated with bacteria that are human pathogens*, and even more inks are contaminated if environmental microbes are included [19, 20]. Labelling inks as 'sterile' makes no difference and cannot be taken as a guarantee. Many inks have no date of production or expiration and no batch number, and often the identity of the manufacturer or country of origin of is not printed on the label. Bacterial strains in inks are *Staphylococci, Streptococci, Pseudomonas*, and *E. coli* species.

The sterility of tattoo needles, despite being prepacked for single use, labeled 'sterilized', and even CE quality stamped, remains obscure, since such markers of quality may easily be false. The best guarantee of sterility is the tattooist's own autoclaving of needles and hand pieces. Tattoo machines cannot be sterilized but disinfected, and many tattooists wrap machines and connections in plastic to make the operation clean. Water for dilution of ink shall be sterile, and not distilled or from the tap. Poor techniques of tattooing, such as using needles with hooks or tattooing the area of skin too much in an operation, may not only cause scarring, but also increase the risk of infection (fig. 3). Traumatic tattooing goes hand in hand with an increased risk of infection.

Infection from the tattoo parlor, from the room, tables, chairs, and other furniture, is a risk depending on the organization of the parlor and the routines of cleaning.

Aftercare during the healing of a tattoo is in the hands of the tattooists, who have a close cooperation with their customers in this phase as well [21]. Tattooists shall have insight in and attention to signs and 'signals' that shall make the tattoo customers consult their doctor. Symptoms of septicemia should be known to the customer and result in prompt treatment in a hospital.

Tracing the reason for infection is an important albeit difficult task. If the reason is poor routines in the tattoo parlor, this should be corrected in the interest of all parties. If the reason is infected ink, the ink should not be used on other customers. It is often difficult for the doctor or the authority to qualify if an infection in a tattoo was caused by inoculation of microbes from a contaminated ink or from other sources. Often the bottle of ink used is not available. Infection in a tattoo starting in one particular color speaks in favor of inoculation from the tattoo ink of that special color. Infection, which involves the entire tattoo from the start, independent of color, is more likely to originate from instruments, persons, or the tattoo parlor. Infection related to inoculation of bacteria causing pyogenic infections and sepsis starts shortly after tattooing, i.e. in a few hours or 1–2 days, and becomes manifested as described above. Infection due to bacterial invasion of the wound during the healing phase starts later. Such infection may be less likely to be related to the ink. Some bacteria, fungi, protozoa, etc. only cause infection after a long latency, with mycobacteria as an example. Hepatitis and HIV also have a longer incubation, and the introduction of these infections by tattooing may easily be overlooked and is difficult to verify.

Control of Infectious Risk by Authorities

In various countries, professional tattooists and their organizations have already taken many initiatives to make tattooing safer. The operation of making a tattoo as practiced in thousands of tattoo parlors and by thousands of tattooists of different professional levels is a primary concern (fig. 5a, b). Disinfection, use of gloves, single-use new needles for each customer, and keeping the parlor and utensils clean already have influenced the situation in a direction where the number of tattoos with infection appears to be decreasing. In 2009, the United European Tattooist Association (UETA) located in Germany published an elaborate guideline on practices and hygiene in tattoo parlors [21–23]. The Swedish tattooist organization SRT published a comprehensive book on the issue [24]. Experiences and guidelines are summarized in two review articles [21, 25]. In some countries, courses in tattoo hygiene have been conducted with tattooists and experts educating tattooists. In some countries, such courses are a formal requirement to become a registered tattooist.

The European Union and the European Center for Standardization (CEN) recently delegated the task to develop European standards on hygiene in tattoo parlors to the German institution

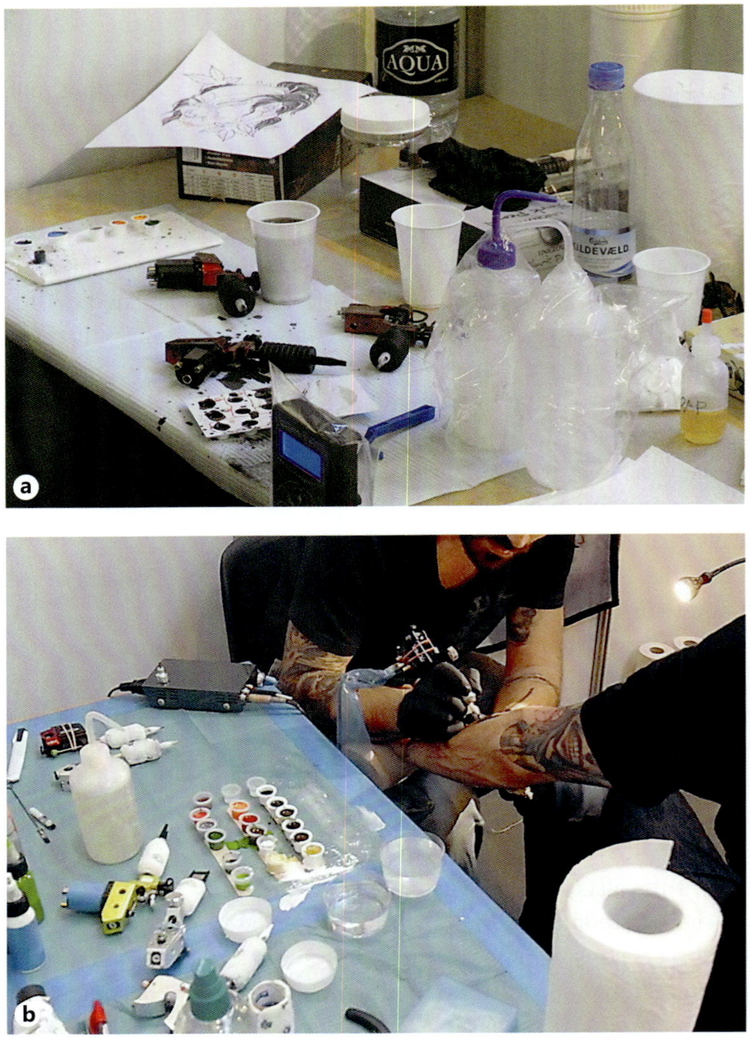

Fig. 5. The tattoo scene and the operation of tattooing. **a** Work table with electric machines, cups with different inks, petrolatum for lubrication of the skin surface, cup of water for cleansing of needle tip between operations, and water for dilution of inks. **b** Same scene as pictured in **a**, with a tattooist using a rotor machine.

Deutsches Institut für Normung (DIN). The work shall harmonize and improve existing standards with the ambition to develop one common guideline. Thus, depending on the success of the guideline, including its general acceptance and implementation, and finally the control of routines in tattoo parlors, a significant improvement of tattoo hygiene might be achieved, which will hopefully result in fewer tattoo infections.

The sterility of tattoo ink stock products remains a pending issue. In resolutions from 2003 and 2008, the Council of Europe recommended tattoo inks to be produced sterile and preferably as mono-dose ampoules replacing the recent use of larger bottles, which are used from one customer to another and over time (fig. 6a–c) [26]. Tattooists are against mono-dose ampoules, see these as impractical, and insist on bottles. The resolution accepts preservation of inks but recommends sterile inks. The European Union and the Directorate-General for Justice and Consumers (DGJUST) addressed the regulation of chem-

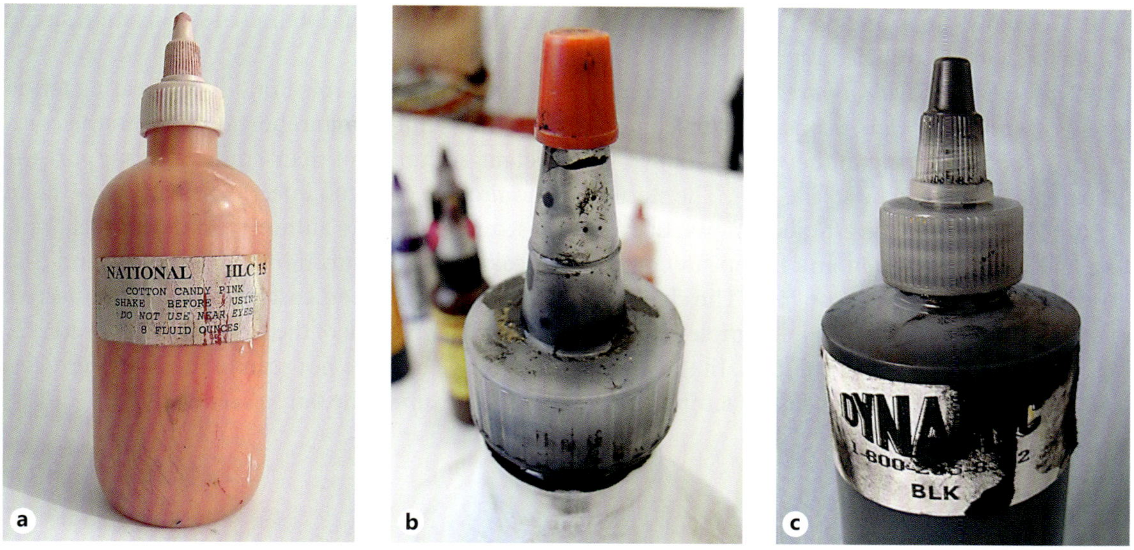

Fig. 6. Unsafe tattoo ink bottles reused a number of times and over some unknown period of time on different customers. Sterility from new, preservation, date of production, date of first use, and date of expiry or end of use after opening were unknown. Bottles were collected by the 'Tattoo Clinic' of Bispebjerg University Hospital. Bottles are not in a shape accordant with recommendations of tattooists' organizations [23].

ical ingredients of tattoo inks, and in their final report also considered bacterial complications [27]. Thus, Europe may be on a move towards tattooing with less risk of infection.

In allied fields, namely in the production of medicines and cosmetics, there are recognized standards for the quality of product manufacturing through good manufacturing practices (GMP). Good clinical practice (GCP) standard was also considered for tattoo ink products and is logic for this type of products, which are injectables [28]. However, being resource demanding and difficult to implement and control, the initiative has been met with pessimism rather than optimism. Most tattoo inks used in Europe are imported from the USA and many come in from Asia.

In the USA, the Food and Drug Administration (FDA), which is responsible for tattooing, decided not to be very active due to the fact that tattooing is causing no measurable number of deaths and since efficient regulation of the field is resource demanding and meets many difficulties due to many knowledge gaps [29]. In the USA, the emphasis is on vigilance, with active intervention once accumulated problems, such as local outbreaks of infection, are reported to the FDA through MedWatch adverse-event reports. In Europe, organized by the European Union, there is a vigilance system covering consumer products of any kind, RAPEX, which sporadically receives reports on tattoo inks but only a few clinical cases of complications [30]. In Europe, doctors' reporting of adverse effects of tattooing, including tattoo infections, shall primarily be directed to the relevant local authority.

National institutions in most European countries have implemented some control of the tattoo business, emphasizing control of hygiene and infections [31]. In most countries, it is now required to be registered as a tattooist and have the parlor inspected before start of business. A few countries require tattooists to have passed a course in tattoo hygiene. The Netherlands, Italy, Switzerland, Germany, and later Spain, France, and other countries, have introduced regulations of tattooing. However, regulations are at very different levels of ambition and inconsistent in content, many of them referring to the ResAp(2008)1, requiring tattoo inks to be sterile [24]. The sterility of tattoo ink has not been fulfilled in practice and to a level of perfection in any European country due to Internet sales of tattoo inks. The challenge of sterile inks, albeit in principle simple to reach, is not facing an immediate solution. In the meantime, inks from established manufacturers, who can document their method of sterilization, are to be preferred.

Doctors have a role not only in treating tattoo infections but also in reporting cases to the competent authority in their country to support the monitoring of tattoo infections at any time, as an instrument for the authority to detect local outbreaks of tattoo infections early enough and prevent that new tattoo customers become infected. It is a potential risk of the future that new and very aggressive bacteria not seen in the past unexpectedly show up in the tattoo scene.

References

1 Zorp J, Boonstra A, Coutinho R-A, van den Hoek J-A-R: Tattooing, permanent make-up and piercing in Amsterdam; guidelines, legislation and monitoring. Euro Surveill 2006;11:34–36.

2 Veenstra T: Tattoo Hygiene Guidelines. National Institute of Public Health and the Environment, The Netherlands, 2014.

3 Veenstra T: The Amsterdam model for control of tattoo parlours and businesses; in Serup J, Kluger N, Bäumler W (eds): Tattooed Skin and Health. Curr Probl Dermatol. Basel, Karger, 2015, vol 48, pp 218–222.

4 Kazandjieva J, Tsankov N: Tattoos: dermatological complications. Clin Dermatol 2007;25:375–382.

5 Kluger N: Complications infectieuses cutanées associées au tatouage permanent. Med Mal Infect 2010;41:115–122.

6 Kluger N: Cutaneous complications related to permanent decorative tattooing. Expert Rev Clin Immunol 2010;6:363–371.

7 Klügl I, Hiller KA, Landthaler M, et al: Incidence of health problems associated with tattooed skin: a nation-wide study in German-speaking countries. Dermatology 2010;221:43–50.

8 Kluger N: Acute complications of tattooing presenting in the ED. Am J Emerg Med 2012;30:2055–2059.

9 Wenzel SM, Rittmann I, Landthaler M, et al: Adverse reactions after tattooing: review of the literature and comparison to results of a study. Dermatology 2013;226:138–147.

10 Tattooing – Health, Risks and Culture. The Council on Health and Disease Prevention, Copenhagen, 2015, pp 1–165. www.vidensraad.dk.

11 Drage LA, Ecker PM, Orenstein R, et al: An outbreak of *Mycobacterium chelonae* infections in tattoos. J Am Acad Dermatol 2010;62:501–506.

12 Kluger N, Muller C, Gral N: Atypical mycobacteria infection following tattooing: review of an outbreak in 8 patients in a French tattoo parlor. Arch Dermatol 2008;144:941–942.

13 Porter CJW, Simcock JW, MacKinnon CA: Necrotising fasciitis and cellulitis after traditional Samoan tattooing: case report. J Infect 2005;50:149–152.

14 Jafari S, Copes R, Baharlou S, et al: Tattooing and the risk of transmission of hepatitis C: a systematic review and meta-analysis. Int J Infect Dis 2010;14:928–940.

15 Doll DC: Tattooing in prison and HIV infection. Lancet 1988;1:66–67.

16 Woelber E, Schrick EJ, Gessner BD, Evans HL: Proportion of surgical site infections occurring after hospital discharge: a systematic review. Surg Infect (Larchmt) 2016;17:510–519.

17 Hellard ME, Aitken CK, Hocking JS: Tattooing in prisons – not such a pretty picture. Am J Infect Control 2007;35:477–480.

18 Baumgartner A, Gautsch S: Hygienic-microbiological quality of tattoo- and permanent make-up colours. J Verbrauch Lebensm 2011;6:319–325.

19 Bonadonna L: Survey of studies on microbial contamination of marketed tattoo inks; in Serup J, Kluger N, Bäumler W (eds): Tattooed Skin and Health. Curr Probl Dermatol. Basel, Karger, 2015, vol 48, pp 190–195.

20 Høgsberg T, Saunte DM, Frimodt-Møller N, et al: Microbial status and product labelling of 58 original tattoo inks. J Eur Acad Dermatol Venereol 2013;27:73–80.

21 Rosenbaum BE, Milam EC, Seo L, Leger MC: Skin care in the tattoo parlor: a survey of tattoo artists in New York City. Dermatology 2016;232:484–489.

22 Schmidt A: Hygiene standards for tattooists; in Serup J, Kluger N, Bäumler W (eds): Tattooed Skin and Health. Curr Probl Dermatol. Basel, Karger, 2015, vol 48 pp 223–227.

23 United European Tattooist Association (UETA): Hygiene standards for tattooists. 2009. http://www.ueta.org/service/guidelines/.

24 Bodlund M (ed): Vägen til at bli tatuerare, rekommendationer och regler för yrkesverksamme tatuerare. Helsingborg, Sveriges Registrerede Tatuerare (SRT), 2013. ISBN 978-91-637-1899-1.

25 Bergström J, Bodlund M: Hygiene standards in the tattoo parlour and practices for prevention of infection; in Serup J, Kluger N, Bäumler W (eds): Tattooed Skin and Health. Curr Probl Dermatol. Basel, Karger, 2015, vol 48, pp 228–235.

26 Council of Europe: Resolution ResAp(2008)1 on Requirements and Criteria for the Safety of Tattoos and Permanent Make-Up (superseding Resolution ResAp(2003)2 on Tattoos and Permanent Make-Up). Strasbourg, 2008.

27 European Commission: JRC Technical Reports. Safety of tattoos and permanent make-up. Final report of work package 3. Administrative arrangement N. 2014-33617 conducted on behalf of DG JUST, 2016. EUR 27247 EN; ISBN 978-92-79-58783-2 (PDF); DOI 10.2788/011817.

28 Michael R: Manufacturing of tattoo ink products today and in future: Europe; in Serup J, Kluger N, Bäumler W (eds): Tattooed Skin and Health Curr Probl Dermatol. Basel, Karger, 2015, vol 48, pp 103–111.

29 LeBlanc P-M, Hollinger K-A, Klontz K-C: Tattoo ink-related infections – awareness, diagnosis, reporting, and prevention. N Engl J Med 2012;367:985–987.

30 Verdier C: Surveillance of tattoo-related adverse events by the EU RAPEX system and by national monitoring; in Serup J, Kluger N, Bäumler W (eds): Tattooed Skin and Health. Curr Probl Dermatol. Basel, Karger, 2015, vol 48, pp 210–217.

31 Laux P, Luch A: The European landscape of national regulations of tattoo inks and businesses; in Serup J, Kluger N, Bäumler W (eds): Tattooed Skin and Health. Curr Probl Dermatol. Basel, Karger, 2015, vol 48, pp 196–200.

Prof. Jørgen Serup, DMSc
Department of Dermatology D41, Bispebjerg University Hospital
Bispebjerg Bakke 23
DK–2400 Copenhagen NV (Denmark)
E-Mail joergen.vedelskov.serup@regionh.dk

Serup J, Bäumler W (eds): Diagnosis and Therapy of Tattoo Complications. With Atlas of Illustrative Cases.
Curr Probl Dermatol. Basel, Karger, 2017, vol 52, pp 42–57 (DOI: 10.1159/000450778)

Diagnostic Tools for Doctors' Evaluation of Tattoo Complications

Jørgen Serup

The 'Tattoo Clinic', Department of Dermatology, Bispebjerg University Hospital, Copenhagen, Denmark

Abstract

Diagnosis of tattoo complications is a multi-facetted field since many clinical entities and disease mechanisms are represented. Infections, allergies, and pigment foreign body reactions with granuloma are the major groups. The clinician needs a structured approach to diagnosis and an armamentarium of standard tests. Diagnosis primarily builds on patient history, objective clinical examination, and punch biopsy, supplemented with microbiology testing, ultrasound scanning, and clinical photography. Evaluation of allergic tattoo reactions and allergy to pigments by patch testing is not applicable and has a falsely negative outcome except for the diagnosis of allergy to metals and preservatives. Simple inspection of raw punch biopsies from chronic tattoo reactions, preferably evaluated with stereo microscopy, provides important information about the density and the local distribution of tattoo pigment in the dermis and changes of microanatomical skin structures. Histology may show subtle structural changes, but traditional patterns (lichenoid reaction, pseudolymphoma, granuloma, and pseudoepitheliomatous epidermal hyperplasia) are of little or no help in the diagnosis since the patterns overlap and have no distinct clinical correlates. Histology cannot separate allergic and nonallergic reactions. However, granulomatous reaction and sarcoid granuloma are significant findings since papulonodular reaction of black tattoos and sarcoidosis are strongly associated with each other. 20-MHz ultrasound scanning is important for noninvasive imaging and characterization of inflammatory tattoo reactions and can be used preoperatively as guide to treatment. Electron microscopy can visualize pigment particles in tissues, cells, and tattoo inks. Chemicals of pigment in tissues and in tattoo inks can be analyzed by high-performance liquid chromatography, mass spectroscopy, and Raman spectroscopy.

Tattoo Complications and Diagnostic Approach

Diagnosing tattoo complications is a challenge since diagnostic entities are numerous [1, 2]. The major groups of complication are as follows:

- Bacterial infections shortly after the tattoo is made.
- Red tattoos with allergic reactions manifested as plaque elevation, excessive hyperkeratosis, or ulceronecrotic reactions developed after a

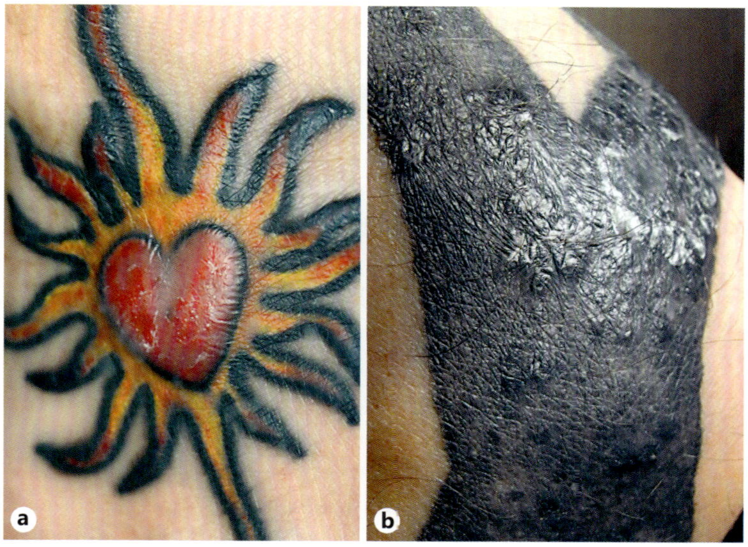

Fig. 1. a Allergic reaction in a red tattoo. Clinical pattern: 'plaque elevation'. Every part tattooed red is affected. **b** Nonallergic reaction in a black tattoo. Clinical pattern: papulonodular reaction. Lesions vary and parts of the tattoo are normal. The pattern is related to black pigment agglomeration in the dermis with formation of pigment foreign bodies.

longer period of sensitization to a hapten (fig. 1a).

- Black tattoos with papulonodular reactions due to pigment foreign bodies formed in the dermis after months or years and causing inflammatory reaction. This can be associated with sarcoidosis (fig. 1b).
- Psychosocial complications.
- A range of miscellaneous complications with many distinct entities representing many different disease mechanisms (30% of complications registered in the 'Tattoo Clinic').

In the diagnostic evaluation, the doctor has to start with a panorama view followed by more precise diagnostic undertakings chosen to confirm or reject a hypothesis and reach a firm conclusion, which can argue for rational therapy. A major distinction to be made is between allergic and nonallergic inflammatory complications and infections.

The armamentarium of diagnostic tools is mostly methods familiar to dermatologists and therefore easily available. By knowing the hints to diagnosis, the clinicians can do most of the job in their office already at the initial consultation.

In the past, there was no established reference or diagnosis system of tattoo complications. Doctors are referred to the chapter by Serup [this vol., pp. 58–73] and to the original article [2]. This new system is submitted to the 11th revision of the World Health Organization's international classification of diseases used globally.

Patient History

In the following, a standard approach to diagnosis is presented, which is used routinely in the 'Tattoo Clinic' of Bispebjerg University Hospital.

Basic information in a patient file shall consider the following issues:

- Allergy to contact allergens especially nickel, chromate, preservatives, and textile dyes.
- Previous diseases of relevance, i.e. psoriasis, eczema, urticaria, photosensitivity, sarcoidosis, hepatitis, HIV, systemic diseases, including autoimmune conditions, and ongoing immunosuppressive treatment.
- The problematic tattoo, i.e. when, where, and how (professional or amateur) was the tattoo acquired, hygiene standard of the tattoo parlor, the tattooist, needle, tattoo inks and other

utensils, precautions taken to avoid infection, bleeding or pain during tattooing indicating tattoo trauma, the healing phase, and after-care.

- Time from tattooing to debut of tattoo problems, progression of symptoms, and fever or other symptoms; treatments taken and the effect of treatments.
- History of photosensitivity locally in the tattoo or generally in the skin.
- Other tattoos, i.e. concomitant or subsequent reaction of other tattoos and debut of reaction relative to the problematic tattoo.
- Other conditions and organs, i.e. fever or general malaise, lymphadenopathy, other reactions in the skin, manifestations of internal organs, eyes, and joints.
- Concomitant reactivity or activity, i.e. signs of associated reaction in another tattoo of the same color *(allergic cross-sensitization)* or widespread reaction in any black tattoos (*'rush phenomenon'*, associated with sarcoidosis) parallel to reaction of the problematic tattoo.
- Pain of neurosensitive tattoo reactions, severe, maybe invalidating and the main symptom.
- Scarring of tattoos on different backgrounds, i.e. traumatization by tattooing, sequel of infection, or sequel from laser removal or removal by chemical caustics.

Objective Findings by Clinical Examination

- Signs of local infection of the tattoo, i.e. the tattoo showing redness, swelling, crusts, or oozing with progression into the surrounding skin or into deeper structures. Are there signs of systemic infection with progression into septicemia and risk of septic shock?
- Is the pathology limited to one, and only one, specific tattoo color?
- If pathology is limited to one color, is it independent of dose of pigment or dose dependent, i.e. fully expressed in any part of the color of the tattoo or diluted or absent in parts of the tattoo tattooed with little pigment?
- Is the pathology monomorphic with flat plaque elevation, hyperkeratosis, or ulceration (indicating allergy) or dimorphic with a mix of papules and nodules and an unaffected tattoo sharing the same color?
- Is the affected color deeply colored with direct signs of overdose with pigment?
- Are there signs of scarring of the tattoo due to traumatic tattooing, previous laser treatments, use of caustics for tattoo removal, or self-inflicted interventions?
- Are there disturbances of neural sensation in the tattoo, in the relevant dermatome, and in the skin?
- Are other and older tattoos affected with similar or with different reactions?
- Are there alterations of the skin with signs of scar sarcoidosis, erythema nodosum, psoriasis, lichen planus, or other dermatological diseases?
- Is the nontattooed skin normal or with signs of concomitant skin disease, which might or might not be manifested in the tattoo?
- Based on objective findings and patient history, a clinical diagnosis shall be concluded as a final or tentative diagnosis awaiting the outcome of other examinations.

Clinical Photography

Tattoos are pictures on the skin canvas made to be seen. Photos of normal and abnormal tattoos can tell more than words. Photos are important elements of the patient file documenting the objective status at the date of the photo. Clinical photography and skin is a specialized field [3–5]. Professional cameras with ring flash prepared for photography of the skin are preferable, but cheap cameras often can do a good job. Light conditions are important for the quality of the photo. Photography using daylight may produce the best pictures and the light, and object may be positioned with incident light under a low angle to highlight skin surface contours, elevation and thickening of a lesion. However, good photographic quality often requires powerful lighting using a flash designed to emit bluish light of the preferred Kelvin temperature. Room lighting and especially operation lamps often are not suited for photography and result in disturbed color. It is always important to choose a proper background, which is neutral, and also avoid irrelevant objects disturbing the photo, such as jewelry, colorful textiles, and shoes. Photos of patients' faces are best taken with their eyes closed.

Close-up photography of small objects as exemplified by a punch biopsy cylinder is preferably made using a tripod limiting blurred photos due to vibrations of the camera. Close-up photography performed free hand can be helped by some improvised method of fixation, i.e. by leaning one's elbow on the table with the object being photographed. In close-up photography, the depth of optical sharpness is narrow and manual control of camera distance to object may be preferred to the autofocus setting. Small movements of the camera and thus fine adjustment of the distance to the object can be navigated with the peak sharpness of focus positioned precisely on the detail of interest in the object. With modern high-resolution cameras it is often advantageous to take photos from a longer distance, then crop and magnify the miniature image, and in this way obtain a photo with wider depth of optical sharpness than close-up photography can provide.

Photography using smartphones has become popular. Often patients who present with tattoo complications took photos of the newly made tattoo. In the case of complications, they often can present serial photos showing the progress of disease. Photos taken with smartphones are often of surprisingly good quality.

Infrared photography was successfully applied to 8 Inuit mummies from Greenland to image old tattoos weak in color but still with significant amount of pigment hidden in the dermis [6]. This photographic technique clearly has a potential for the study of the effectiveness of tattoo removal by lasers.

It is necessary that the patients provide their consent if photos are used for educational and scientific purposes. Release of photos to the free press shall be made with full attention to the situation a publication of the photo might foster.

Bacterial Culture and Other Methods for Identification of Microbial Pathogens

Sampling the bacteria of the skin may seem simple, but it is not [7]. Swaps taken from the skin surface may or may not isolate the pathogen responsible for a tattoo infection. In infections of deeper structures, i.e. in erysipelas, cellulite, and necrotizing fasciitis, culture of bacteria directly from the infected tissue may be necessary, and a swap taken from the skin surface may easily be misleading. Culture from tissues may be not enough sensitive to allow isolation of the specific bacteria causing the infection, and the bacteria can also be anaerobic. In septicemia, of course, culture from the blood shall be performed. With the polymerase chain reaction (PCR) technique, even few colonies and fragments of bacteria can be measured and characterized by their DNA sequence. PCR diagnostics is applicable to killed bacteria and thus useful for the period after antibiotic treatment has been initiated. Mycobacteria can be identified in biopsies with the Ziehl-Neelsen stain (a.m.) and cultured on special media. Characterization of different subtypes of mycobacteria by PCR with reference to international libraries is possible. Fungal infections can be diagnosed by microscopy of skin surface scrapes and by culture on Sabouraud agar or another appropriate medium [8]. Microbiological diagnostics is best performed after consultation with the local department of microbiology, particularly if rare and endemic infections are suspected. In most countries routine bacteriology includes screening for bacteria resistant to antibiotics.

In many cases verification of the precise pathogen behind a tattoo infection may not be possible or feasible in practice. Doctors shall institute antibiotic treatment based on their clinical diagnosis and general knowledge about the bacteria typically causing that particular type of infection. The treatment later may be adjusted guided by the outcome of microbiological examination, if the microbiology outcome is available and relevant. Information indicating infection to bacterial strains resistant to antibiotics is important and may necessitate isolation of the patient.

Punch Biopsy

Punch biopsy using a 3-mm standard punch is an important tool with different purposes. Local anesthesia with injection of carbocaine or another local anesthetic is often unpleasant and sometimes painful, and, surprisingly, many tattooed individuals declare 'needle fear' in the doctor's office. Depending on the patient, it may be preferable to perform a quick biopsy without anesthesia, which is often easy because of the inflammatory edema of the skin. Cooling of the outer skin with a liquid nitrogen spray is another alternative to injection anesthetics.

In the diagnostic evaluation of tattoo reactions, punch biopsy can serve different aims, which are presented below.

Visual Inspection of the Raw Biopsy Cylinder

Visual inspection of the raw biopsy cylinder by the naked eye, under a magnifying lens, or in the stereomicroscope immediately after the biopsy is taken to see the density of tattoo pigment in the dermis, the vertical level of the pigment layer, the relative thickening of the skin, excessive hyperkeratosis and thickening of the epidermis, and special abnormal findings such as sarcoid granulomas and epidermoid inclusions (fig. 2a–f).

The raw biopsy displays the microanatomy of the skin, and dermal thickening due to inflammation and epidermal thickening is easily seen, the latter as a yellowish band on the top of the biopsy cylinder. Scar formation in the dermis can sometimes be seen as a porcelain-white layer. Epidermoid cysts can occasionally appear as onion-like structures, if the biopsy is cut between razor blades. Importantly, the lateral cutting edge of the biopsy cylinder may have a number of small dome-shaped protrusions representing sarcoid granulomas, a finding called the 'bunch of grape' sign (fig. 2e) [2, 9]. This sign is strongly indicative of sarcoid granuloma manifested directly in the tattoo [9, 10]. The raw biopsy is the preferred specimen for quick estimation of density and location of tattoo pigment in the skin. Tattoo pigments are selected as materials especially colorful to the human eye, which in color perception is nonlinear in comparison with a spectrophotometer. In the optically transparent 3-mm raw biopsy cylinder, much more dermal tissue holding pigment can be viewed than in a routine dermatome slice of tissue only a few microns thick. Moreover, the specimen for routine histology is stained, which may disturb the assessment of pigment. *Visual inspection of the raw biopsy, ideally under a stereo microscope, is a quick, easy, and efficient tool to assess the microanatomy of the skin as well as the density and local distribution of tattoo pigment in the dermis.*

Histology of the Skin

Histology of the skin is done by routine methodology with hematoxylin-eosin staining or studied with advanced methods such as immunohistochemistry, and a range of special staining methods is used to display tissue details, pathological reactions, as well as reaction patterns and clusters of pigment particles (fig. 3a, b). The conventional light microscope works with magnifications up to about ×800.

Routine histology is important in the evaluation of cellular infiltration and inflammatory reaction of tattoos with a chronic complication. Histology is especially important because it provides

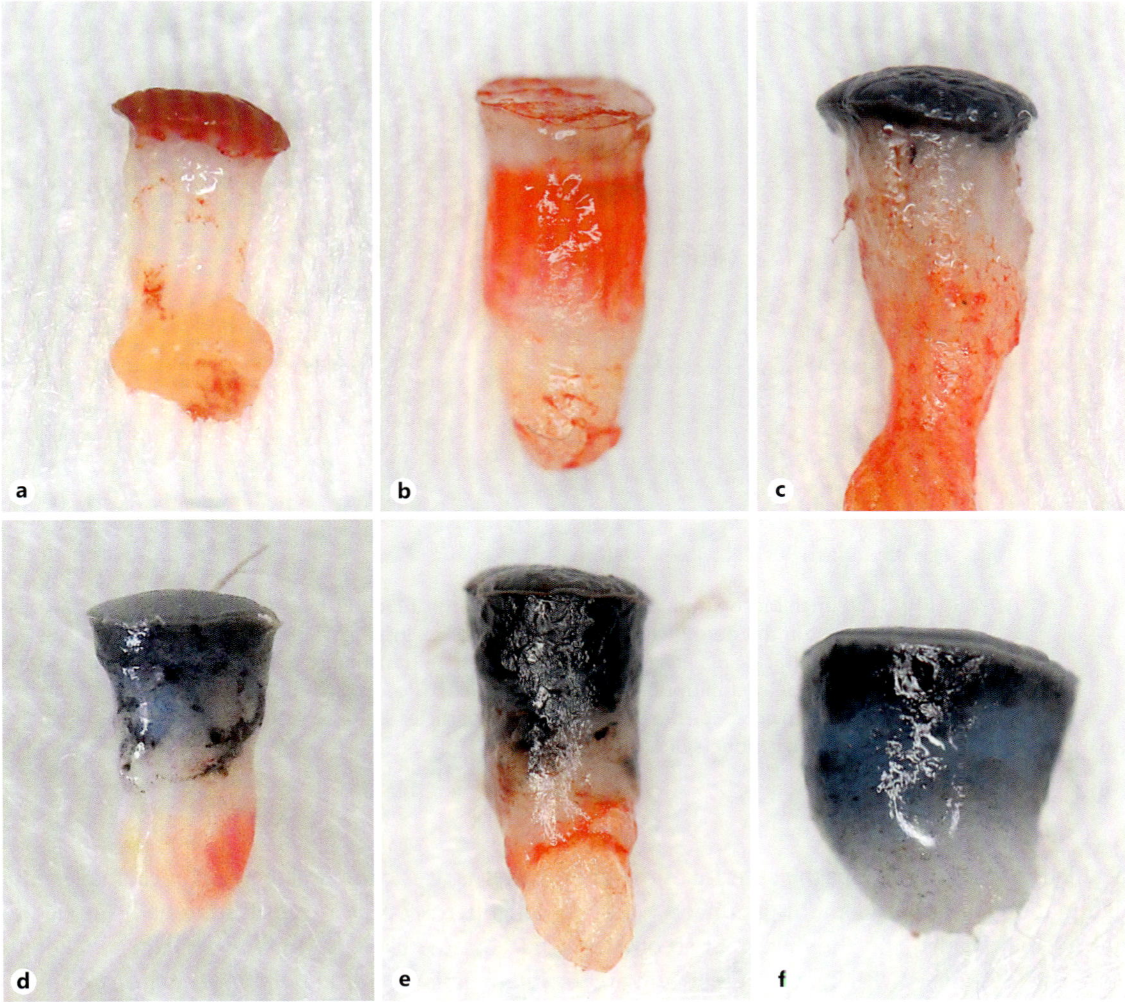

Fig. 2. Raw punch biopsies from various chronic tattoo reactions. **a** Red pigment concentrated in the papillary dermis; normal epidermis. **b** Broad zone of pigment in the outer two thirds of the dermis; thickened epidermis with excessive hyperkeratosis. **c** Black pigment concentrated in the papillary dermis; normal epidermis. **d** Black pigment in the outer dermis concentrated in the papillary layer, with agglomerated pigment following the vasculature, i.e. supposedly the lymphatics deep in the dermis. The mid-dermal porcelain-white shadow indicates fibrosis. Epidermis is flattened and possibly with minute thickening. Interface to fat is normal. **e** Excessive black pigment and dense clusters of black pigment in most of the dermis indicating sarcoid granulomas, i.e. 'bunch of grape' sign. **f** Dense black pigment in the dermis, but diffused with no sign of granulomas. Small pigment bodies are drifting to the bottom of the dermis. The porcelain-white shadow indicates mid-dermal fibrosis. Further information and illustrations are shown in the atlas, pp. 150–152, 155, 156, 158–160, 163, 167, 173, 175, 176, 186, 190, 195–197, 199, 201, 203, 204.

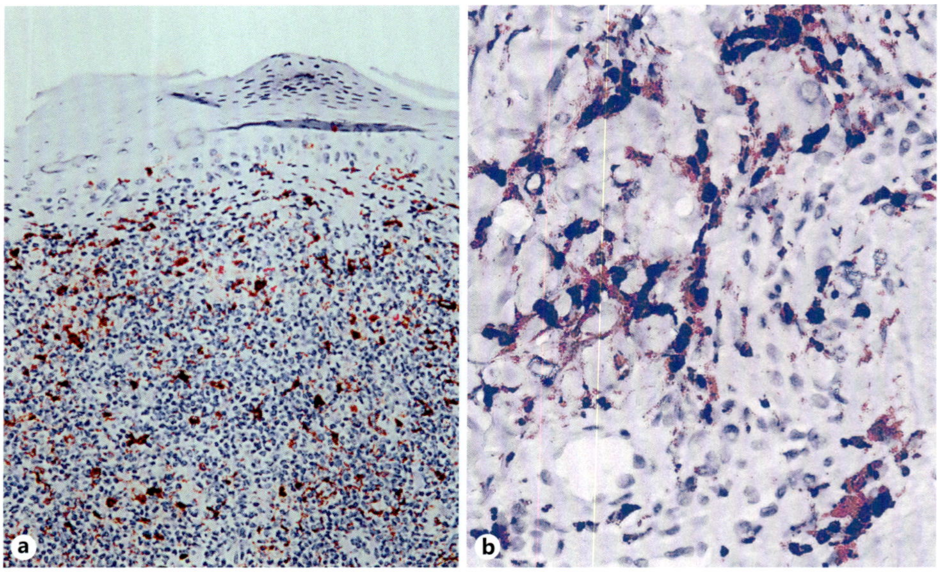

Fig. 3. a Punch biopsy from a red tattoo with allergic reaction, by transmission light microscopy. The pigment in the dermis is seen as brown or black foreign bodies when the pigment clusters are large and thick. Small-sized pigment clusters are transparent and thus display their genuine color, i.e. red. Heavy infiltration with lymphocytes. **b** Close-up with details. Hidden under the resolution of the microscope are primary pigment particles sized smaller than about 1 μm and chemical breakdown products of pigments.

detailed information about the severity of the inflammation, the level of the inflammatory reaction in the dermis, and the degree of secondary epidermal responses with hyperkeratosis and other markers of abnormal epidermal function. Subtle details such as pimples with microabscess formation and excessive hyperkeratosis with notches and epidermoid inclusions can be verified. Also, the degree of subclinical dermal fibrosis seen as a sequel of needle trauma can be described. Histopathology offers a range of special staining methods including immunochemistry. Histology, however, has major limitations when it comes to clarification of mechanisms behind tattoo reactions. Histology is pattern recognition guided by tradition. The conclusion is made by the individual pathologist and by his/her subjective eye when making a qualitative assessment through the microscope ocular, referenced to a library of recognized patterns. It is comparable to a clinical inspection. The microscopic patterns traditionally applied to tattoos are *lichenoid reactions, pseudolymphomatous reactions, granulomatous reactions, and pseudoepitheliomatous epidermal hyperplasia* [11–14]. However, reactions overlap and may be present in the same biopsy, and reactions have not found distinct correlates in specific clinical entities linked with individual microscopic patterns, except for granulomatous reactions associated with sarcoid granuloma and the sarcoidosis disease. Histology is indispensable in the diagnosis of fully developed sarcoid granuloma and also in the delineation of the forerunner, granulomatous inflammation [9, 10]. Pathologists are often reluctant in their distinction of the two patterns and thus may appear imprecise. They have a difficult job and often see their role as being supportive to the clinician, who is expected to make the final di-

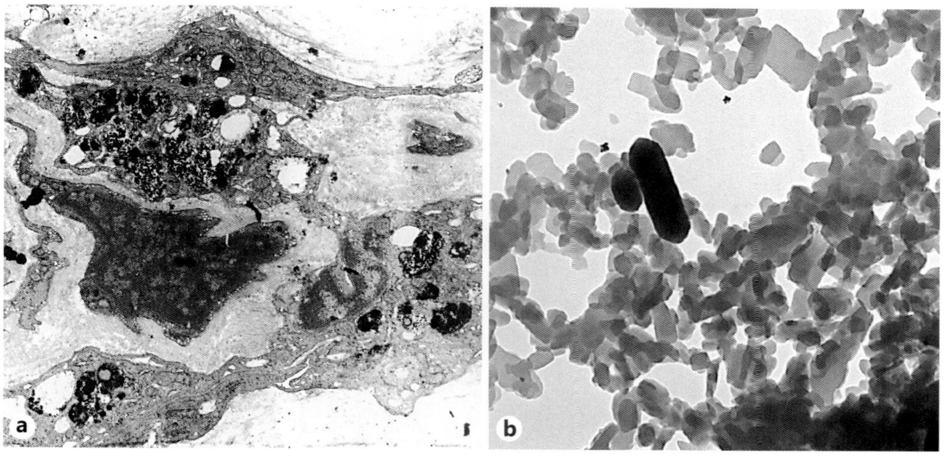

Fig. 4. Electron microscopy. **a** Transmission electron microscopy from a mast cell-storing tattoo pigment in intracellular inclusions with vesicles. The pigment has undergone variable degrees of physical disruption. The image probably illustrates a state of permanent deposition. The pigment is also deposited extracellularly between collagen fibrils. **b** Scanning electron microscopy from a commercial tattoo ink product made with Pigment Red 17 (Color Index number 12390, single azo chemical structure). Note the spontaneous variability of pigment particle size and shape. Courtesy from T. Kobayasi, Bispebjerg University Hospital, and T.B. Sejersen, Panum Institute, Copenhagen, Denmark.

agnosis. Sarcoidosis is not a well-defined disease entity, and there is no established set of internationally recognized diagnosis criteria.

In chronic tattoo reactions the distinction of allergic and nonallergic reactions is important. Histology applied neither to tattoo reactions nor to contact dermatitis cannot distinguish allergic reactions from irritant reactions and other types of noninfectious dermal inflammation. However, it has recently been shown in a systematic analysis of several individual histologic features and study by immunohistochemistry that interface dermatitis is common in reactions of red tattoos concluded allergic [15]. Allergic tattoo reactions and lichen planus have some similarity in the clinic. Interface dermatitis manifested partly or fully in red tattoos with an allergic reaction may have been overlooked in the past and may in the future be used as a marker of allergy.

Tattoo pigments range in size from nanoparticles under 100 nm to microparticles sized up to 6–800 nm. Some pigments, especially carbon black, tend to agglomerate and aggregate and form larger clusters sized microns. The resolution of light microscopy is not high enough to see nanoparticles and smaller microparticles; thus, light microscopy can only display clusters of aggregated pigment in the dermis, and for optical reasons the method will not be able to detect all tattoo pigments present in the skin. Particles that are smaller than the resolution of the light microscope are not seen, and chemical breakdown products of pigments are also invisible. There is limited experience with tattoo pigments viewed with dark field and polarization microscopy, but these methods might be useful for a more detailed study of tattoo pigments in the skin.

In summary, histology is a useful tool and sometimes indispensable in the clarification of tattoo reaction. However, it is a major limitation that histology patterns traditionally applied to

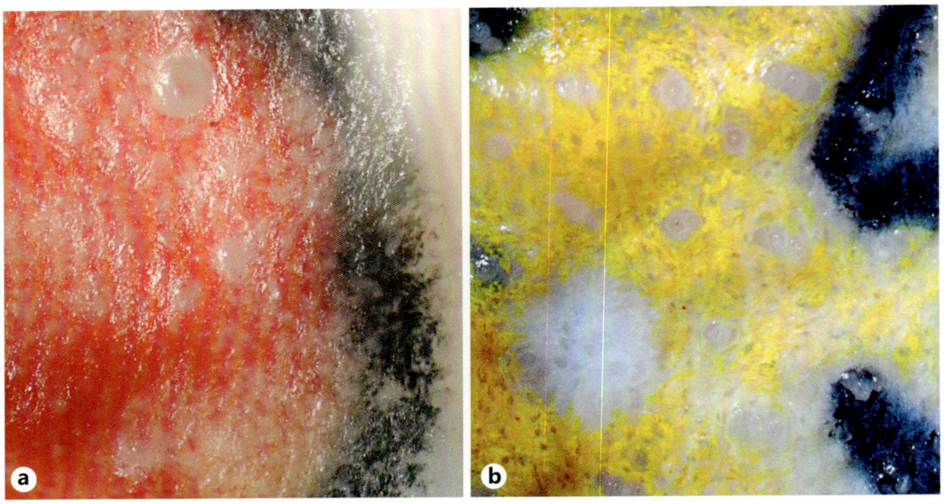

Fig. 5. Horizontal dermatome sections from chronic allergic tattoo reactions. **a** Red tattoo with dense and diffuse dermal pigment and aggregated black pigment in the lining. Hair sheets with their epidermis are without pigment. **b** The same situation in a yellow tattoo, with minor fibrosis. Dermatome shave cuts from the papillary dermis are ideal for the biochemical analysis of pigment and pigment metabolites since clean anatomical specimens can be prepared by microdissection. Pigments are concentrated.

tattoo reactions have not found meaningful clinical correlates, and histology cannot support the distinction of allergic and nonallergic tattoo reactions. Therefore, histology is mainly positioned as a tool of supplementary information useful for the grading of cellular infiltration and with the capacity to display subtle tissue structures and specific lesions of interest. Histology is indispensable in the assessment of sarcoidosis albeit the separation of granulomatous inflammation and sarcoid granuloma is variable and observer dependent, as is the sarcoidosis diagnosis.

Electron Microscopy

Electron microscopy to see cellular and subcellular details including pigments in mast cells in the transmission electron microscope working at magnifications up to ×75,000 is the method of choice for visualization of tattoo pigments in tissues, i.e. the skin, lymph nodes, and the liver (fig. 4a). The method is available at some university clinics but not part of normal routine and requires special samples and special media. Pigments, pigment crystals, and their physical fragments in mast cells can be displayed [16]. Pigments in tattoo ink stock products can be visualized with scanning electron microscopy (fig. 4b). Pigment particles and crystals can have many shapes, and the same chemical pigment can have different shapes depending on production. The size of the pigment can be measured with the electron microscope and more conveniently by laser diffraction [16].

Scientific Purposes

Scientific purposes include in particular chemical analysis of tattoo pigments and their breakdown products locally in the dermis. Chemical analysis of pigment chemicals and the many impurities and chemical breakdown products in dermal tissue is difficult due to the generally low solubility of pigments [17, 18]. Punch biopsies and horizontal biopsies from the papillary dermis harvested with a dermatome or a shaver blade are proper samples for chemical analysis (fig. 5a, b). High-performance liquid chromatography and mass spectrometry were introduced for the analysis of red azo pigments and other types of tattoo pigment [19–21]. Chemical analysis of tattoo pigments in the skin, in organs, and in ink stock products is hampered by a lack of validation and standardization of methods, as recently concluded in the extensive report of the European Union on methods applicable to chemical analysis of tattoo inks [22]. Analysis of metals distinguishing between total amounts, including inert metal and soluble amounts such as ionic nickel and chromate VI, causing allergy has not found a solution [23]. Acidic microwave treatment of samples is far away from physiological conditions of metal metabolism. It remains an obstacle that tattoo pigments are industrial and not refined chemicals of high purity thus with many other chemicals surrounding the main chemical of the pigment. Safety issues, such as the potential to sensitize, may not be an effect of the main pigment itself. The many challenges of measuring pigments in the skin and in tattoo ink stock bottles have recently been reviewed [24]. Raman spectroscopy available at many laboratories deserves a special mention since this method can be applied to intact skin, skin biopsies, and tattoo inks at the same time. Thus, information on spectra related to for example allergic tattoo reactions in the skin can be bridged to other sources of information, including libraries of spectra available on the Internet [25]. The method is qualitative and semiquantitative and not a priori limited by shortage of specific knowledge about what to search in the sample being measured. Risk spectra found in allergic tattoo reactions have been published [25].

When studying the dose of tattoo pigment per surface area unit, it is worth knowing that the piece of dermis punched with a biopsy punch, despite elastic retraction during cutting and tissue distortions during histological processing, accurately represents the vertical cylinder of dermal tissue defined by the diameter of the punch [26, 27].

Examination for Microbial Pathogens in the Dermis

After thorough disinfection of the skin surface before and after serial tape strips with abrasion of the stratum corneum, punch biopsies can be used for culture of bacteria and other microorganisms in the dermis, and for PCR measurement of DNA fragments of bacteria. This may be of special interest if infection with mycobacteria is suspected.

High-Frequency Ultrasound Examination and Other Noninvasive Methods

The different methods of skin structure evaluation based on punch biopsy ranging from visual inspection of raw punch biopsies over light microscopy to electron microscopy has the inbuilt dilemma that a higher resolution and a smaller tissue sample do not automatically mean increased information when information is extrapolated from a small sample to the entire lesion of a tattoo reaction and when useful information does not depend on detail. High-frequency ultrasound scanning of the skin using 20-MHz scanners was introduced more than 30 years ago, and the method is well known in university dermatology [28]. The method is applied to many clinical and experimental skin conditions and established internationally [29, 30]. Images of the skin and inflammatory edema in the dermis can be analyzed by computer technology [30]. With histological processing, water is extracted and thus also the tissue edema. Ultrasound works directly on intact skin and is not intrusive to tissue water.

With ultrasound, the full thickness of the skin and typically a cross-sectional vertical scan line of 10–15 mm can be imaged, i.e. a tissue sample in

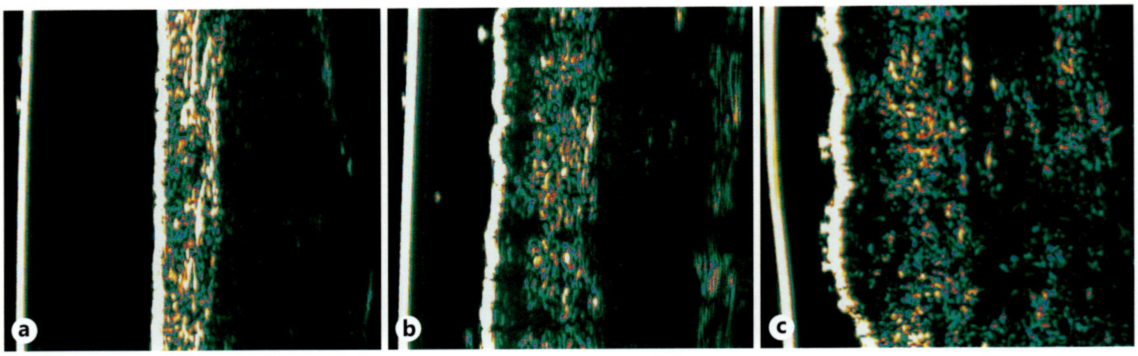

Fig. 6. 20-MHz ultrasound scanning of an allergic reaction in a red tattoo. **a** Normal skin oriented vertically. From left to right: membrane of probe, black layer of coupling gel, epidermis and entrance echo, and dermis with variable echo density illustrating the undisturbed collagen network/interstitial water acoustic structure. **b** Less active site of the tattoo reaction towards the periphery, with dermal thickening and a subepidermal low echogenic band indicating inflammatory edema. **c** More active site in the center, with major dermal thickening, a broad low echogenic band, and also disturbance of the lower dermis and the subcutaneous fat to the level of the muscle fascia (right) [31].

width corresponding to 3–5 biopsy punches. The ultrasound probe can be moved freely over the skin and the skin lesion, and any part of interest can be selected for scanning independent of anatomical site [29]. Commercial dermal scanners have inbuilt software for measurement of distances in the tissue, area of regions of interest, and computerized image analysis of echo density, with defined low echogenic fields or bands in the dermis representing inflammatory edema or another change of tissue depending on the situation.

20-MHz ultrasound scanning of inflammatory tattoo reactions was studied in detail (fig. 6a–c) [31]. Tattoo pigment is normally concentrated in the outer dermis. Inflammatory tattoo reactions show a low echogenic band in the dermis corresponding to the active reaction with the thickness of the band correlating with histological assessment of severity of cellular infiltration. Ultrasound is the method of choice in the noninvasive diagnosis of chronic tattoo reactions. The method can be used preoperatively before dermatome shaving, excisional surgery, or laser treatment to indicate the depth of the pathology in the dermis.

Confocal microscopy using a fluorescent confocal microscope was applied to normal tattoos, and black pigment in the outer dermis can be visualized [32]. It is not known if reflectance confocal microscopy can be used. However, confocal microscopy has the limitation that only the epidermis and the very outer dermis are seen. Optical coherence tomography has the same limitation and a resolution that does not allow visualization of tattoo pigments and their aggregates. Dual photon tomography has a very high resolution, allowing subcellular structures to be displayed, and this method might be used as 'optical biopsy' and for the study of tattoo pigments in the outer dermis or in tissue samples.

Tattoos with chronic inflammation are supposed to have an altered vascularization. Colorful tattoo pigment and hyperkeratosis are bound to interfere with the colorimetric measurement of redness of reactions. Laser Doppler flowmetry will not have the same limitation and could be applied to tattoo reactions to quantify the vascular component of reactions and to evaluate the vasomotor rhythm. Infrared thermography has not been applied to tattoo reactions, but the method is potentially useful for monitoring the development of inflammatory tattoo reactions during treatment.

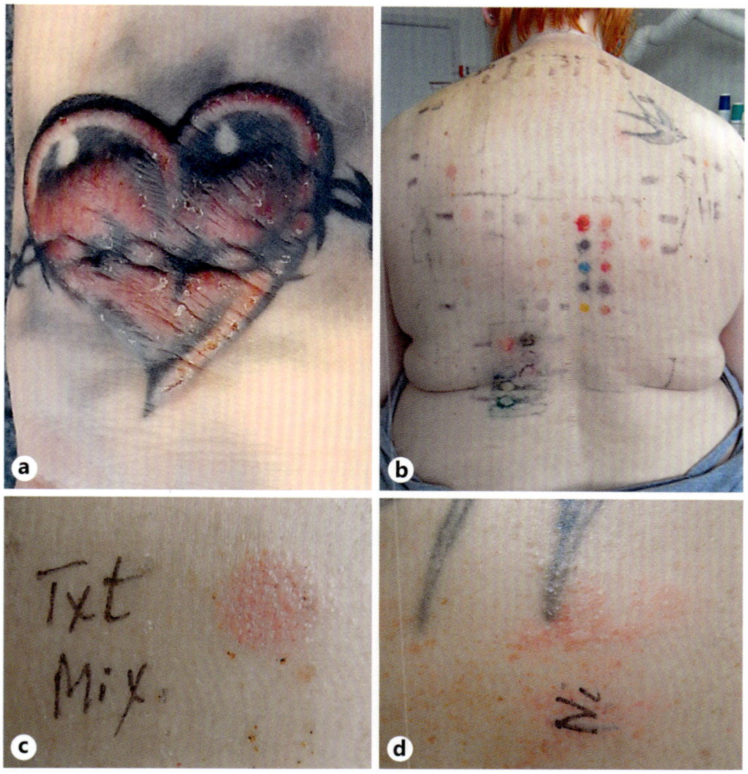

Fig. 7. A case with a very strong allergic reaction in a red tattoo on the wrist. Type: 'plaque elevation'. Histology showed heavy lymphocytic infiltration of the entire dermis given the diagnosis pseudolymphoma. **a** Clinical photo of the reaction. **b** Patch test on the back with the European standard of 32 allergens, a standard textile dye panel of 42 allergens, a BBH risk panel of 7 tattoo inks, and additionally the culprit ink she was tattooed with (color name 'True Magenta') [33]. **c, d** The patient reacted to textile mix (2+), to disperse yellow 3 (1+) in the textile panel, and to tattoo red ink (2+) in the BBH panel, but there was no reaction to the culprit ink. Nickle reaction was 3+. The test allowed no precise conclusion.

Noninvasive methods for measurement of epidermal functions, i.e. transepidermal water loss and electrical conductance and capacitance and visualization of skin surface relief and scaling, have not been applied to tattoos but might be used in research of chronic reactions and epidermal change.

Ultrasound is presently the only noninvasive instrumental method, which is introduced and shown to be directly applicable to tattoo and tattoo reactions. The method providing easy access to structural information from any site of a tattoo is especially useful in the preoperative evaluation of inflammatory tattoo reactions before dermatome shaving or laser surgery. With a very broad band of inflammation involving the deep part of the dermis, both treatments have increased risk of treatment failure and scar sequel.

Allergy Patch Test

Allergic reactions of the tattooed have different manifestations and scenes of testing.

Allergic Reaction in a Red Tattoo

Allergic reaction in a red tattoo or tattoos made with inks of nuances of red and sometimes even green, blue, and yellow manifested as chronic inflammation of the tattoo and sometimes with cross-reactivity of other tattoos made in the past with an ink sharing chemical property with the ink of the recent tattoo is a logic object for patch testing. Reactions are chronic. The dominating class of pigments causing allergy is azo pigments, and occasionally quinacridones [33, 34]. The allergy becomes manifested after months or years and is supposed to be caused by a hapten formed in the dermis. Thus, the allergen is not directly in the tattoo ink bottle and is unknown. A study of 90 patients with allergic reactions of tattoos found a negative outcome of patch testing with a battery of tattoo inks, with individual culprit inks, and with dispersed textile dyes [33]. Thus, *patch testing in tattoo allergies from tattoo inks and pigments is not applicable and likely to produce falsely negative outcomes despite the allergy being convincing according to clinical criteria.* A case illustrating tattoo allergy and patch testing is shown in figure 7a–d. There may be different reasons, i.e. poor percutaneous permeation of the test substance and, importantly, the precise allergen not being present in the test application since the allergen is a hapten. Tattooists now and then perform predictive intradermal testing of allergy by making minute test tattoos on the skin of persons wishing guarantee that a new tattoo with some desired color is allergy safe. Such intradermal testing has no rationale in nonsensitized individuals since the test dose may be too small and because it can take years to become sensitized. It is unknown if intradermal testing with the specific culprit ink in individuals with an allergic reaction to the same color in a tattoo is useful. Also, in the already sensitized individual challenged with a miniature tattoo intradermal test, it can take a long time for the local metabolism to foster the specific chemical breakdown product which contributes to the hapten as an epitope or a determinant.

Allergic Rash in a Newly Tattooed Individual

Newly tattooed individuals already strongly allergic to nickel are prone to develop a severe and widespread allergic rash. *An allergy patch test with a standard battery* of common allergens is indicated, preferably with application of the nickel test chamber for only 1 h. Metallic nickel is a very common contaminant in tattoo inks typically originating from stainless steel vessels used in production [17]. Inks may also be contaminated with chromium. The frequency of contamination with chromium VI, the active allergen, is not known but supposed to be exceptional as patch testing of tattooed individuals indicates [33]. Metals may also originate from tattoo needles. The precise role of low-grade allergy to nickel and chromate in tattooed individuals with and without reactions is unknown. A standard patch test in tattooed individuals with active inflammatory tattoo reactions seems comparable to the background population, with no special positive finding and no indication of increased allergy to paraphenylenediamine. Preservatives may be added to tattoo inks and sensitize the tattooed individual, causing a severe rash. The standard *patch test should include preservatives.*

Abnormal Healing of a Tattoo

Abnormal healing of a tattoo with inflammation booming within a few days after the tattoo is made and with delayed healing mimicking infection is a scenario little studied. The frequency of this kind of reaction, which may be seen as comparable to a challenge from a nickel patch test or another allergen in the already sensitized person, is unknown. Patients should be evaluated by *patch testing with the standard battery of common allergens including preservatives.* The individuals are supposed to have been sensitized at some previous occasion, with low-grade allergy as the outcome, and active allergic contact dermatitis in their newly acquired tattoo overlapping spontaneous healing and probably often misinterpreted as bacterial infection in the tattoo. No elevated body temperature and no increase of blood parameters of infection may speak in favor of this special allergic manifestation. So may the development of hand dermatitis or some other local eczema occurring during or after the reaction.

Wheal-and-Flare and Urticarial Reactions

Tattoo reactions can be fluctuating, urticarial, and associated with or followed by general urticaria lasting weeks and months. The initial tattoo needle trauma is histamine driven, and local wheal and flare in the tattooed skin during and a few hours after tattooing is normal. In individuals with factitial urticaria, the needle-induced wheal-and-flare reaction is supposed to be more advanced; nevertheless, it is supposed to disappear after a few hours or a day.

In individuals reporting recurrent urticarial swelling of a tattoo, an *urticaria scratch test* can be performed by scraping the tattoo and the surrounding skin with a sharp instrument. Wheal and flare in the tattoo indicates active histamine release in the tattooed skin possibly related to the pigment. *Provocation of the tattoo with light or a sun simulator* can illustrate if the reaction is a photosensitivity reaction possibly related to the photochemical breakdown of tattoo pigment in the dermis. Such a reaction can be immediate and driven by reactive oxygen species or delayed with a cellular response. Use of sun blocker is rational, and it can be tested if pretreatment with the blocker eliminates the reaction.

In urticaria involving major parts of the skin, the urticarial reactions may be by coincidence, acquired with the tattoo due to an unknown sensitizer in the tattoo ink, or related to drug intake during the healing of the tattoo. A *standard prick test of common allergens and measurement of specific antibodies in the blood* guided by information about oral intakes and other exposures can be performed. It is not known if prick testing with the specific tattoo ink used for tattooing is a valid test; the test will leave a punctual tattoo.

Photosensitivity Testing

Photosensitivity is commonly observed in tattoos as a mild and often acceptable complaint but also as a chronic complication or as photosensitivity on top of another type of reaction such as an allergic reaction in a red tattoo.

Standard photosensitivity testing to daylight and selectively to UVB and UVA can be performed depending on the severity of the problem. Not only test spots on the back shall be tested, and testing shall include the tattoo.

Systemic Complication, Cross-Sensitization, 'Rush Phenomenon', and Testing

Chronic inflammatory tattoo reactions may be followed by two different types of remarkable reactions in the skin outside the tattoo.

Cross-sensitization, with reactions in older tattoos induced by a new tattoo of visually the same color, shares difficulty of testing with allergic reactions in red tattoos, as mentioned above.

Black tattoos with papulonodular reactions and granulomatous reaction or sarcoid granuloma by histology can be associated with or followed by similar reactions all over the skin in black tattoos tolerated in the past, a reaction called the 'rush phenomenon'. Such reactivity is due to the combination of black pigment aggregates in tattoos causing local foreign body reactions with inflammation, granulomas, and systemic activation, which is supposed to be autoimmune. Similarly, and parallel to activity in the skin, pulmonary sarcoidosis, eye affection, joint problems, scar sarcoidosis, and erythema nodosum can be triggered. Examinations shall include skin biopsies as described above, and screening of major organs of predilection especially the lungs by X-ray or high-resolution computerized tomography. Sarcoidosis has no internationally recognized system of diagnostic criteria and apparently is a spectrum of overlapping disease entities having different triggers but with autoimmunity and granulomatous tissue responses at least in some organs in common [36]. It has recently been documented that the association between black tattoos with papulonodular reaction is strong and 500-fold, with sarcoidosis in the background population as the reference. Black tattoos are able to trigger systemic sarcoidosis and 'rush phenomenon' in any other black tattoo hitherto tolerated [9, 35]. Thus, sarcoidosis shall always be considered in reactions of black tattoos, and relevant diagnostic evaluation shall be instituted.

References

1 Serup J, Hutton Carlsen K, Sepehri M: Tattoo complaints and complications: diagnosis and clinical spectrum; in Serup J, Kluger N, Bäumler W (eds): Tattooed Skin and Health. Curr Probl Dermatol. Basel, Karger, 2015, vol 48, pp 48–60.

2 Serup J, Sepehri M, Hutton Carlsen K: Classification of tattoo complications in a hospital material of 493 adverse events. Dermatology 2017, in press. DOI 10.1159/000452148.

3 Kentorp N: General aspects in medical/clinical photography; in Serup J, Jemec GBE, Grove G (eds): Handbook of Non-Invasive Methods and the Skin, ed 2. Boca Raton, CRC Taylor and Francis Group, 2006, pp 81–88.

4 O'Goshi K: Use of compact digital camera for snap photography; in Serup J, Jemec GBE, Grove G (eds): Handbook of Non-Invasive Methods and the Skin, ed 2. Boca Raton, CRC Taylor and Francis Group, 2006, pp 89–94.

5 Hawkins S: Computerized image analysis of clinical photos, in Serup J, Jemec GBE, Grove G (eds): Handbook of Non-Invasive Methods and the Skin, ed 2. Boca Raton, CRC Taylor and Francis Group, 2006, pp 95–100.

6 Kromann NP, Kapel H, Løytved ER, Hart Hansen JP: The tattooings of the Qilakitsoq Eskimo mummies; in Hart Hansen JP, Gulløv HC (eds): The Mummies from Qilakitsoq – Eskimos in the 15th Century. Meddr Grønland, Man and Soc, 1989, pp 168–71. Nyt Nordisk Forlag, Arnold Busk A/S, Copenhagen, 1989. ISBN 87-17-05963-1.

7 Eady EA: Sampling the bacteria of the skin; in Serup J, Jemec GBE, Grove G (eds): Handbook of Non-Invasive Methods and the Skin, ed 2. Boca Raton, CRC Taylor and Francis Group, 2006, pp 457–466.

8 Faergemann J: Mapping the fungi of the skin; in Serup J, Jemec GBE, Grove G (eds): Handbook of Non-Invasive Methods and the Skin, ed 2. Boca Raton, CRC Taylor and Francis Group, 2006, pp 467–470.

9 Sepehri M, Hutton Carlsen K, Serup J: Papulo-nodular reactions in black tattoos as markers of sarcoidosis, study of 92 reactions from a hospital material. Dermatology 2017, in press. DOI 10.1159/000453315.

10 Kluger N: Sarcoidosis on tattoos: a review of the literature from 1939 to 2011. Sarcoidosis Vasc Diffuse Lung Dis 2013; 30:86–102.

11 Thum CK, Biswas A: Inflammatory complications related to tattooing: a histopathological approach based on pattern analysis. Am J Dermatopathol 2015;37:54–66.

12 Gutermuth J, Hein R, Fendt F, et al: Cutaneous pseudolymphoma arising after tattoo placement. J Eur Acad Dermatol Venereol 2007;21:566–567.

13 Kluger N, Durand L, Minier-Thoumin C, et al: Pseudoepitheliomatous epidermal hyperplasia in tattoos: report of three cases. Am J Clin Dermatol 2008;9: 337–340.

14 Porter CJ, Simcock JW, MacKinnon CA: Necrotising fasciitis and cellulitis after traditional Samoan tattooing: case reports. J Infection 2005;50:149–152.

15 Høgsberg T, Thomsen BM, Serup J: Histopathology and immunohistochemistry of red tattoo reactions: interface dermatitis is the lead pathology, with increase of T-lymphocytes and Langerhans cells suggesting an allergic pathomechanism. Skin Res Technol 2015;21:449–458.

16 Høgsberg T, Loeschner K, Löf D, Serup J: Tattoo inks in general use contain nanoparticles. Br J Dermatol 2011;165: 1210–1218.

17 Jacobsen E, Tønning K, Pedersen E, Bernth N, Serup J, Høgsberg T, Nielsen E: The Danish Environmental Protection Agency. Report on Chemical Substances in Tattoo Ink, 2012, report 216 (English version). ISBN 978-87-92779-87-8. www.mst.dk/publications/English.

18 Laux P, Tralau T, Tentschert J, Blume A, Al Dahouk S, Bäumler W, Bernstein E, Bocca B, Alimonti A, Colebrook H, de Cuyper C, Dähne L, Hauri U, Howard PC, Janssen P, Katz L, Klitzman B, Kluger N, Krutak L, Platzek T, Scott-Lang V, Serup J, Teubner W, Schreiver I, Wilknіß E, Luch A: A medical-toxicological view of tattooing. Lancet 2016;387:395–402.

19 Engel E, Santarelli F, Vasolid R, Ulrich H, Maisch T, König B, Landthaler M, Gopee NV, Howard PC, Bäumler W: Establishment of an extraction method for the recovery of tattoo pigments from human skin using HPLC diode array detector technology. Anal Chem 2006; 78:6440–6447.

20 Engel E, Vasolid R, Santarelli F, Maisch T, Gopee NV, Howard PC, Landthaler M, Bäumler W: Tattooing of skin results in transportation and light-induced decomposition of tattoo pigments – a first quantification in vivo using a mouse model. Exp Dermatol 2010;19:54–60.

21 Høgsberg T, Jacobsen NR, Clausen P, Serup J: Black tattoo inks induce reactive oxygen species production correlating with aggregation of pigment nanoparticles but not with polycyclic aromatic hydrocarbon content. Exp Dermatol 2013;22:464–469.

22 European Commission: JRC Technical Reports. Safety of tattoos and permanent make-up. Compilation of information on legislative framework and analytical methods. Report of work package 1. Administrative arrangement N. 2014-33617 conducted on behalf of DG JUST. 2015.EUR 27528 EN; ISBN 978-92-79-50394-8 (PDF); DOI 10.2788/542617.

23 Prior G: Tattoo Inks, Analysis, Pigments, Legislation. Berlin, Epubli GmbH, 2014. ISBN 978-3-8442-8611-3

24 Olsen O: The challenges and limitation of chemical analysis of particulate pigments of very low solubility; in Serup J, Kluger N, Bäumler W (eds): Tattooed Skin and Health. Curr Probl Dermatol. Basel, Karger, 2015, vol 48, pp 158–163.

25 Hutton Carlsen K, Køcks M, Sepehri M, Serup J: Allergic reactions in red tattoos: Raman spectroscopy for 'fingerprint' detection of chemical risk spectra in tattooed skin and culprit tattoo inks. Skin Res Technol 2016;22:460–469.

26 Serup J: Punch biopsy of the skin by electric power drill: effect of speed. A post-mortem study. Dan Med Bull 1985; 32:189–191.

27 Serup J: Punch biopsy of the skin: effect of tissue fixation with CO2-freezing. An experimental study. J Dermatol 1984;11: 465–470.

28 Serup J, Keiding J, Fullerton A, Gniadecka M, Gniadecka R: High-frequency ultrasound examination of skin: introduction and guide; in Serup J, Jemec GBE, Grove G (eds): Handbook of Non-Invasive Methods and the Skin, ed 2. Boca Raton, CRC Taylor and Francis Group, 2006, pp 473–491.

29 Olsen LO, Takiwaki H, Serup J: High-frequency ultrasound characterization of normal skin. Skin thickness and echographic density of 22 anatomical sites. Skin Res Technol 1995;1:74–80.
30 Gniadecka M, Gniadecki R, Serup J, Søndergaard J: Ultrasound structure and digital image analysis of the subepidermal low echogenic band in aged human skin: diurnal changes and interindividual variability. J Invest Dermatol 1994; 102:362–365.
31 Carlsen KH, Tolstrup J, Serup J: High-frequency ultrasound imaging of tattoo reactions with histopathology as a comparative method. Introduction of preoperative ultrasound diagnostics as a guide to therapeutic intervention. Skin Res Technol 2014;20:257–264.
32 O'goshi K, Suihko C, Serup J: In vivo imaging of intradermal tattoos by confocal scanning laser microscopy. Skin Res Technol 2006;12:94–98.
33 Serup J, Hutton Carlsen K: Patch test study of 90 patients with tattoo reactions: negative outcome of allergy patch test to baseline batteries and culprit inks suggests allergen(s) are generated in the skin through haptenation. Contact Dermatitis 2014;71:255–263.
34 Gaudron S, Bouēdec MCF, Franck F, D'Incan M: Azo pigments and quinacridones induce delayed hypersensitivity in red tattoos. Contact Dermatitis 2015;72: 97–105.
35 Haimovic A, Sanchez M, Judson MA, Prystowsky S: Sarcoidosis: a comprehensive review and update for the dermatologist. J Am Acad Dermatol 2012; 66:699–716.

Prof. Jørgen Serup, DMSc
Department of Dermatology D41, Bispebjerg University Hospital
Bispebjerg Bakke 23
DK–2400 Copenhagen NV (Denmark)
E-Mail joergen.vedelskov.serup@regionh.dk

Serup J, Bäumler W (eds): Diagnosis and Therapy of Tattoo Complications. With Atlas of Illustrative Cases.
Curr Probl Dermatol. Basel, Karger, 2017, vol 52, pp 58–73 (DOI: 10.1159/000450780)

How to Diagnose and Classify Tattoo Complications in the Clinic: A System of Distinctive Patterns

Jørgen Serup

The 'Tattoo Clinic', Department of Dermatology, Bispebjerg University Hospital, Copenhagen, Denmark

Abstract

Tattoo complications represent a broad spectrum of clinical entities and disease mechanisms. Infections are known, but chronic inflammatory reactions have hitherto been inconsistently reported and given many interpretations and terms. A clinical classification system of distinct patterns with emphasis on inflammatory tattoo reactions is introduced. Allergic reactions prevalent in red tattoos and often associated with azo pigments are manifested as the 'plaque elevation', 'excessive hyperkeratosis', and 'ulceronecrotic' patterns. The allergen is a hapten. Nonallergic reactions prevalent in black tattoos and associated with carbon black are manifested as the 'papulonodular' pattern. Carbon black nanoparticles agglomerate in the dermis over time forming foreign bodies that elicit reactions. Many black tattoos even develop sarcoid granuloma, and the 'papulonodular' pattern is strongly associated with sarcoidosis affecting other organs. Tattoo complications include a large group of less frequent but nevertheless specific entities, i.e. irritant and toxic local events, photosensitivity, urticaria, eczematous rash due to soluble allergen, neurosensitivity and pain syndrome, lymphopathies, pigment diffusion or fan, scars, and other sequels of tattooing or tattoo removal. Keratoacanthoma occurs in tattoos. Carcinoma and melanoma are rare and occur by coincidence only. Different tattoo complications require different therapeutic approaches, and precise diagnosis is thus important as a key to therapy. The proposed new classification with characteristic patterns relies on simple tools, namely patient history, objective findings, and supplementary punch biopsy. By virtue of simplicity and broad access, these methods make the proposed classification widely applicable in clinics and hospitals. The system is reported to the 11th revision of the WHO diagnosis classification used as international standard.

This chapter presents a guide for doctors, who are confronted with new cases of tattoo complications in their practice. The chapter shall be read as a vade mecum using the atlas at the end of the book to illustrate the many different conditions each with their special and characteristic traits. The conditions have a degree of specificity in the clinic. The chapter primarily builds on the experience and the original publication of the 'Tattoo

Clinic' of Bispebjerg University Hospital, Copenhagen, Denmark, recently published in *Dermatology* [1]. The clinical material of tattoo complications collected from 2008 to 2015 includes 405 consecutive cases with 493 complications. The new concept of diagnosing tattoo complications relying on patient history and objective findings referenced to distinctive patterns, which can be recognized by dermatologists by simple means, was outlined in the report 'Tattooing – Health, Risks and Culture' of the Danish Council on Health and Disease Prevention [2]. Broad information including basic research is found in the same report and in the book *Tattooed Skin and Health* published by Karger, the whole book serving as an introductory volume to the present book dedicated to diagnosis and therapy [3]. A recent review by Laux et al. [4] published in *The Lancet* presents an updated analysis of the medical-toxicological view of tattooing with emphasis on the state of tattoos and toxicology versus clinical and epidemiological observations.

The present chapter is also referenced to the medical literature with a few hundred individual cases of tattoo complications reported over a century, reviewed by Nicolas Kluger and others [5–11]. However, older reports may easily be obsolete. The tattoo industry underwent major changes, which included the introduction of organic pigments that have been used for decades. Recent practices, inks, and pigments have become more refined and are very different from those used in the old times, when cinnabar crude powder was dispersed in sputum and tattooed directly into peoples' skin using dirty self-made needles. A review by Wenzel et al. [12] especially on newer cases and an Internet-based study with open entry performed in German-speaking countries with over 3,000 spontaneous reports by the public may better illustrate the present situation of tattoo complications and complaints [12, 13].

Clinical research dominated by case reports is hampered by lacking international classification of tattoo complications, which are thus reported variably. For example, out of the literature, it is not possible to distinguish allergic from nonallergic cases. Reports of infectious complications follow general diagnostic standards and are clearer and already better understood, and this chapter therefore shall primarily address tattoo complications with chronic inflammation of the dermis and a chronic course.

The World Health Organization's diagnosis coding system used globally has only one code for 'tattoo' (L81.8E) with no distinction between type of tattoo and complication. Tattoo complications can also be coded under infections and other established major entities. The diagnostic classification described in the present chapter was submitted to the World Health Organization as a proposal to the 11th revision of the international classification of diseases to promote international consensus with precise diagnosis and registration of tattoo complications by health systems.

Tattoo complications are defined as advanced adverse effects in tattoos (or resulting from tattoos), which manifest themselves as objective pathological/clinical changes, as well as subjective symptoms to a degree that they have the nature of disease or disablement, and which typically make the tattooed person seek medical treatment. This contrasts complaints, which are mild and often do not make the tattooed person contact the health system.

Chronic tattoo complications with itching as the lead symptom are cumbersome and were shown to influence quality of life to a degree comparable to the known pruritic disease of the skin [14]. Patients' burden with tattoo complications often appears to be underrated by politicians and the medical community.

The Clinical Material of Bispebjerg University Hospital

The proposed new classification builds on the clinical material of patients with tattoo complications seen in the 'Tattoo Clinic' of Bispebjerg

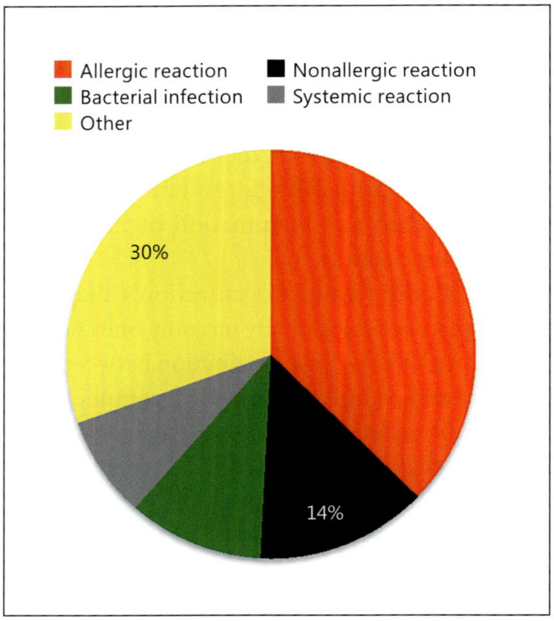

Fig. 1. Distribution of commonly observed tattoo complications by main diagnosis (n = 493). Allergic reactions primarily in red tattoos, nonallergic reactions primarily in black tattoos, bacterial infections, and systemic reactions are large groups. There is a large segment of other complications covering many special and distinct complications as exemplified by neurosensory, traumatic, and other complications.

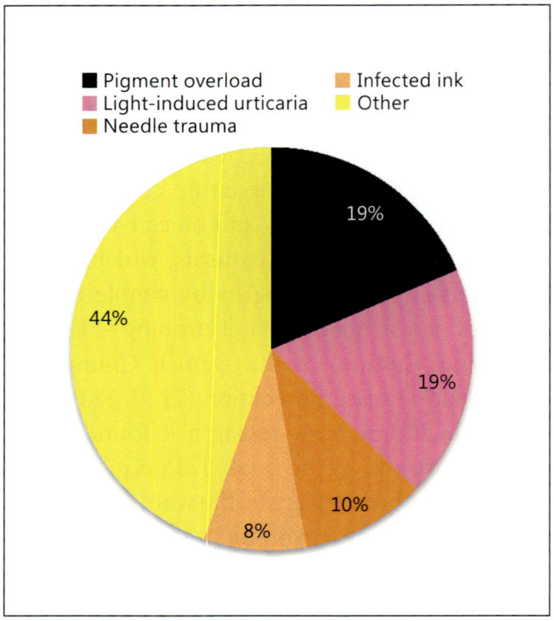

Fig. 2. Distribution of tattoo complications by secondary or supplementary diagnosis illustrating the cause of complications, i.e. a case may have a main and a supplementary diagnosis (n = 231). Pigment overload indicates that too much pigment was injected, mostly associated with black pigment and more than the skin can tolerate. Needle trauma is associated with infection and scarring, and infected ink with infection maybe starting in one colour. The segment 'Other' represents many different conditions as exemplified by tattoo removal with lactic acid and lasers causing scarring or burn.

University Hospital from 2008 to 2015 [1]. The spectrum of tattoo complications registered in the material is illustrated in figures 1 and 2. Infections, allergic reactions of primarily red tattoos, and papulonodular reactions of black tattoos (associated with sarcoidosis or not) are the large groups, but a big segment includes many different conditions, which all are distinct.

The *simplified diagnosis tree* of tattoo complications summarizing the experience of the 'Tattoo Clinic' is given below as an introduction, with definitions and details presented later in the text:

- Bacterial and other infections
- Allergic reactions primarily in red tattoos, with 'plaque elevation', 'extensive hyperkeratosis', or 'ulceronecrotic' reaction, caused by pigment-associated allergic sensitization
- Papulonodular reactions primarily in black tattoos with papules and nodules and possibly sarcoid granuloma/associated sarcoidosis, with pigment foreign body reaction as the trigger and individual predisposition as a prerequisite
- Psychosocial complications
- Miscellaneous complications including many distinct entities representing different disease mechanisms

Tattoo reactions and the typical patterns of reactions mentioned above are shown in figures 3a–d and 4a–d. Readers are referred to the extensive atlas at the end of this book for more detailed illustrations (see pp. 139–229).

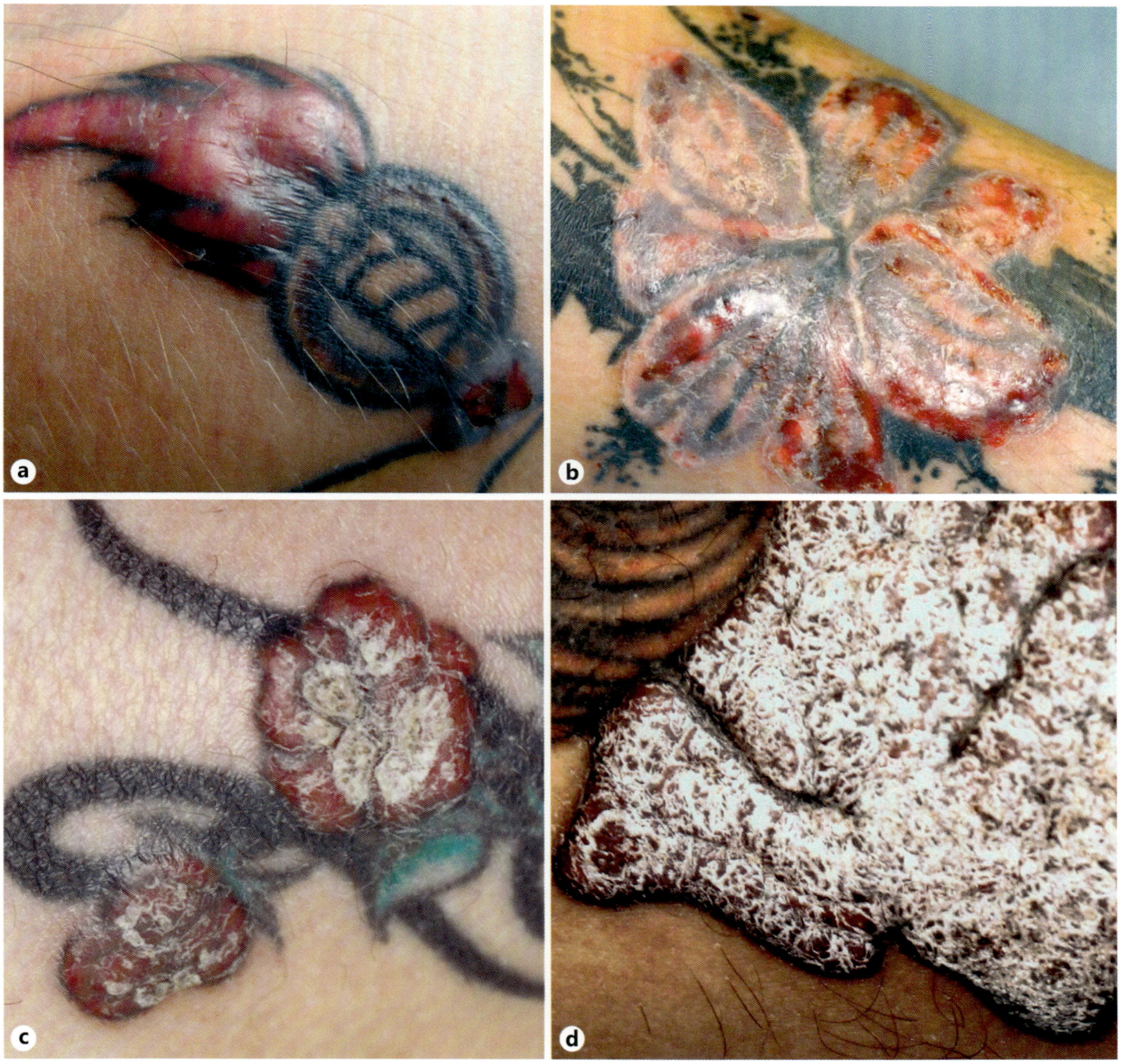

Fig. 3. Allergic tattoo reactions by clinical type. **a** 'Plaque elevation'. **b** 'Plaque elevation' with variable thickening and mild keratosis. **c** 'Excessive hyperkeratosis' with major thickening. **d** 'Excessive hyperkeratosis' with major thickening and furrows, dominated by epidermal hyperplasia. Further information and illustrations are shown in the atlas, pp. 149–176.

Doctors' *direct inspection of the raw biopsy punch by the naked eye, using a lens or a surface microscope*, provides important supplementary information, as shown in figure 5a–d. The density of pigment is stronger in the cylinder punch as compared to thin tissue specimens cut for histology, and pigment in the dermis albeit of visible colour macroscopically may easily fall under the resolution of light microscopy, whereby only larger aggregates are seen, with pigment colour possibly modified by histological processing and overshined by staining.

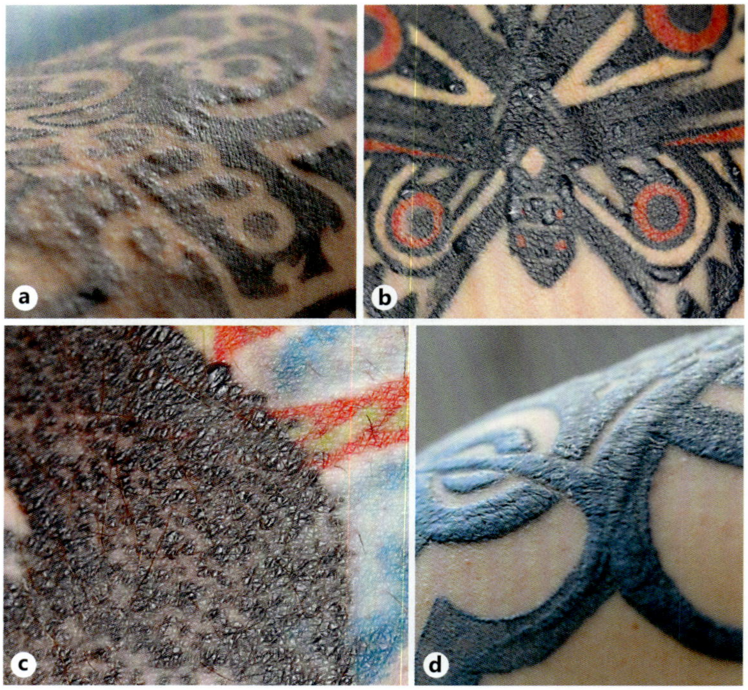

Fig. 4. Nonallergic tattoo reactions: papulonodular type of different variants. **a** Papules and pimples. **b** Nodules with sarcoid granuloma. **c** Papules and nodules, manifestations of the 'rush phenomenon' in sarcoidosis. **d** Papulonodular swelling, more prominent in sites with dense pigment. Further information and illustrations are shown in the atlas, pp. 184–202.

Entities, Patterns of Inflammatory Reactions, and Their Definitions

In the *distinction of inflammatory tattoo reactions being allergic or nonallergic*, patient history and objective findings are the main tools, since patch testing of tattoo inks and pigments was shown to be not reliable and merely produce falsely negative outcomes [15]. The following information speaks in favour of allergy:

- Reactions are monomorphic; that is, consistent in one and only one colour and everywhere this colour is used in the tattoo.
- There is a latency period; that is, a sensitization period, which may last for weeks, months, and maybe years from the time the tattoo is made until the occurrence of the reaction.
- The reaction is chronic and constant in appearance and degree of discomfort, and usually it is resistant to treatment with local steroids.

A more definitive sign of allergy of type IV is the development of *cross-sensitivity reaction* in another tattoo, i.e. an active reaction in a newer tattoo results in a concomitant reaction in some older tattoo(s) made with the same or nearly the same colourant but localized in another anatomic region and carried out independently of that problematic new tattoo, which activated secondary reaction(s).

The *definitions of distinct inflammatory reaction patterns explained by allergy or foreign body reaction* introduced as new entities are as follows [1–3].

Plaque elevation or plaque-like patterns (allergic) show consistent thickening and elevation of the entire tattoo at any site of the tattoo where the problematic colour was injected (fig. 3a–d). The skin surface may be rough and scaly or smooth and shiny with loss of skin markings, or in between. Histology shows cellular infiltration with T-lymphocytes of the outer dermis and some-

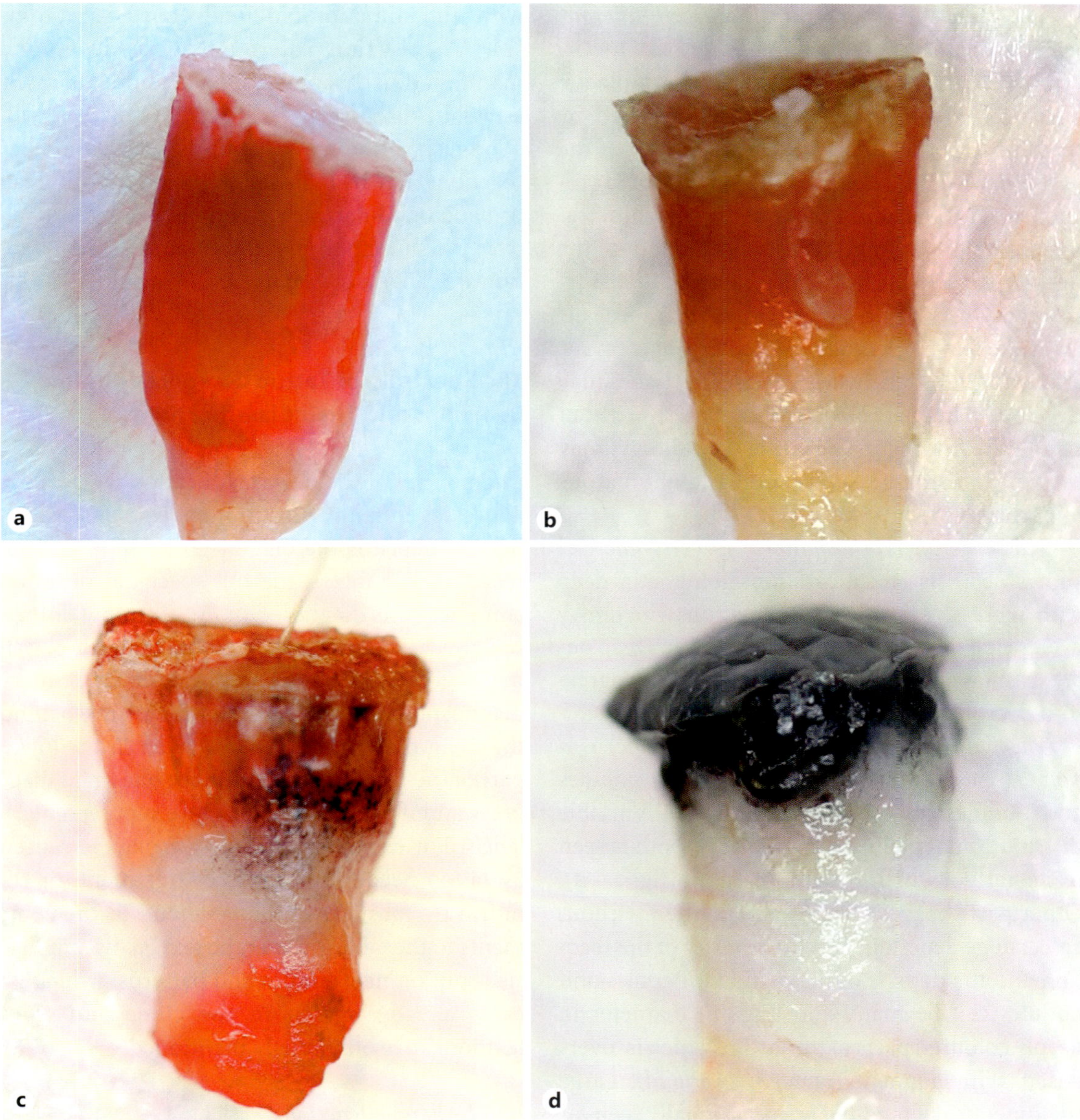

Fig. 5. Raw punch (3 mm) biopsies. **a** Allergic reaction with red pigment in the entire dermis. **b** Allergic reaction with hyperkeratosis and epidermoid inclusions in the dermis. **c** Allergic reaction with excessive hyperkeratosis and drift of black pigment. **d** Nonallergic reaction with 'bunch of grape' sign and sarcoid granuloma. Further information and illustrations are shown in the atlas, pp. 150–152, 155, 156, 158–160, 163, 167, 173, 175, 176, 186, 190, 195–197, 199, 201–204.

times the whole dermis concluded as pseudolymphoma, which is benign [16]. There may be secondary reaction of the epidermis, fibrosis in the dermis and disturbances of the dermoepidermal junction with interphase dermatitis [17, 18]. Histology with immune histochemistry showed activation of Langerhans cells, which supports allergic mechanism [17].

The excessive hyperkeratosis pattern (allergic, with an epidermal response with reactive hyperproliferation) shows the basic features of plaque elevation. However, lesions are dominated by massive hyperkeratosis and cornification of the surface with an extraordinary epidermal response of proliferation provoked by the underlying dermal inflammation and the pigment in the dermis (fig. 3d). The surface may be flat, furrowed, whitish, and occasionally with local ulceration due to necrosis. Notches, ducts, cysts, and epidermoid inclusions deeper in tissues may develop. The pathologist sometimes, without seeing the finding in the context of allergy, may interpret histology as pseudoepitheliomatous hyperplasia [18, 19].

The ulceronecrotic pattern (severe allergic) shows necrosis and ulceration, going skin deep with aggressive dermal inflammation, which may even reach the level of the muscle fascia. Deep necrosis may also be infectious and even progress into necrotizing fasciitis [20].

The papulonodular pattern (nonallergic) is a nonallergic inflammatory reaction with papules and nodules by clinical examination. Variable distribution of papules or nodules or both is seen in the tattoo, which is typically black (fig. 4a–d). Other parts of the same tattoo are often without any change depending on the severity of the reaction and the density of the pigment. Papules and nodules can be many and large in diameter in deeply coloured parts of the tattoo, which is 'overdosed' with pigment *(pigment overload)*. Large agglomerates of pigment are occasionally seen directly by the naked eye in a raw punch biopsy taken from the tattoo seen as a 'bunch of grape' surface of the biopsy cylinder. Subject to individual predisposition, papules and nodules may have the histology of plain inflammation and foreign body reaction, granulomatous inflammation, or sarcoid granuloma (fig. 4b). Tattoo ink that aggregates in water was shown to induce formation of reactive oxygen species, and aggregation of black pigment in the tissue thus may be linked with inflammation and subjective symptoms [21]. The reaction pattern is associated with or a manifestation of sarcoidosis in a number of cases, as will be discussed later [8, 22]. Associated with a predisposition to sarcoidosis, papulonodular reactions may be followed by an abrupt outbreak of papulonodular activity in any black tattoo all over the skin booming at the same time, a reaction we call *'rush phenomenon'* (fig 4c) [22].

The Spectrum of Tattoo Complications and Reactions and Their Classification

The novelty of the new classification we propose addresses inflammatory tattoo reactions, which by prevalence is the biggest group in a hospital material. In table 1, the full spectrum of tattoo complications diagnosed in the 'Tattoo Clinic' is reviewed. The upper part of the table shows all major groups of tattoo complications by primary diagnostic entity, with the mechanisms behind the main patterns and events given in the lower part of the table. A case may have one main diagnosis and if relevant one or more supplementary labels. For example, a tattoo scar may be caused by tattoo needle trauma, laser treatment, or removal by caustics. In the table and in the comments to the table given in the text below, emphasis is put on new entities and patterns, while diseases already known in the clinic and from textbooks are only briefly mentioned.

Local Allergic Reactions

Local allergic reactions in the tattoo depend on the severity of the allergy and the proliferative response of the epidermis to the underlying dermal inflammation manifested as 'plaque elevation', 'excessive hyperkeratosis', and 'ulceronecrotic' reactions. The vast majority of plaques with allergy are red, but allergy also may appear in red nuances, green, blue, violet, yellow, and orange. Black tattoos and white tattoos do not develop allergy against the pigment. In 'plaque elevation',

Table 1. Summary of clinical diagnoses of tattoo complications by clinical entity, mechanism, and type of allergy according to the 'Tattoo Clinic' of Bispebjerg University Hospital

Local allergic reactions in the tattoo[1]	*Plaque elevation*, with flat elevation of one specific colour and in any site with that colour, type IV allergy *Excessive hyperkeratosis* (possibly with notches and epidermoid structures skin deep), type IV allergy Ulceration/deep reaction with necrosis, type IV allergy Allergic reactions may show *cross-sensitivity reactions* with activation of older tattoos
General allergic reactions	Dermatitis/rash, primary sensitisation or by challenge (nickel, preservative, etc.), type IV allergy Urticaria, widespread, type I allergy Anaphylaxis (latex), type I allergy
Local and systemic[2] papulonodular reactions (pigment agglomeration/ foreign body induced)	*Nonallergic inflammatory reaction*, limited to parts of the tattoo that are more densely tattooed Sarcoid inflammation/cutaneous sarcoidosis, limited to the tattoo and the skin and associated with scar sarcoidosis/erythema nodosum; older tattoos may react abruptly due to autoimmunity, *rush phenomenon* Sarcoidosis of internal organ(s) also afflicting the tattoo
Bacterial infections	*Local, regional*, and possibly systemic; various G+/G– bacteria, and TB and environmental mycobacteria
Viral and other infections/ infestations	Papilloma and herpes simplex viruses Hepatitis B and C and HIV Leprosy, syphilis, leishmaniosis, etc.
Reactions induced by external factors including light (includes phototoxicity and photoallergy)	*Light-induced urticaria-like reaction*, locally and mostly in dark tattoos Urticaria-like reactions by heat, trauma, alcohol intake, etc. affecting any tattoo
Neurosensitive reactions	Local in the tattoo or regional/in the dermatome including chronic pain syndromes induced by tattooing
Lymphopathy	Local, regional, and affecting regional nodes, lymphedema, and/or swollen node(s)
Tumours	Keratoacanthoma, fibroma, pyogenic granuloma Malignant skin tumours by coincidence only
Scars and keloids	By predisposition or sequel of tattooing/tattoo removal
Tattoo pigment diffusion or fan	Superficial in skin or deep into underlying tissues
Irritant and local toxic events	*Common during tattoo healing causing delayed healing* but uncommon as a chronic event
Tattoo technique failure and hazards (by mechanism)	Needle trauma Overdose with tattoo ink Infections from an identified source (needle, machine, inks)
Tattoo removal failures and hazards (by mechanism and techniques)	Tattoo removal by laser, intense pulsed light, etc. Removal by chemicals/caustics/dermabrasion/salabrasion Surgery and any other physical approach
Miscellaneous	Local events (pimples and other minor manifestations) Manifestations of other disease of the skin and body (Köbner phenomenon in psoriasis, etc.)
Psychosocial complications with and without associating psychiatric disease	A broad spectrum of individual cases ranging from mild to severe dissonance with society, with tattooing of the face/tongue/eyes/extensive skin fields and piercings, scarification, implants, and body modifications as associated high-risk adornments

Prevalent complications are indicated in italics. [1] Dominated by red tattoos. [2] Dominated by black tattoos. Individual cases may be given a main diagnosis (upper part of table) and an additional diagnosis indicating the mechanism of the complication (lower part of table). TB = Tuberculosis.

the surface is smooth or with adherent scales and what was traditionally called a 'lichenoid' look. The term 'lichenoid tattoo reaction' is imprecise and was variably used, referring to the lichen plant family of many species each with different colours and exophytic appearances. The term shall be considered obsolete when applied to tattoo reactions. In 'excessive hyperkeratosis', the epidermis has proliferated excessively and presents as very thick elevation of the tattoo with a rough, stiff and horny surface, which may have minor spots or islands of necrosis due to nutritional deficiency caused by the thickening. Lesions may also be furrowed with notches by histology, the notches going deep and sometimes with herniation planting epidermoid inclusions in the dermis. Notches and inclusions may even have an acneiform appearance resembling acne cysts and fistulas. The acneiform variant of excessive hyperkeratosis is difficult to treat with dermatome shaving because of epidermoid tissue, which may be found deeply in the dermis and prolong or inhibit healing. 'Ulceronecrotic' reactions have a sudden onset with heavy dermal inflammation that soon turns into deep necrosis. Such lesions may heal slowly over several months. Excision surgery is contraindicated, since the pigment behind the allergy may have propagated to the level of the muscle fascia and even deeper and wider. The patient's general condition is fair, in contrast to necrotizing fasciitis and infection with aggressive bacteria, a situation which may require acute surgery.

Allergic reactions are mostly not responding to treatment with topical corticoids. The first-line treatment of allergic reactions of the type 'plaque elevation' and 'excessive hyperkeratosis' is dermatome shaving performed to a horizontal level in the dermis when visible tattoo pigment has been removed and the white colour of naïve dermal collagen appears [23]. Laser removal of allergic tattoo reactions is, independent of the type of reaction, relatively contraindicated since the allergy may be boosted [24, 25]. Photochemical breakdown of pigment upon laser light exposure is unforeseeable.

Some allergic tattoo reactions may provoke a *cross-allergic reaction* of older tattoos of the same colour acquired months or years before, despite the tattoo inks used unlikely to be perfectly identical. Such a cross-reaction especially occurs with red tattoos performed with azo pigments. It typically takes a few weeks or months for the newly acquired tattoo to provoke a cross-reaction in older tattoos. Patch testing is not useful for evaluation of allergy to tattoo ink final products and pigments since the particulate pigment is little soluble. Moreover, the active allergen eliciting the reaction is not the pigment directly but a hapten formed in the skin over weeks, months, or years [15]. Allergy test of tattoo inks and pigments is not applicable due to falsely negative outcomes, unless the problem is related to soluble materials in the inks, i.e. nickel, chromate, and preservatives. This can be studied using a panel of standard allergens, as will be discussed below.

General Allergic Reactions

General allergic reactions in the skin include dermatitis/rash caused by type IV allergy to soluble ingredients of the tattoo ink formulation, in particular nickel and preservatives but also with other allergens such as chromate VI as a possible allergen. If the person is already sensitized to the allergen, as exemplified by persons allergic to nickel, a severe exanthema can develop abruptly within 1–2 days and involve the tattoo and most of the skin including the face and neck with a need for oral treatment with prednisone. The rash will fade over a period of a few weeks or months depending on the rate of elimination or inactivation of the allergen and the severity of the reaction. Nearly all tattoo inks are contaminated with metallic nickel in low concentration, but only a few contain larger amounts [26]. The risk group of severe rash appears to be persons who already had a strong allergy to nickel before they were tattooed, i.e. positive patch test 3+ and possibly 2+, while persons with a lower-grade allergy to nickel are unlikely to develop a rash despite the use of tattoo ink contaminated with nickel. Some might develop a local reaction with delayed healing of their tattoo misinterpreted as infection but actually caused by nickel provocation from the new tattoo. Ionic nickel has a short half-life in the body and such local reaction in a new acquired tattoo is supposed to heal parallel to a positive patch test reaction to nickel, i.e. in 1–2 weeks. Nickel in tattoo inks is primarily metallic, originating from stainless steel vessels used in production; however, exceptional inks may contain soluble nickel in higher concentrations. Metallic nickel in surgical implants, such as artificial joints, in general does not sensitize. Tattooed persons as a whole, and despite piercings and other metal contacts being popular in this group, apparently and contrary to expectations have not a more prevalent allergy to nickel than the background population, and tattooing may not induce primary sensitization to nickel to any significant degree despite exposure to tattoo inks that very often are contaminated with nickel. Preservatives added to tattoo inks exemplified by parabens can cause primary sensitization and elicit severe generalized dermatitis, which may persist for months and require immunosuppressive treatment. Paraphenylenediamine is not present in tattoo inks, and there is no cross-reactivity between henna tattoo allergy and permanent tattoo allergy [26]. There is no indication from the clinic, accordant with experiences with red textile dyes, that primary aromatic amines seen as breakdown products of azo pigments are relevant as allergens neither in local tattoo reactions nor in generalized rash events.

Urticaria associated with tattoos is not very uncommon and apparently neglected in the medical literature. Independent of a history of urticaria, patients may develop urticarial wheal-and-flare reactions in any part of the skin a few weeks or months after the tattoo is performed, indicating primary sensitization induced with the new tattoo. The condition, which may fade over some months, can require oral prednisone for a period. The allergy is likely to be induced by a soluble ingredient of the tattoo ink rather than the pigment. Other types of allergens may be introduced with new tattoos and cause type I allergy. Severe anaphylactic reactions of the tattooed occurred due to latex particles from tattooists' gloves and motivated many tattooists to use latex-free gloves [27]. Tattooists may acquire type IV allergy and hand dermatitis due to rubber chemicals.

Local and Systemic Papulonodular Reactions

Local and systemic papulonodular reactions are associated with black tattoos and represent a spectrum from mild to severe, with acute and chronic reactions. Reactions are not allergy of type IV, and activity only affects parts of the tattoo, while other parts are normal. Carbon black is composed of carbon particles in the nanoparticle range, and with contaminants depending on raw materials and production of the pigment. Acute reactions with papules may already arise during the healing of new tattoos. Such reactions are more frequent and stronger with overdose of the ink. Needle trauma may contribute. Reactions resolve over weeks or months and may sometimes respond to topical corticoids. Chronic reactions appear after months or years and may affect selected tattoos or many tattoos. Reactions may depend on the particular ink used and on the tattooist. Reactivity may be widespread affecting many tattoos made on different occasions. The basic mechanism behind reactions is the tendency of especially black pigment particles to aggregate and agglomerate and thus form larger clusters of particles reaching a size in the range of 1–10 μm. Such clusters represent foreign bodies and may elicit an inflammatory reaction of the dermis possibly with induction of reactive oxygen species [21]. Chronic papulonodular reactions by histology typically show inflammation of the outer dermis where the pigment is concentrated. Inflammation, papules, nodules, and clinical symptoms with itch and sometimes sensitivity to sun are prominent at those sites of the tattoo where the pigment is dense or excessive. A black tattoo with a reaction may have papules ranging from miniature papules to large-sized nodules contrasting parts of the same tattoo without any visible change.

In some papulonodular reactions, a special tissue reaction with *granulomatous reaction or fully developed sarcoid granuloma* may come up. A study from the 'Tattoo Clinic' of Bispebjerg University Hospital found sarcoid granuloma in 1/4 of papulonodular reactions, with sarcoidosis limited to the tattoo as final diagnosis in 1/4, associated with cutaneous sarcoidosis (scar sarcoidosis and erythema nodosum) in 1/10, and associated with systemic sarcoidosis in as many as 6/10 with affection of the lungs, eyes, and joints [22]. Development of sarcoid reactions of tattoos depends on individual predisposition. The association is likely to be explained by an autoimmune mechanism. Clusters of black pigment in the dermis may apparently trigger sarcoid reactions in the skin and also systemic activity, and systemic sarcoidosis in the active state or as a subclinical predisposition vice versa may trigger reactions in a newly acquired black tattoo. The surface of carbon black particles is chemically active and may, as aluminium added to vaccines forming tissue foreign bodies as well, function as an adjuvant promoting immunization. *Due to the association between papulonodular reactions of black tattoos and sarcoidosis, patients with papulonodular reactions shall be screened for sarcoidosis of other organs.* The risk of sarcoidosis of the skin and internal organs in persons with black tattoos with papulonodular reactions is in a hospital material estimated to be 500 times higher as compared to the risk of the general population [22]. Sarcoidosis was also reported in red tattoos in older reports, but today and with modern organic pigments sarcoid granuloma in red tattoos is exceptional [8, 22]. Nevertheless, red tattoos with inflammatory reactions often have minor traits of granuloma with granulomatous inflammation by histology found in 1/3 of red tattoos versus 1/2 of black tattoos [22]. The association of granulomatous inflammation and clinically manifested sarcoidosis of any organ is rather weak, and the association with sarcoidosis is much stronger if a biopsy from the reacting tattoo convincingly shows sarcoid granuloma.

A new black tattoo with papulonodular reaction may trigger a sudden onset of inflammatory reaction with papules and nodules of other black tattoos hitherto tolerated, what we call the *'rush phenomenon'* (fig. 4c). The reaction may be a minor rush affecting a few other tattoos or a major rush affecting every or nearly every black tattoo in any part of the skin, independent of the tattoo ink used, the density of pigment in the skin, and the tattooist [22]. The rush phenomenon is a strong denominator of sarcoidosis and likely to be a direct manifestation of sarcoid autoimmunity. Reactions due to rush phenomenon activity are chronic, however with a tendency to heal over several months. Oral prednisone is efficient. Patients with rush phenomenon shall be screened for systemic sarcoidosis.

Bacterial Infections

Bacterial infections with *Staphylococcus aureus* and other bacteria are common and manifested as local infections in the tattoo, regional infections involving the surrounding tissues, and systemic infections as described in detail in the chapter by Serup [this vol., pp. 30–41] and in the literature [5, 6]. Pyogenic bacterial infections have their debut shortly after the tattoo is made. Infections may become systemic and even fatal with blood poisoning and endocarditis [28]. Some infections are unusual and only relevant in some countries where the infection is endemic. Infection with *Mycobacterium chelonae* from a contaminated environment, including tap water used to dilute tattoo ink, is rare but may occur as local outbreaks affecting a number of customers of a tattoo parlour [29, 30]. It shall be bared in mind that about 10% of new tattoo inks were shown to be contaminated with bacteria pathogenic to humans, and the same prevalence was found in inks labelled 'sterile' [31–33]. Thus, tattoo ink as the source of infection is logic in many cases.

Viral and Other Infections
Viral and other infections may be seen as local infections in the tattoo as exemplified by warts, papillomas, and condylomas [5, 6]. Herpes simplex virus can be introduced in the skin by tattooing and cause a primary infection or activated by tattooing with a secondary outbreak, especially seen in cosmetic tattooing of the lips. Systemic infection with hepatitis B and C are known risks; however, tattooists' use of gloves has reduced but not eliminated this risk [34]. The risk of viral inoculation and infection depends on the inoculum of a specific virus needed to cause infection in the recipient. The risk of transferring HIV is apparently not high, and only sporadic cases were reported [35]. Viruses live in live cells, and infection by inoculation normally will require biologic material along with the virus, thus a route with direct transfer from person to person by critical utensils as exemplified by the reuse of tattoo needles. Other infections include fungal, protozoal, spirochaetal, and endemic infections from the local environment as described in the chapter by Serup [this vol., pp. 30–41].

Reactions Induced by External Factors
Reactions induced by external factors including light are common. Photosensitivity is remarkably common as a mild complaint. It is also common as a significant clinical problem, thus as a complication in an otherwise normal looking tattoo, or secondary to an inflammatory tattoo reaction. In photosensitivity reactions, itch and pain are major symptoms. Inflammation makes the tattoo more vulnerable to light exposure. Photosensitivity reactions with itch and pain may switch on and off in seconds on sun exposure with reactive oxygen species as a possible mechanism or show a protracted course over a few days with polymorphous clinical manifestations of the exposed tattoo, which becomes inflamed. Reactions to sun generally are phototoxic, and photoallergic manifestations in tattoos apparently appear exceptional. Dark tattoos, i.e. black, red, and blue colours, are more prone to photosensitivity reactions. Local increase of skin temperature with vasodilatation may sometimes explain solar reactions. However, in some colourful tattoos, sensitivity to sun is related to one specific colour only and thus a result of a physical or photochemical reaction in that special pigment. Warm environment, hot climate, and intake of alcohol also may induce itch and swelling of tattoos at the level of complaint.

Neurosensitive Reactions
Neurosensitive reactions are characterized by severe itch, pain, and discomfort in a tattoo without significant inflammation of the tattoo. Symptoms also may affect a dermatome or be more widespread and classified as a pain syndrome [36]. Neurosensitive reactions are chronic and can be invalidating. Reactions are probably caused by some neurostimulatory chemical released from the pigment with direct effect on the C-fibres of peripheral neurons. Indeed, also tattoo reactions with inflammation such as allergic reactions are remarkably itchy, and neurosensitive activation might be relevant in a broad range of inflammatory tattoo reactions even if other features such as plaque elevation and hyperkeratosis may dominate objective findings.

Lymphopathies
Lymphopathies are of two kinds. Lymphatics draining a tattoo on the arm or the leg may have become insufficient with lymphedema of the tattoo, the surrounding skin, and even the distal extremity. The condition is chronic and supposed to be caused by clusters of pigment particles blocking or damaging the lymphatics draining the field of the tattoo where the pigment was installed. The tattoo itself may be without any other abnormality than signs of swelling. A similar condition from Ethiopia, Africa, known as 'podoconiosis' with

lymphedema and swollen legs due to bentonite clay particles from the soil, which has entered through fissures under the feet while walking barefooted. The clay particles block lymphatics and reach the inguinal lymph nodes. Another type of lymphopathy in the tattooed affects the regional lymph nodes, which are intermittently or chronically swollen due to reactive inflammation of the node caused by reaction to tattoo pigment deposits accumulated in the node. In case of an allergic reaction of the tattoo and concomitantly of the node, the swelling of the node will continue after the tattoo with allergic reaction has been excised and it may also be necessary to excise lymph nodes with painful reactions. Tattoo pigment in lymph nodes may not cause lymphedema.

Tumours

Tumours arising in the epidermis and normally seen in the skin, such as basal cell carcinoma, squamous cell carcinoma, and malignant melanoma, of course may affect any tattoo by coincidence, independent or potentially dependent of the tattoo pigment in the dermis. The epidermis protecting the basal cell membrane barrier normally is devoid of pigment. Clinical evidence and an extensive literature review conclude that tattoo pigments do not cause skin cancer in man, despite some tattoo inks containing potential carcinogens known from toxicology [37]. This was supported by a photocarcinogenicity study of mice tattooed on the back with an ink withdrawn from the market due to a high content of carcinogen [38]. In contrast to expectation, the tattooed mice showed delayed skin cancers on UV light exposure in comparison with nontattooed controls. Black pigment in the dermis was speculated to absorb light, thus with less backscattered light towards the epidermis.

Keratoacanthoma, which is clinically benign and a 'pseudomalignant' tumour that easily may mimic squamous cell carcinoma by histology, is associated with tattoos. A large study has recently confirmed that keratoacanthoma is clinically benign [39]. Keratoacanthoma often has a characteristic clinical appearance with major keratosis in the centre and a circular basis, but lesions also may be less typical. Suspected keratoacanthoma may, depending on the doctor's opinion, be followed without excision and histology, which may only confuse the diagnosis.

There is a special problem of benign nevi tattooed with black colour since observation of malignant change of such over-tattooed nevi makes early detection of malignant melanoma difficult. Also, black tattoo pigment accumulated in regional lymph nodes originating from a black tattoo in the draining field of the node may complicate the diagnosis of melanoma involvement of the node in sentinel node surgery of malignant melanoma, when the tattoo and the melanoma are nearby and share lymphatic drainage [40, 41].

Hypertrophic Scars and Keloids

Hypertrophic scars and keloids in tattoos are surprisingly uncommon. Some anatomical sites are at potential risk: the breast and shoulders as well as the wrists and the ankles over the joints. Persons with predisposition to keloid and with traumatic or excisional keloids on the breast even may carry tattoos on shoulders and the breast without having abnormal scarring in the tattoo. Abnormal scarring in relation to tattoos mainly is found over or nearby the wrist and ankle joints seemingly triggered by the stretch stimuli of joint motions. The commonest reasons of abnormal scarring locally in a part of the tattoo or involving the entire tattoo are needle trauma, amateurism, and attempts to remove the tattoo with lasers not suited for this purpose or used incorrectly. Caustic chemicals, such as lactic acid 20–40% used to remove tattoos, very often cause severe scarring with hypertrophic scars and even keloid formation in a characteristic pattern with multiple 4–8 mm circular scars where the acid initially was injected [42]. Tattoo removal by caustic chemicals is unrestricted in many countries and can be provided by any lay person.

Tattoo Pigment Diffusion (Blowout) or Fan
Tattoo pigment diffusion, also called blowout, or fan with tattoo pigment visibly staining the surrounding normal skin occurs a few weeks or months after a new tattoo. The stain may distribute following the direction of the lymphatic drainage or move in the tissues under the influence of gravity. Pigment also may diffuse to the subcutaneous tissue and near joints causing bursitis with tenderness, pain, and swelling over the joint. Fan to deeper structures is not automatically paralleled by visual fan horizontally in the skin. Pigment diffusion is a special problem in cosmetic tattoos, when tattooing of eye surroundings, such as eye liner of the lower lids, is complicated with dark shadows under the eye extending to the rim of the orbital margin. Laser removal is helpful even if pigment in deeper tissues cannot be reached with the laser.

Irritant and Local Toxic Events
Irritant and local toxic events are common, natural, and to be expected in tattooing involving both a major needle trauma and exposure to tattoo inks made as industrial products and bought on an open market out of control. Clinical manifestation is dominated by inflammation directly in the tattoo and often seen as what is conveniently called 'delayed healing'. Tattooists practice very different aftercare treatments, and there is no consensus [43]. Failure of aftercare may worsen the condition, as may secondary infection. In severe reactions with long healing time, scarring may be the outcome. Also, pigment failure of the tattoo with irregular pigment loss or general weakening of colour in the tattoo may occur and need repair with a cover-up tattoo.

Tattoo Technique Failures and Hazards
Tattoo technique failures and hazards by mechanism and techniques are the responsibility of the tattooist. Causes are manifold, i.e. use of needles of poor quality, damaged needles with hooks, too intense tattooing of a skin site with cuts and major needle trauma, poor quality and incorrect setting of the tattoo machine with a too deep injection of the dermis relative to anatomical site and skin stiffness, dosing too much tattoo ink into the skin, or inoculation of bacteria and other microbes from skin not properly disinfected. In addition, such failures and hazards can also originate from the tattooist, the needle, the tattoo ink, the parlour, the person being tattooed, etc. The results are delayed healing, infections, scars, pigment loss, and tattoo customers obtaining a permanently damaged tattoo.

Tattoo Removal Failures and Hazards
Tattoo removal failures and hazards by mechanism and techniques represent a broad group of hazards. Lasers used for tattoo removal can cause scarring, depigmentation and hyperpigmentation, and exceptionally sensory disturbance. Also, change of pigment can be seen, as exemplified by white titanium dioxide changing to dark after laser removal. Using inappropriate laser equipment or intense pulse light systems unlikely to produce acceptable results shall be seen as failure of technique. Overdose of laser light as an acute hazard results in vesicles and haemorrhagic blisters and leaves scars. Attempts to remove tattoos by caustic chemicals represent a special hazard as mentioned above [42].

Miscellaneous
Miscellaneous events and complications represent a broad group of separate entities and problems, some minor and some major, determined by geography as well as the local tradition and practice of tattooing. Some examples are given. *Pimples* are pinhead-round elements with local inflammation in the very outer dermis occurring a few months after tattooing. Pimples also may occur after laser removal. They resolve spontaneously. Tattooing may precipitate known skin diseases such as *necrobiosis lipoidica* and *psoriasis*, in the latter seen as a Köbner reaction directly in the new tattoo due to the mechanical trauma of tattooing, with tattoos inducing psoriasis directly in and around the tat-

too mentioned in the original publication from 1876 [44]. Tattooing does no provoke major or general outbreak of psoriasis. Despite similarities of clinical findings of *lichen planus* and allergic reactions in red tattoos, both with interface dermatitis by histology, there seems to be no coincidence and no individual predisposition shared by the two conditions. The strong association between black tattoos, papulonodular complication, and *sarcoidosis* is described above. The many aspects of sarcoidosis have been reviewed, and also other types of foreign body than black tattoo pigment can induce sarcoid granuloma [45].

Psychosocial Complications

Psychosocial complications, with and without associating psychiatric disease, are a huge theme with psychological, psychiatric, and anthropologic aspects reviewed in the Danish report of the Council on Health and Disease Prevention and addressed in a number of original publications [2, 46–49]. There is no clear cut between normal and abnormal, and societies and trends vary considerably over time. Acceptability of tattoos may have an overall mean or median value, but there are always different segments of very different views. Nevertheless, tattoos acquired by youngsters as a snapshot of young age and spirit are permanent and many tattoos cannot be removed. Obviously, tattooing seen in the lifelong perspective creates many cases of psychosocial problems and invalidity. Some tattooed persons become addicted and acquire extensive tattoos covering most of their skin. Some add piercings, implants, and body modifications to their adornment in the irresistible endeavour to be the most deviant in the room at any time. It is individual and up to psychiatrists and other specialists to conclude if a given tattoo at a given time is an expression of psychiatric disease, deviant character, borderline personality, or simply a normal acquirement of a person, who just wishes to have a lifelong personal signature on the skin, such as the day he or she was married or maybe divorced.

References

1 Serup J, Sepehri M, Hutton Carlsen K: Classification of tattoo complications in a hospital material of 493 adverse events. Dermatology 2017, in press. DOI 10.1159/000452148.

2 Tattooing – Health, Risks and Culture. The Council on Health and Disease Prevention, Copenhagen, 2015, pp 1–165. www.vidensraad.dk.

3 Serup J, Kluger N, Bäumler W (eds): Tattooed Skin and Health. Curr Probl Dermatol. Basel, Karger, 2015, vol 48.

4 Laux P, et al: A medical-toxicological view of tattooing. Lancet 2016;387:395–402.

5 Kluger N: Complications infectieuses cutanées associées au tatouage permanent. Med Mal Infect 2010;41:115–122.

6 Kluger N: Cutaneous complications related to permanent decorative tattooing. Expert Rev Clin Immunol 2010;6:363–371.

7 Kluger N: Acute complications of tattooing presenting in the ED. Am J Emerg Med 2012;30:2055–2063.

8 Kluger N: Sarcoidosis on tattoos: a review of the literature from 1939 to 2011. Sarcoidosis Vasc Diffuse Lung Dis 2013; 30:86–102.

9 Goldstein N: Complications from tattoos. J Dermatol Surg Oncol 1979;5: 869–878.

10 Jacob CJ: Tattoo-associated dermatoses: a case report and review of the literature. Dermatol Surg 2002;28:962–965.

11 Kazandjieva J, Tsankov N: Tattoos: dermatological complications. Clin Dermatol 2007;25:375–382.

12 Wenzel SM, Rittmann I, Landthaler M, et al: Adverse reactions after tattooing: review of the literature and comparison to results of a study. Dermatology 2013; 226:138–147.

13 Klügl I, Hiller KA, Landthaler M, et al: Incidence of health problems associated with tattooed skin: a nation-wide study in German-speaking countries. Dermatology 2010;221:43–50.

14 Hutton Carlsen K, Serup J: Patients with tattoo reactions have reduced quality of life and suffer from itch: Dermatology Life Quality Index and Itch Severity Score measurements. Skin Res Technol 2015;21:101–107.

15 Serup J, Hutton Carlsen K: Patch test study of 90 patients with tattoo reactions: negative outcome of allergy patch test to baseline batteries and culprit inks suggests allergen(s) are generated in the skin through haptenation. Contact Dermatitis 2014;71:255–263.

16 Gutermuth J, Hein R, Fendt F, et al: Cutaneous pseudolymphoma arising after tattoo placement. J Eur Acad Dermatol Venereol 2007;21:566–567.

17 Høgsberg T, Thomsen BM, Serup J: Histopathology and immunohistochemistry of red tattoo reactions: interface dermatitis is the lead pathology, with increase of T-lymphocytes and Langerhans cells suggesting an allergic pathomechanism. Skin Res Technol 2015;21:449–458.

18 Thum CK, Biswas A: Inflammatory complications related to tattooing: a histopathological approach based on pattern analysis. Am J Dermatopathol 2015;37:54–66.
19 Kluger N, Durand L, Minier-Thoumin C, et al: Pseudoepitheliomatous epidermal hyperplasia in tattoos: report of three cases. Am J Clin Dermatol 2008;9: 337–340.
20 Porter CJ, Simcock JW, MacKinnon CA: Necrotising fasciitis and cellulitis after traditional Samoan tattooing: case reports. J Infect 2005;50:149–152.
21 Høgsberg T, Jacobsen NR, Clausen P, Serup J: Black tattoo inks induce reactive oxygen species production correlating with aggregation of pigment nanoparticles but not with polycyclic aromatic hydrocarbon content. Exp Dermatol 2013;22:464–469.
22 Sepehri M, Carlsen K, Serup J: Papulo-nodular reactions in black tattoos as markers of sarcoidosis: study of 92 tattoo reactions from a hospital material. Dermatology 2017, in press. DOI 10.1159/000453315.
23 Sepehri M, Jørgensen B, Serup J: Introduction of dermatome shaving as first line treatment of chronic tattoo reactions. J Dermatolog Treat 2015;26:451–455.
24 England RW, Vogel P, Hagan L: Immediate cutaneous hypersensitivity after treatment of tattoo with Nd:YAG laser: a case report and review of the literature. Ann Allergy Asthma Immunol 2002;89: 215–217.
25 Kuperman-Beade M, Levine VJ, Ashinoff R. Laser removal of tattoos. Am J Clin Dermatol 2001;2:231–25.
26 Jacobsen E, Tønning K, Pedersen E, Bernth N, Serup J, Høgsberg T, Nielsen E: The Danish Environmental Protection Agency. Report on Chemical Substances in Tattoo Ink, 2012, report 216 (English version). ISBN 978–87–92779–87–8. www.mst.dk/publications/English.
27 Hutton Carlsen K, Serup J: Tattooing may cause life-threatening latex allergy. J Eur Acad Dermatol Venereol 2016;30: 1242–1244.
28 Armstrong ML, DeBoer S, Cetta F: Infective endocarditis after body art: a review of the literature and concerns. J Adolesc Health 2008;43:217–225.
29 Kluger N, Muller C, Gral N: Atypical mycobacteria infection following tattooing: review of an outbreak in 8 patients in a French tattoo parlor. Arch Dermatol 2008;144:941–942.
30 Drage LA, Ecker PM, Orenstein R, et al: An outbreak of *Mycobacterium chelonae* infections in tattoos. J Am Acad Dermatol 2010;62:501–506.
31 Høgsberg T, Saunte DM, Frimodt-Møller N, et al: Microbial status and product labelling of 58 original tattoo inks. J Eur Acad Dermatol Venereol 2013;27;73–80.
32 Baumgartner A, Gautsch S: Hygienic-microbiological quality of tattoo- and permanent make-up colours. J Verbrauch Lebensm 2011;6:319–325.
33 Bonadonna L, Briancesco R, Coccia AM, et al: Microbiological quality and product labelling of tattoo inks (abstract). Proc 1st Eur Congr Tattoo Pigment Res, Copenhagen, November 2013.
34 Jafari S, Copes R, Baharlou S, et al: Tattooing and the risk of transmission of hepatitis C: a systematic review and meta-analysis. Int J Infect Dis 2010;14: 928–940.
35 Doll DC: Tattooing in prison and HIV infection. Lancet 1988;1:66–67.
36 Morte PD, Magee M: Hyperalgesia after volar wrist tattoo: a case of complex regional pain syndrome? J Clin Neuromuscul Dis 2011;12:118–121.
37 Kluger N, Koljonen V: Tattoos, inks and cancer. Lancet Oncol 2012;13:e161–e168.
38 Lerche C, Sepehri M, Serup J, Poulsen T, Wulf HC: Black tattoos protect against UVR-induced skin cancer in mice. Photodermatol Photoimmunol Photomed 2015;31:261–268.
39 Takai T, Misago N, Murata Y: Natural course of keratoacanthoma and related lesions after partial biopsy: clinical analysis of 66 lesions. J Dermatol 2015;42: 353–362.
40 Moehrle M, Blaaheta HJ, Ruck P: Tattoo pigment mimics positive sentinel lymph node in melanoma. Dermatology 2001; 203:342–344.
41 Friedman T, Westreich M, Mozes SN, et al: Tattoo pigment in lymph nodes mimicking metastatic malignant melanoma. Plast Reconstr Surg 2003;111: 2120–2122.
42 Wolina U: Depigmentation and hypertrophic scars after application of a fluid lactic acid tattoo eraser. Wien Med Wochenschr 2015;165:196–198.
43 Rosenbaum BE, Milam E, Seo L, Leger MC: Skin care in the tattoo parlor: a survey of tattoo artists in New York City. Dermatology 2016;232:484–489.
44 Köbner H: Zür Aetiologie der Psoriasis. Viertel Jahresschrift für Dermatologie und Syphilis 1876;3:559–561.
45 Haimovic A, Sanchez M, Judson MA, Prystowsky S: Sarcoidosis: a comprehensive review and update for the dermatologist. J Amer Acad Dermatol 2012; 66:699–716.
46 Khosla V, Verghese J, Harvey G: Tattoos: what is their significance? Adv Psychiatr Treat 2010;16:281–287.
47 Preti A, Pinna C, Nocco S, et al: Body of evidence: tattoos, body piercing and eating disorder symptoms among adolescents. J Psychosom Res 2006;61:561–566.
48 Dhosseche D, Snell KS, Larder S: A case-control study of tattoos in young suicide victims as a possible marker of risk. J Affect Disord 2000;59:165–168.
49 Hellard ME, Aitken CK, Hocking JS: Tattooing in prisons – not such a pretty picture. Am J Infect Control 2007;35: 477–480.

Prof. Jørgen Serup, DMSc
Department of Dermatology D41, Bispebjerg University Hospital
Bispebjerg Bakke 23
DK–2400 Copenhagen NV (Denmark)
E-Mail joergen.vedelskov.serup@regionh.dk

Serup J, Bäumler W (eds): Diagnosis and Therapy of Tattoo Complications. With Atlas of Illustrative Cases.
Curr Probl Dermatol. Basel, Karger, 2017, vol 52, pp 74–81 (DOI: 10.1159/000450804)

Medical Treatment of Tattoo Complications

Jørgen Serup

The 'Tattoo Clinic', Department of Dermatology, Bispebjerg University Hospital, Copenhagen, Denmark

Abstract

Tattooing is a skin trauma and involves a special vulnus punctatum (with inserted tattoo ink, a vulnus venenatum), which should heal with no infection and no local complication. Local treatment in the healing phase ideally builds on the 'moist wound' principle using plastic film, hydrocolloids, silver dressing, and compression. Bacterial infections during healing are treated with oral antibiotics, and a list of first-line antibiotics is proposed. Notice is given to severe infections with affected general condition, and it is emphasized that intravenous antibiotic treatment must be instituted as early as possible to prevent septic shock and death. Hydrophilic antibiotics shall be given in high load and maintenance dose due to increased renal clearance of such antibiotics. Chronic allergic reactions of red tattoos respond little to local corticoids and are best treated with dermatome shaving. Laser removal is contraindicated due to the risk of photochemical activation of the allergy with anaphylaxis or worsening. Chronic reactions in black tattoos can be treated with local corticoids, dermatome shaving, and lasers as well. Systemic corticoid is used in allergic reactions in red tattoos and in cross-allergic reactions of other red tattoos as well as in black tattoo reactions associated with sarcoidosis and with cutaneous 'rush phenomenon' affecting any black tattoo. Systemic corticoid is also indicated in generalized eczema due to nickel allergy or another allergy challenged through tattooing or introduced by tattooing as a primary sensitization. The use of intralesional corticoid, antihistamines, and immunosuppressive medicines is discussed. A warning against the use of lactic acid and other caustic chemicals for tattoo removal is given, since such chemicals and commercial products cannot be dosed properly and very often result in disfiguring scarring.

Medical treatment of tattoo complications is complex and has many different targets and modalities. Treatment needs adjustment relative to the change of scene over time. Prescription of drugs, of course, is restricted to doctors. Skin care during the healing of the tattoo wound is undertaken by tattooists and the tattooed individuals. There is no team of providers of care and treatment, and there is in practice only limited coordination across sectors.

The pivotal starting point of the course of tattoo complication(s) is the tattoo operation in the tattoo parlor. Tattooing involving several hundreds of needle punctures to the mid-dermal level is a special wound. In classical medicine and according to the historical synopsis of nosologies

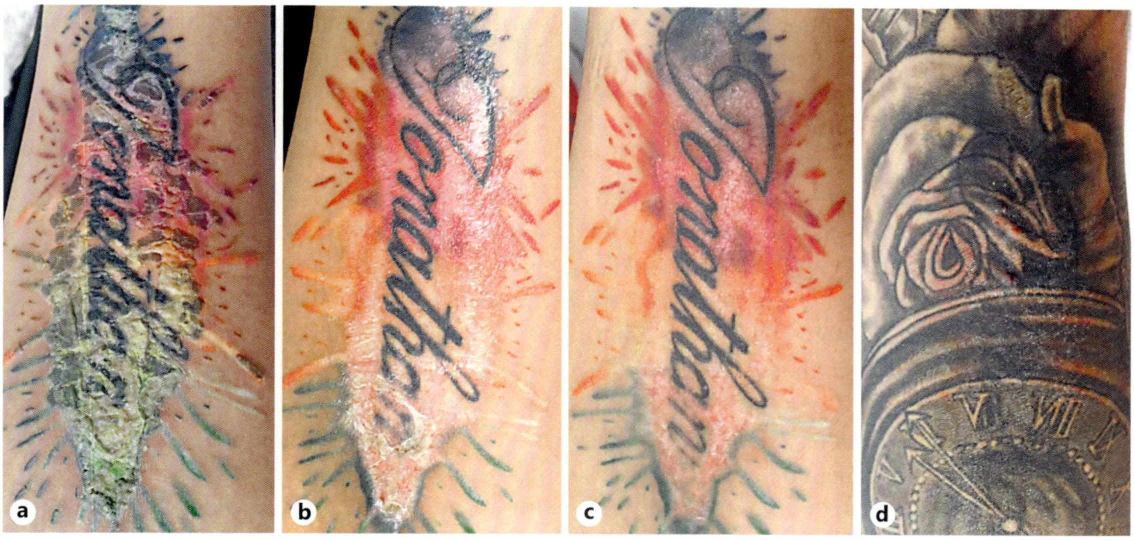

Fig. 1. A history of major tattoo trauma leading to a sequence of complications with relative inadequacy of treatment, illustrated with the patient's own smartphone photos (reproduced with permission). **a** Tattoo a few days after tattooing with a lacerated wound covered with crusts holding pigment extruded form the skin and the tattoo. The tattoo was performed by an amateur, who attempted to make a special effect with different colors overlapping each other, resulting in overworked and traumatized skin. **b** After 4 weeks, loss of pigment, active inflammation, and early scarring; complicated healing, the patient received antibiotics and local corticoid. **c** After 10 weeks, ongoing inflammation and scarring, itch and pain, and with virtually no response to local corticoid and another course of antibiotics. **d** After 18 months, symptoms were less but still cumbersome, despite treatment with corticoid under occlusion followed by intralesional corticoid, all without significant clinical effect. The patient regretted the tattoo and was offered surgical excision covered with a transplant, but she decided to have a black tattoo cover-up, this time made by a professional tattooist. Inflammation, scarring, and some discomfort remained.

of David Hosack from 1818, the uncomplicated tattoo wound is a vulnus punctatum [1]. With particles and chemicals of inks (the nosology, which was published before the era of modern medicine, uses the word 'poisons') introduced with the punctures and exerting various unwanted effects, the wound is more correctly of the type vulnus venenatum. If the tattoo needle and machine produce linear lesions and cuts, the wound is a vulnus incision, and if the physical traumatization of the skin is more extensive, it is a vulnus laceratum. This distinction remains relevant even today. Tattooists, who have learned the craftsmanship and art of tattooing, of course, do their job aiming at a minimum risk, and so do responsible manufacturers of tattoo ink.

Traumatic tattooing as well as the dose and brand of some tattoo inks predispose to delayed healing, infections, and various other complications and sequels, which cannot always be alleviated, as exemplified in figure 1a–d. The figure shows a case of traumatic tattooing with some vulnus laceratum followed by a cascade of adverse events, i.e. poor healing with recurrent infections, pigment loss, chronic inflammation and scarring, tattoo regret, cover-up tattoo but still having underlying chronic inflammation, and scarring causing itch and chronic discomfort. It also exemplifies the relative inadequacy of treatment, which cannot overcome hazards by tattooing. However, proper treatment of tattoo complications now and then can do much and even save lives, but damaged skin cannot be made natural again and regain its normal structure and function. Damage can be permanent and incurable, which is worth to be informed about and recognize before the tattoo is decided.

To the best of my knowledge, there is no published systematic study of care and medical treatment of tattoos and tattoo complications, and the formal level of medical evidence, thus, is rather low. Research in medical treatment was hampered by lacking diagnostic classification of reactions and complications, a problem discussed in the chapter by Serup [this vol., pp. 58–73]. In this chapter on medical treatment of tattoo complications, the clinical experience of the 'Tattoo Clinic' of Bispebjerg University Hospital, based on a patient material of over 500 patients diagnosed according to the new diagnostic classification system, is presented. In our hospital, the 'Tattoo Clinic', the laser surgery unit and surgery of wound in the 'Wound Healing Center' are integrated in the same dermatology department and building.

Tattoo Healing and Aftercare

Tattooists routinely treat the tattooed skin and advice the customer on how to treat the wound during uncomplicated tattoo healing, which takes a few weeks [2]. Tattooists practice many different treatments, and there is no consensus. It is common to perform 'moist wound healing' for a couple of days by covering the tattooed skin with a wrap of transparent foil, followed by moisturizing ointments or creams.

Doctors probably would prefer the more expensive hydrogels, hydrocolloids, foams, and hydrogels, agreeing to the principle of 'moist wound healing'. In suspected bacterial infection, antiseptics with iod-starch, silver, chlorhexidine, chloramine, acetic acid, and hydrogen peroxide may be considered, but chlorhexidine and chloramine may damage granulation tissue. Silver dressings work by release of silver ions, which may damage cell walls of bacteria and interfere with RNA/DNA and replication. In suspected infection with *Pseudomonas aeruginosa* aluminum subacetate can be used. Local antibiotics are little used because of the risk of selecting strains resistant to antibiotics. Compressive bandages may be applied to control edema of the wound and the surrounding skin, which may be a problem with tattoos on the legs. Compressive bandage also may be helpful in tattoos over joints, such as the wrists, to reduce stretch and bending of the skin during healing. Tattoo healing is dynamic, and the individual state of healing shall argue treatment at any time. There are many ways of treatment and many opinions and preferences about how to treat. The tattoo will remain vulnerable for some time after it is visually healed, with increased sensitivity to sun.

Tattooists may or may not recommend their customers long-term care of their tattoos. The primary concern may be cosmetic, namely bleaching of the tattoo color over time. Tattoos are sensitive to light, which may induce the photochemical breakdown of pigment associated with complaints, especially swelling and itching of the tattoo [3–6]. Thus, regular use of sun blockers in the summertime, at the beach, and on special exposure to sun is rational. If sensitivity to light is advanced and a medical complication, of course, treatment with sun blockers is mandatory, with detailed instructions on the correct application and use.

Treatment of Infectious Complications

Bacterial infections the day after tattooing or a few days later manifested as local infection in the tattoo or as infection spread to the surrounding skin or to deeper structures are described in the chapter by Serup [this vol., pp. 30–41]. Such infections, depending on the doctor's evaluation, require treatment with oral or intravenous antibi-

Table 1. Bacterial tattoo infections and systemic antibictics, proposed first-line treatments and oral dose unless otherwise indicated

Hemolytic streptococci group A, C, and G Fenoxymethyl penicillin (1 million units/660 mg thrice daily)
Staphylococci (commonly penicillinase producing) Dicloxacillin (1 g 4 times daily), clindamycin (600 mg thrice daily)
Methicillin-resistant staphylococci (MRSA)[1] Vancomycin (1g twice daily, intravenously) or linezolid (600 mg twice daily)
Gram-negative bacteria Amoxicillin (1g thrice daily), ciprofloxacin (500 mg twice daily), or cefuroxime (750 mg thrice daily, intravenously)
Pseudomonas aeruginosa Ciprofloxacin (500 mg twice daily)
Severe infection and affected general condition[1] Cefuroxime (1,500 mg thrice daily, intravenously) or gentamycin (intravenous dose adjusted to body weight and renal function) Anaerobic bacteria, metronidazole (500 mg thrice daily)

Local hospitals or departments of microbiology may have other recommendations on treatment. Length of treatment course is individual and decided by the doctor in charge.
[1] Shall always be coordinated with microbiologists; early treatment is imperative and can be started according to a guideline. A higher loading and maintenance dose than indicated in the table can be given depending on the patient's condition and the solubility of the antibiotic in watery media.
This table is adapted from the guidelines 'Rational use of antibiotics', Region Copenhagen Hospitals, and from 'Pharmacologic treatment of problematic chronic wounds', Institute of Rational Pharmacotherapy (IRF), The Medicines Agency, Denmark.

otics [7]. The choice of antibiotic, route of administration, and duration of treatment depends on the severity of the infection, the circumstances, the spontaneous resistance of the person, and certainly, the suspected or verified causative bacteria and the choice of antibiotic(s), which may be selected after consultation with the local department of microbiology. If the infection is not under control within 1–3 days, a switch form oral to intravenous treatment or a switch of antibiotic shall be considered. Table 1 shows antibiotics, which may be considered drugs of first priority in the treatment of bacterial tattoo infections.

Severe infection and affected general condition with septicemia and systemic inflammatory response syndrome is a life-threatening condition, which within a few hours may develop into septic shock with a high mortality [8, 9]. Development of shock depends on early start of intravenous treatment with a combination of antibiotics. Increased loading dose and maintenance dose shall be considered from the start since creatinine clearance may be increased, known as augmented renal clearance [10, 11]. As a consequence, hydrophilic antibiotics are eliminated faster and blood concentrations lowered. Hydrophilic antibiotics include beta-lactam and carbapenem antibiotics, aminoglycosides and glycopeptides. Penicillin is in the hydrophilic group. Lipophilic antibiotics, which are not subject to increased renal clearance, include fluoroquinolones, macrolides, metronidazole, and others. There is a direct correlation between survivals and start of effective treatment of septic shock and a mortality of 90% if treatment is started later than 24 h after the shock started [10]. Antibiotic treatment instituted early according to a guideline and without the causative bacteria being identified also prevents shock, which supports the strategy of earliest possible treatment on the existing premises of availability and recognition [11].

Thus, when treating bacterial tattoo infections, the patient shall be closely monitored, and worsening with affected general condition considered alarming, with the patient urgently remitted to the casualty department of the hospital. In the past and also today sepsis and septic shock is the main reason of death from tattooing.

Surgery only has little place in the treatment of tattoo infections. The exception is necrotizing fasciitis and infection with 'flesh-eating' bacteria, which may require urgent excisional surgery and even amputation. Thus, infection going deep and with rapid progression is alarming and calls for action.

Treatment of Noninfectious Complications

Inflammatory tattoo complications is a field with many distinctive patterns and types of chronic reactions [see chapter by Serup, this vol. pp. 58–73]. Being of high complexity, careful diagnostic evaluation is necessary as described in the chapter by Serup [this vol., pp. 42–57]. The dominating groups are allergic reactions in red tattoos and papulonodular reactions in black tattoos, the latter without or with associated sarcoidosis in the skin or in internal organs [12, 13]. Another large group of chronic complications is represented by a number of specific conditions, which may not be inflammatory and thus require special treatments depending on the nature of the complication.

Allergic tattoo reactions of red tattoos and other colors require the pigment in the outer dermis to be effectively removed, since effective elimination of the hapten in the skin is the only fundamental cure. Dermatome shaving is the first-line treatment [see chapter by Sepehri and Jørgensen, this vol., pp. 82–93]. With dermatome shaving the horizontal cut is sharp and performed sequentially slice by slice until white dermal collagen network is reached and the pigment thus removed [14]. Laser treatment with pulses of light scattered in the treated field with uncertainty about the horizontal distribution of spots, with uncertainty about the width of the conus of light in the tissue in a given depth of the skin, and also the decline of laser intensity versus dermal depth make laser treatment applied to inflammatory tattoo reactions imprecise and a dubious endeavor. For those reasons, laser treatment is not rational in the treatment of inflammatory tattoo reactions. In allergic tattoo reactions, laser treatment is highly controversial because of the risk of type I allergic reactions including anaphylaxis and the risk of flare-up of chronic allergic reactions because of photochemical breakdown of pigment exposed to powerful laser light and activation of ongoing allergy in the tattoo, as described in reports from the clinic and in other chapters of the book [15]. *Allergy in a tattoo, urticarial or delayed, shall be considered a contraindication of lasers.*

Having performed diagnostic evaluation, excluded infection, and considered surgical treatment as an option, the need for medical therapies come into consideration. Corticoids, local and systemic, and other local or immunosuppressive treatments can be used.

Local corticoids of medium class or high potency often are tried and may be beneficial in some indications. Allergic reactions in red tattoos exceptionally can be relieved and improved by local corticoids if the amount of pigment in the skin is limited and concentrated in the very outer dermis in a tattoo small in size. However, the rate of recurrence is high, and the treatment is limited in time because of the risk of skin atrophy. Allergic reactions mostly do not respond to local corticoids, and many are resistant even to corticoid under occlusion. Some reactions spontaneously may decrease in activity over time, but this can take years. Treatment attempts resulting in skin atrophy can create surgical problems when dermatome shaving is performed to finally eradicate the problem. This problem is especially relevant when tattoos are located over the wrist and foot joints, on the back of the hands and on the dorsum of the foot.

Nonallergic inflammatory reactions in black tattoos of the papulonodular type may respond to local corticoids and respond better than allergic reactions do. Some reactions coming up shortly after tattooing and explained by an overdose of black ink may respond well and only may need treatment for some few months. Excessive black pigment sometimes can relocate in the tissue and become acceptable and nonreactive. Reactions in black tattoos developed after a latency of months or years and related to pigment agglomeration over time with foreign body formation and inflammation show a poorer response to local corticoids, albeit the response is better than seen in allergic reactions. Again, the duration of treatment and risk of skin atrophy in practice limits the treatment. If reactions represent a significant problem to the patient, despite proper use of local corticoids, dermatome shaving or laser removal are therapeutic options. Dermatome shaving can remove the pigment, and since reactions are not allergic, it may suffice just to reduce some excessive amount of pigment and thereby limit the risk of scarring following the operation. Scarring can be a problem if shaving is performed to the depth of the lower one third of the dermis. Reactions in black tattoos can be treated with lasers without concerns about allergic reaction induced by the treatment. In addition, with lasers, partial removal of the pigment can be enough to eliminate the problem. Black pigment absorbs laser light more efficient than any other color.

Sarcoid reaction in black tattoos is a special therapeutic challenge and shall be seen as a local manifestation of a systemic disease and individual predisposition [15]. Nodular tattoo reactions with sarcoid granuloma often do not respond to local corticoid since a potent background factor of autoimmune stimulation is active, which cannot be treated with a topical. Therapy depends on diagnostic evaluation and systematic mapping of the different risk organs of sarcoidosis affliction. Dermatome shaving and lasers somehow have a limited role in the treatment because of the risk of scar sarcoidosis in the treated field.

In local treatment of tattoo reactions, it shall be taken into account that adherence to local treatment often is low and very disappointing. About 1/3 of new prescriptions to dermatology patients are not redeemed in the pharmacy, and if redeemed, about 95% of the patients apply the remedy only occasionally and in a much smaller dose than expected [16, 17]. There is no expectation that sufferers of tattoo complications have better adherence to local therapy.

Intralesional injection of protracted corticoid is used with some success for the treatment of scarring and hypertrophic scars in tattoos. There is limited experience with such drugs used to treat allergic reactions. The treatment might be practiced in small-sized tattoos located in anatomical sites with thicker skin and not over the joints. The risk of skin atrophy of the surrounding skin in the direction of the lymph flow is rather high. Injection can be painful, and in allergic tattoo reactions with fiery inflammation and urticaria, anaphylactic shock can be provoked, possibly caused by unspecific release of vasoactive amines from the inflammation to the blood stream rather than elicited by a specific allergy to the injected drug (Serup, pers. observation). Thus, care is needed when allergic reactions with very active inflammation are injected, and maybe such treatment is best performed in a hospital clinic. There is no experience with 'dermojet' pneumatic high-pressure injection of allergic tattoo reactions, but it may be an option worth exploring.

Oral corticoid and immunosuppressive treatments have a few indications. Oral prednisone exceptionally can be used in severe and very cumbersome allergic reactions of red tattoos awaiting more fundamental treatment. Some reactions itch day and night [18]. *Allergic reactions with cross-reactivity in other red tattoos* can also indicate prednisone for a period. There is limited but positive experience with cyclosporine used for allergic tattoo reactions (S. Van der Bent, Rijnland Ziekenhuis, Dermatology, Leiderdorp, The Netherlands, 2016, pers. observation).

Similarly, sarcoid reactions in black tattoos with *'rush phenomenon'* and outbreak of inflammatory reactions in other black tattoos tolerated in the past indicates oral prednisone, in this case used as first-line treatment with high efficiency in relieving symptoms [13]. Depending on screening for sarcoidosis in other organs, prednisone shall be maintained for months, taped out gradually, and substituted by methotrexate or another immunosuppressant as recommended by internists.

Generalized allergic eczema occurring shortly after tattooing and involving large skin fields is a straightforward indication of oral prednisone. Such a rash may be severe and appear within a day if the tattooed already has a severe allergy to nickel and through tattooing is challenged with tattoo ink contaminated with nickel in a soluble form. The rash will fade over a few months. Another scenario and indication for oral prednisone is a new allergy acquired through tattooing, with the rash coming up after a few weeks, preceded by a period of primary sensitization, for example to preservatives contained in the tattoo ink. In aggressive allergy, generalized dermatitis can persist and require cyclosporine or another immunosuppressant.

Antihistamines are the treatment of choice in urticarial tattoo reactions. Urticaria provoked by tattooing and local or widespread in the skin can be relieved by antihistamines; however, the treatment is not very effective and often oral treatment with prednisone is required for a period of months until the activity may spontaneously decline.

Miscellaneous treatments and other indications: in the range of tattoo complications, there are many special entities and needs of treatments, which can be instituted after a doctor's individual assessment.

Nonsurgical Tattoo Removal Using Chemicals and Caustics

Many remedies have been used for nonsurgical removal of tattoos, i.e. salicylic acid, chloroacetic acids, phenol, sulfuric acid, nitric acid silver nitrate, tannic acid, zinc chloride, and sodium chloride abrasion (salabrasion) [19]. Cryosurgery, dermabarasion, and thermal cautery by fulguration were also tried. The treatments were given up because of side effects, particularly scarring and difficulties of controlling dose versus effect and hazard, curves which obviously are not linear but individual for the person and with a very narrow therapeutic window, if any. Salabrasion actually sometimes may produce good results, and the treatment has the advantage that any color can be removed with a gradual visual transition zone towards normal skin (A. Alomar, Department of Dermatology, Hospital de Sant Pau, Barcelona, Spain, 2016, pers. observation).

Recently, removal of tattoos with 20 and 40% lactic acid and removal with high concentrations of a mix of metal oxides and possibly enzymes were marketed in a number of countries. Applications are made sequentially by repeated tattoo needle puncturing of the skin in small circular fields bridged by untreated skin. This treatment has the same limitations as other caustics have. A number of very severe cases of scarring have been treated in hospital with no acceptable outcome [20]. The treatment is disfiguring, leaving scars for the rest of life, and shall be warned about. The treatment principle is old, dating back to 1888, when Variot described the so-called French method of Variot for tattoo removal [21]. Solutions of tannic acid and silver nitrate were successively applied after breaking the skin barrier with linear incisions, scratches or punctures.

References

1 Hosack D: A system of practical nosology, to which is prefixed a synopsis of the systems of Sauvages, Linnæus, Vogel, Sagar, MacBride, Cullen, Darwin, Crichton, Pinel, Parr, Swediaur, and Young with references to the best authors on each disease, ed 2. New York, C.S. van Winkle, 1821, p 290.

2 Rosenbaum BE, Milam EC, Seo L, Leger MC: Skin care in the tattoo parlor: a survey of tattoo artists in New York. Dermatology, 2016;232:484–489.

3 Bäumler W, Eibler WT, Hohenleutner U, Sens B, Sauer J, Landthaler M: Q-switch laser and tattoo pigments: first results of the chemical and photophysical analysis of 41 compounds. Lasers Surg Med 2000;26:13–21.

4 Vasold R, Naarmann N, Ulrich H, Fischer D, König B, Landthaler M, Bäumler W: Tattoo pigments are cleaved by laser light – the chemical analysis in vitro provide evidence of hazardous compounds. Photochem Photobiol 2001;80: 185–190.

5 Høgsberg T, Carlsen KH, Serup J: High prevalence of tattoo complaints among a young population tattooed with recent organic pigments. J Eur Acad Dermatol 2013;27:846–852.

6 Carlsen KH, Serup J: Photosensitivity and photodynamic events in black, red and blue tattoos are common. A 'beach study'. J Eur Acad Dermatol Venereol 2014;28:231–237.

7 LeBlanc P-M, Hollinger K-A, Klontz K-C: Tattoo ink-related infections – awareness, diagnosis, reporting, and prevention. N Engl J Med 2012;367:985–987.

8 Vincent JL, Opal SM, Marshall JC, et al: Sepsis definition: time for change. Lancet 2013;381:774–775.

9 Angus DC, van der Poll T: Severe sepsis and septic shock. N Engl J Med 2013; 369:840–851.

10 Kumar A, Roberts D, Wood KE, et al: Duration of hypotension before initiation of effective antimicrobial therapy is the critical determinant for survival in human septic shock. Crit Care Med 2006;34:1589–1596.

11 Ferrer A, Martin-Loeches I, Phillips G, et al: Empiric antibiotic treatment reduces mortality in severe sepsis and septic shock from the first hour: results from a guideline based performance improvement program. Crit Care Med 2014;42:1749–1755.

12 Serup J, Sepehri M, Hutton Carlsen K: Classification of tattoo complications in a hospital material of 493 adverse events. Dermatology 2017, in press. DOI 10.1159/000452148.

13 Sepehri M, Carlsen K, Serup J: Papulo-nodular reactions in black tattoos as markers of sarcoidosis: study of 92 tattoo reactions from a hospital material. Dermatology 2017, in press. DOI 10.1159/000453315.

14 Sepehri M, Jørgensen B, Serup J: Introduction of dermatome shaving as first line treatment of chronic tattoo reactions. J Dermatol Treat 2015;26:451–455.

15 Gaudron S, Bouëdec MCF, Franck F, D'Incan M: Azo pigments and quinacridones induce delayed hypersensitivity in red tattoos. Contact Dermatitis 2015;72: 97–105.

16 Storm A, Andersen SE, Benfeldt E, Serup J: One in 3 prescriptions are never redeemed: primary nonadherence in an outpatient clinic. J Am Acad Dermatol 2008;59:488–496.

17 Storm A, Andersen SE, Benfeldt E, Serup J: A prospective study of adherence to topical treatments: 95 of patients underdose. J Am Acad Dermatol 2008;59: 975–980.

18 Hutton Carlsen K, Serup J: Patients with tattoo reactions have reduced quality of life and suffer from itch: Dermatology Life Quality Index and Itch Severity Score measurements. Skin Res Technol 2015;21:101–107

19 Goldstein N, Penoff J, Price N, Ceilley RI, Goldman L, Hay-Roe V, Miller TA: Techniques of tattoo removal. J Dermatol Surg Oncol 1979;5:901–910.

20 Wolina U: Depigmentation and hypertrophic scars after application of a fluid lactic acid tattoo eraser. Wien Med Wochenschr 2015;165:196–198.

21 Variot G: Nouveau procédé de destruction des tatouages. Compte Rencu de la Société de Biologie (Paris) 1888;8:836–838.

Prof. Jørgen Serup, DMSc
Department of Dermatology D41, Bispebjerg University Hospital
Bispebjerg Bakke 23
DK–2400 Copenhagen NV (Denmark)
E-Mail joergen.vedelskov.serup@regionh.dk

Serup J, Bäumler W (eds): Diagnosis and Therapy of Tattoo Complications. With Atlas of Illustrative Cases.
Curr Probl Dermatol. Basel, Karger, 2017, vol 52, pp 82–93 (DOI: 10.1159/000450808)

Surgical Treatment of Tattoo Complications

Mitra Sepehri • Bo Jørgensen

The Wound Healing Centre and The 'Tattoo Clinic', Department of Dermatology, Bispebjerg University Hospital, Copenhagen, Denmark

Abstract

With a continuing increase in the number of tattoos performed worldwide, the need to treat tattoo complications is growing. Earlier treatments of chronic inflammatory tattoo reactions were dominated by a medical approach, or with no active intervention. In this chapter, we will address modern surgical approaches applied to situations when medical treatment is inefficient and lasers are not applicable. Dermatome shaving is positioned as first-line treatment of allergic tattoo reactions and also indicated in a number of other tattoo reactions, supplemented with excision in selected cases. The methods allow fundamental treatment with removal of the culprit pigment from the dermis. The different instruments, surgical methods, and treatment schedules are reviewed, and a guide to surgeons is presented. Postoperative treatments and the long-term outcomes are described in detail. An algorithm on specialist treatment and follow-up of tattoo reactions, which can be practiced in other countries, is presented.

Tattooing is mainstream, and this is paralleled by an increasing need to treat tattoo complications by surgery. Earlier treatments were dominated by a medical approach, including topical corticosteroids, antihistamines, and laser surgery as empiric first-line treatments.

Laser surgery primarily positioned for tattoo removal in persons who regret their tattoo is little documented when applied to chronic tattoo reactions. These reactions are inflamed and often allergic in nature. In fact, laser treatment of allergic tattoo reactions may be considered contraindicated since allergic reactions can worsen and become serious with anaphylaxis [1–3]. Lasers, especially Q-switched lasers, are universally used for removal of *nonreacting* tattoos and considered the gold standard in this indication. The outcome of laser removal in tattoo regret, however, is variable and may range from excellent to poor, depending on a number of factors such as the tattoo color being treated [4–8].

In this chapter, we will focus on the surgical approach, mainly applied to chronic tattoo complications dominated by inflammatory reaction of the outer dermis, i.e. when a medical approach

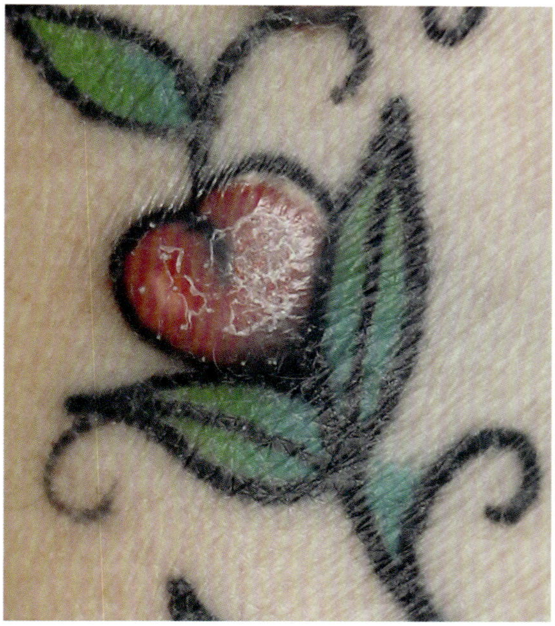

Fig. 1. Plaque elevation: allergic reaction in a red tattoo.

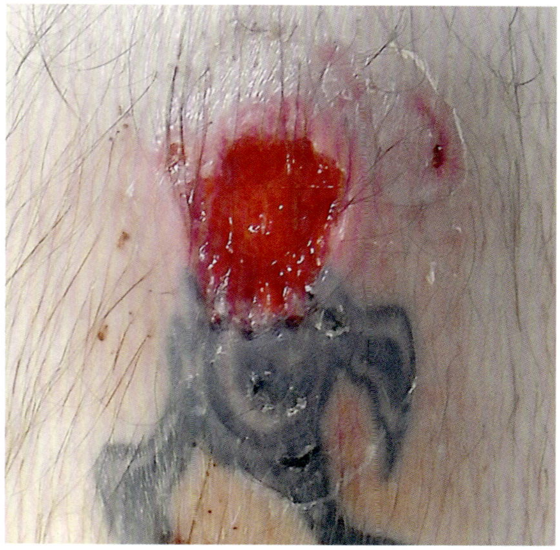

Fig. 2. Ulceronecrotic reactions: allergy exclusively in previously red parts of the tattoo.

is not applicable or likely to fail. As described in this chapter, we operate with two main categories of chronic tattoo complications, which seem to benefit from surgical intervention: *allergic reactions* and *nonallergic reactions* (the latter manifested as *papulonodular reactions*), predominant in red and black tattoos, respectively.

Tattoo Complications Suitable for Surgical Intervention

Allergic reactions show three different clinical patterns:

Plaque elevation or plaque-like patterns (allergic) occur primarily in red tattoos with consistent thickening and elevation of the entire tattoo at any site of the tattoo where the problematic color is injected. Large adherent scales may be present or the surface may be entirely smooth and slightly glistening (fig. 1) [9].

The *ulceronecrotic pattern (severe allergic)*, with necrosis and ulceration, may progress deeply in the dermis with aggressive dermal inflammation. The reaction affects any site of the tattoo where a particular color is injected [9] (fig. 2).

The *excessive hyperkeratotic pattern (allergic, with a special epidermal response)* is dominated by massive hyperkeratosis and cornification of the surface with an extraordinary epidermal response of proliferation elicited by the underlying inflammation. Surface may be flat, furrowed, whitish, and occasionally with local ulceration due to necrosis of an excessively hyperkeratotic epidermis. Notches, ducts, cysts, and epidermoid inclusions deeper in the tissue may develop [9] (fig. 3).

The nonallergic reactions are described as follows:

Papulonodular pattern (nonallergic): papules or nodules, or both, are variably distributed in the tattoo and typically confined to the problematic

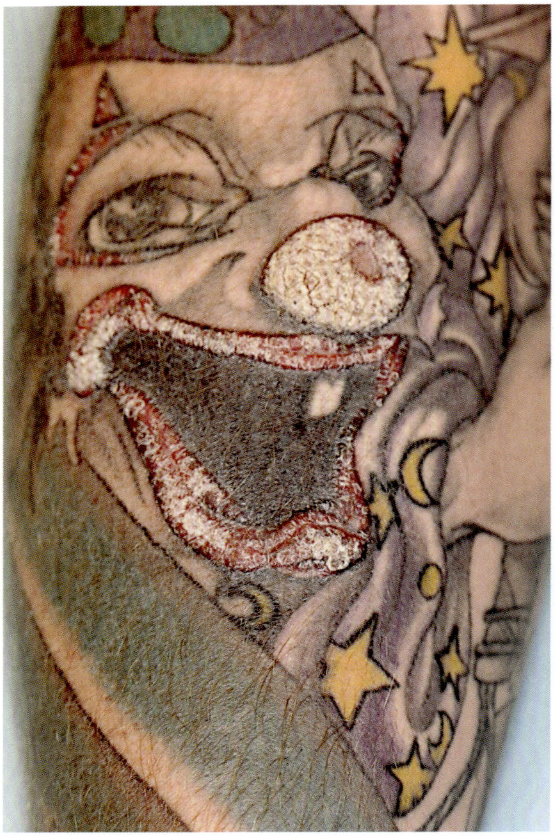

Fig. 3. Excessive hyperkeratotic pattern: allergic reactions exclusively in red parts of the tattoo.

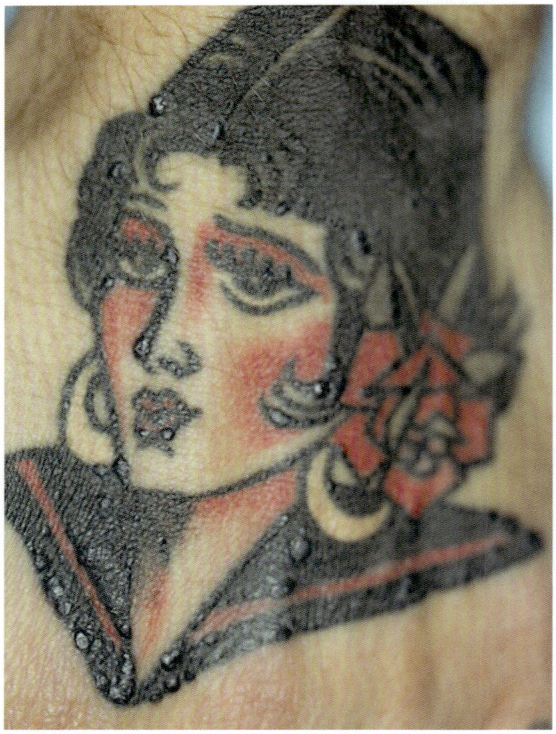

Fig. 4. Papulonodular reaction, with isolated nodules contrasting other parts of the black tattoo with no reaction. The reaction is nonallergic and caused by foreign body reaction to agglomerated black pigment in the dermis. Nodular reaction is indicative of sarcoidosis.

color, which is typically black. Elements are denser and larger in diameter in deeply colored parts of the tattoo, which may be 'overdosed' with pigment *(pigment overload)*. Large agglomerates of pigment may occasionally be seen directly by the naked eye in a raw punch biopsy. Other parts of the same tattoo containing the same color and made with the same tattoo ink product, however dosed more sparsely, may appear completely normal. Subject to individual predisposition, papules and nodules may have the histology of plain inflammation, granulomatous inflammation or sarcoid granuloma. Reaction may possibly be an isolated local manifestation of sarcoidosis exclusively in the tattoo or part of widespread sarcoidosis even involving the lungs and other organs [9, 10] (fig. 4).

Indications for Surgical Treatment

In chronic inflamed tattoo reactions not responding or unlikely to respond to medical treatment, surgical treatment should be considered. The patient's symptoms, often with severe itching and reduced quality of life, are essential for

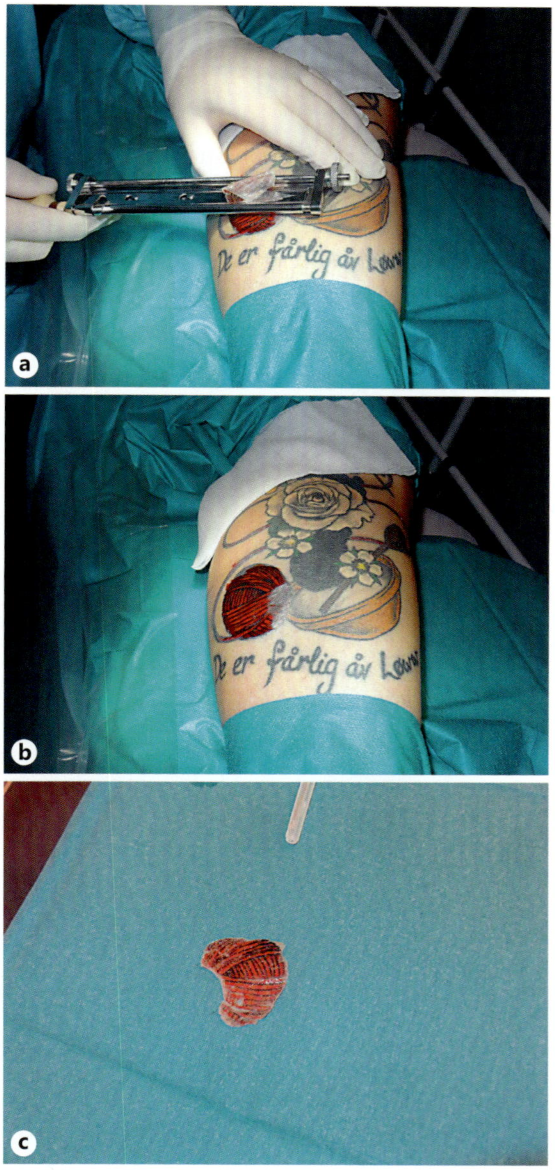

Fig. 5. a–c Dermatome shaving with the Watson® hand-operated dermatome. The bulk of pigment in the outer dermis is removed with a clean horizontal cut, repeated until dermis free of visible pigment is reached.

the decision whether to recommend surgery [11]. Sometimes severe itching and scratching results in excoriations, superficial wounds, and infections.

Table 1. Indications and type of surgery in tattoo complications

Indication / recommendation
Chronic inflammatory tattoo reactions[1]
Allergic, type plaque elevation and excessive hyperkeratosis
Nonallergic, type papulonodular reaction
Therapy-resistant tattoo reactions, other types
Severe persistent symptoms, including local pain syndrome
Recommendation: dermatome shaving (1st line), excision with/without split-skin transplant (2nd line)[2]
Pigment 'overload' (overdosed tattoo pigment) with inflammation and intermittent symptoms
Recommendation: dermatome shaving, depending on severity and case
Skin tumors in tattoos (benign or malignant)
Recommendation: excision, possibly by punch excision[3]
Critical necrosis, caused by severe and deep infection
Recommendation: excision without or with split-skin transplant[4]

[1] Beyond a healing phase of 3 months. [2] Excision preferred if pigment and inflammation involves the very low part of the dermis. [3] In keratoacanthoma the tumor is benign and normally resolves spontaneously over time. [4] If the general condition is deteriorated, surgery may be required.

Based on the experience at the Wound Healing Center (a surgical department), affiliated with the 'Tattoo Clinic' and the Department of Dermatology of Bispebjerg University Hospital in Copenhagen, the following indications for surgery are used, as listed in table 1.

Instruments

In the following section, the different surgical instruments and indications of their specific use will be described.

The *Watson*® hand-operated dermatome was the instrument first used by us for dermatome shaving of tattoo reactions back in 2009. In our

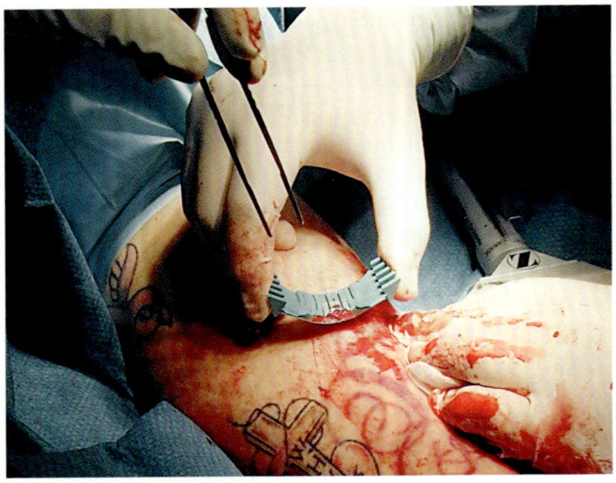

Fig. 6. Dermatome shaving with a flexible knife, Miltex®.

surgical unit it is routinely used for harvesting skin in split-skin transplantation and necrectomies. It is preferred for dermatome shaving on the extremities (fig. 5).

Flexible knives (Miltex® and DermaBlade®) are convenient and useful instruments suited for small- and medium-sized reactions, well-defined lines, and borders. Depending on the 'pressure' you put on the tool manually with your fingers, you decide the flexibility, width, and depth of the shaving (fig. 6).

The *Zimmer Dermatome*® is routinely used as well, when harvesting skin for split- skin transplantation. It is recommended for dermatome

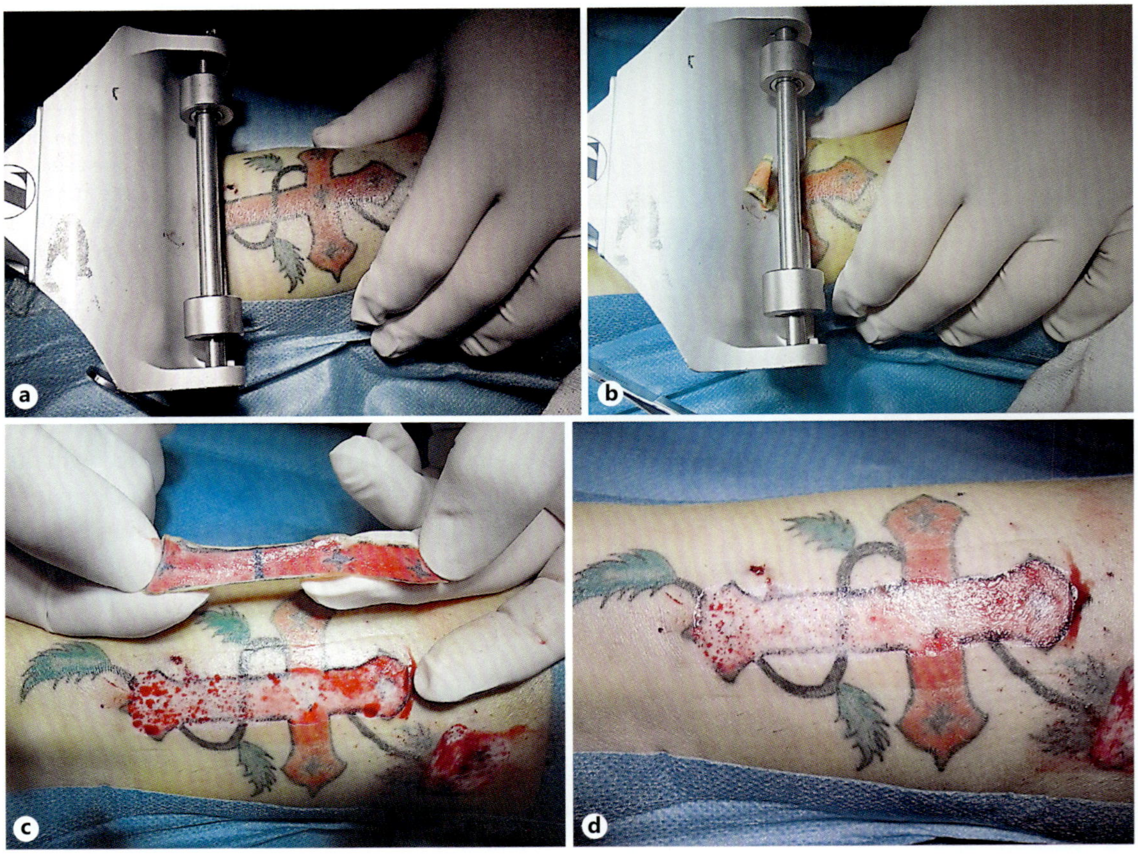

Fig. 7. a–d Dermatome shaving with the Zimmer Dermatome®. **c** The removed slice of skin holding red pigment is presented, with the dermal cut of the slice turned upwards. **d** The shave bed after sequential shaving displays white dermis devoid of visible pigment, and with punctual bleedings.

shaving of big tattoos. This dermatome is primarily applicable to extremities (fig. 7a–d).

Punch excision is recommended for removal of very small and well-defined tattoo reactions and lesions in tattoos (single nodules, small skin tumors, gun powder tattoo, graphite tattoo, tattoo markers of radiation field, etc.) causing discomfort (fig. 8).

Surgical Techniques

We published our experiences and the results obtained with dermatome shaving of tattoo reactions in an original publication [12]. The publication documents the effectiveness of dermatome shaving of tattoo reactions. In this chapter we explain the main results updated with present experiences.

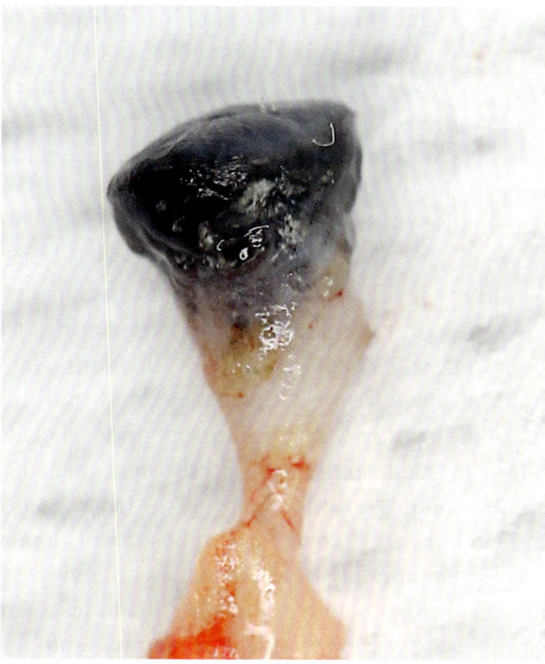

Fig. 8. Punch excision of a nodule in a black tattoo. Visually and directly on the raw biopsy the intensity and depth of pigment in the dermis is seen. In this case, the raw biopsy has an irregular surface with a 'bunch of grapes' appearance. Histology showed sarcoid granuloma.

The main goal of surgery is to remove the pigment of the reacting tattoo. Pigment is concentrated in the outer dermis. Ideally, the field must be cleared from visible pigment, and this is typically achieved at the mid-dermal level and occasionally lower in the dermis [12].

However, in some cases, the pigment may approach the interface to the subcutis, and the surgeon shall compromise with effectiveness to minimize operative sequels and help secure healing. If going too deep and even into the subcutis, prolonged healing and major scarring will be the result. If ever possible, it is recommended to limit shaving to the dermis at the mid-dermal level or just below.

Granulomatous reactions and skin tumors going deep into the dermis towards the interface to the subcutis may require full thickness excision.

In very severe tattoo complication with deep infection with critical necrosis and affected general condition of the patient, a deep excision of the tattoo and the entire necrosis performed to the muscle fascia can be necessary, performed as an acute operation.

Practical Guide to Surgery of Tattoo Reactions

Dermatome Shaving

Indications

Dermatome shaving is indicated in chronic tattoo reactions, especially allergic or papulonodular reactions, not responding to medical treatment (corticoids, antihistamine). Dermatome shaving can be applied to larger tattoo reactions and is altogether a quick and rational approach in the treatment of chronic tattoo reactions [12].

Instruments

Miltex® (fig. 6) or DermaBlade® flexible knives, Watson® dermatome (fig. 5) and Zimmer Dermatome® (fig. 7).

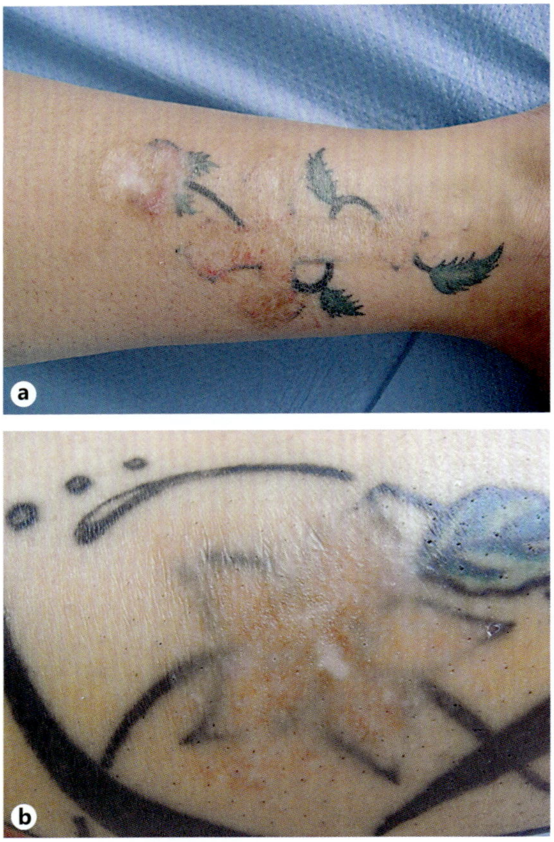

Fig. 9. a, **b** Scars after dermatome shaving after 1 year. In both cases, the patients had suffered allergic reactions of red tattoos of the plaque elevation type. Discomfort and symptoms were relieved, and the patients were very satisfied with the operation. There remains discrete hyperpigmentation, and local scars are seen where pigment deep in the dermis necessitated a deeper cut with the dermatome aiming at complete eradiation of the hapten. The case shown in **a** is also illustrated in figure 7, showing the operation.

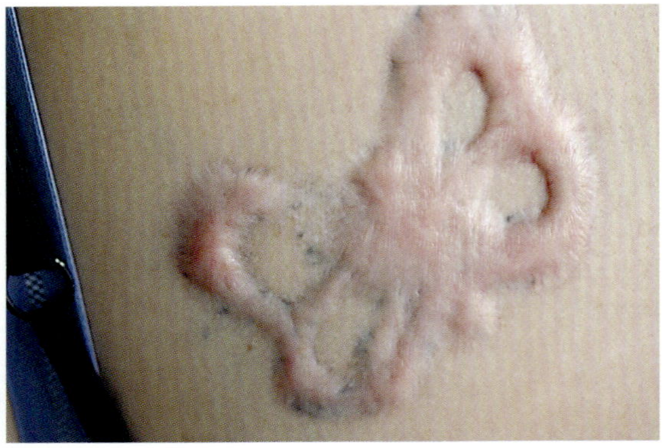

Fig. 10. Hypertrophic scarring after dermatome shaving in a patient who unexpectedly was predisposed to abnormal scarring. The figure also illustrates remnants of pigment at the tattoo margin, thus, shaving had not been performed aggressively. Abnormal scarring and anatomical sites predisposed to scarring are relative contraindications of dermatome shaving.

Procedure

The reacting tattoo is shaved in thin slices ranging from 0.25 to 1 mm, with thicker slices cut initially if the area is elevated over the surrounding skin. The surgery is individualized and also dependent on anatomical site. The depth of shaving is guided by visual inspection of tattoo pigment and color of slices removed from the dermis, and the visual pigment remnants in the wound bed. The procedure is continued until whitish collagen tissue devoid of any visual pigment is obtained in the entire field of the reaction. The depth of shaving typically reaches the mid-dermis level; however, if indicated due to pigment remnants, the level may come close to the interface to the subcutis. The shave level is as superficial in the dermis as ever possible. Shaving is limited to the affected area of the tattoo and the particular color giving rise to the problem. Depending on the case and the tattoo, the shave field is widened 1–3 mm into the surrounding skin to ensure efficient removal of all tattoo pigment and to physically smoothen the contour of the transition zone [12]. After surgery, the wound bed is covered with absorbent dressings, preferably alginate covered with semipermeable film, to obtain a humid environment. An elastic compression bandage is applied and removed after 1 week.

Postoperative Treatment

One week after surgery, absorbent foam and elastic compression are applied and continued until complete healing occurs. The bandages are changed once or twice weekly during this period. When healing occurs, a hypopigmented area is seen. The healed field must not be exposed to sun for at least 12 months or treated eagerly with a sun blocker (fig. 9a, b).

Postoperative sequels, such as *hypertrophic scarring*, are prevented and can also be treated with prolonged use of elastic compression bandage (fig. 10) [13]. Otherwise, intralesional injection of a corticoid, triamcinolone acetonide, in a 10 mg/ml slow release formulation can be used. The injected volume is individualized. *Prolonged inflammation* is treated with topical corticoids. If *pigment remnants* persist in the scar, a secondary operation might be indicated.

Outcome
Our results of dermatome shaving studied in a larger series with follow-up and measurement of patient satisfaction showed the operation to be efficient and safe for the treatment of chronic tattoo reactions, and we propose this operation is used as first line. A follow-up study showed that the burden of operation was rated low and patient satisfaction was high [12].

Excision
Indications
Selected cases of granulomatous tattoo reactions (i.e. nodular elements, sarcoid granuloma,) and well-defined skin tumors extending deep into the dermis towards the interface to the subcutis may need surgical removal with excision of the entire pathology.

Instruments
Punches normally used for punch biopsy of the skin of diameters 2–8 mm (small, delimited lesions) or a surgical scalpel, occasionally supplemented with flexible knives (Miltex® and DermaBlade®) or the Watson® dermatome.

Procedure
Deep excision to the fat and muscle fascia, including the affected area and surrounding tissue in toto. If possible, a suture to adapt the wound margins is used, made guided by the Langer lines of skin tension. After surgery, a simple dressing or absorbent foam is applied for 1 week or until healing.

Postoperative Treatment
When healed, a small scar possibly with hyper- or hypopigmentation may be seen. Sun shall be avoided for at least 12 months.

Outcome
The symptoms, such as itching and soreness, often decline rapidly and significantly. If histopathology shows malignancy, the patient may candidate to a second and more radical operation.

Excision Combined with Split-Skin Transplant
Indications
Selected cases of *severe allergic reactions* with deep pigment deposition even into the subcutis, when excisional surgery is not contraindicated because of broad deposition of allergenic pigment in the surrounding tissues, which shall be allowed to escape through the open wound and over a prolonged period of time of spontaneous healing, which can take several months. In severe allergy, with pigment widespread in the tissues, excisional surgery may worsen the allergy and cause progressive necrosis. Thus, depending on the case, surgery can be contraindicated and risky. As discussed, *severe and critical tattoo infection* going deep into the subcutis may indicate acute excision. Fortunately, both conditions are rare events.

Instruments
Primarily scalpel, sometimes also flexible knives (Miltex® and DermaBlade®) or the Watson® dermatome for excision of the area *(recipient site)*, depending on the case. The Zimmer derma-

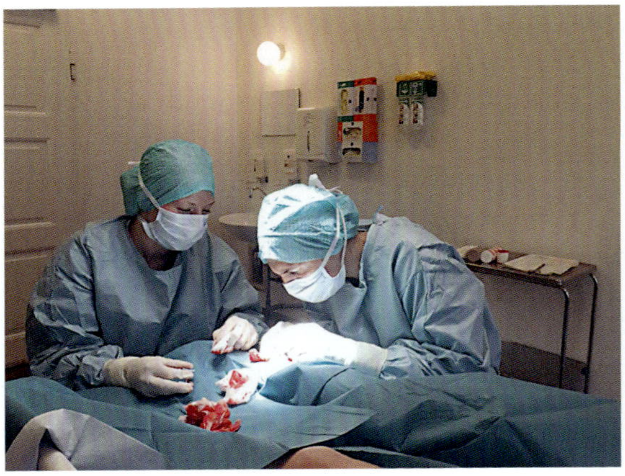

Fig. 11. Standard operation setting. Dermatome shaving with flexible knives.

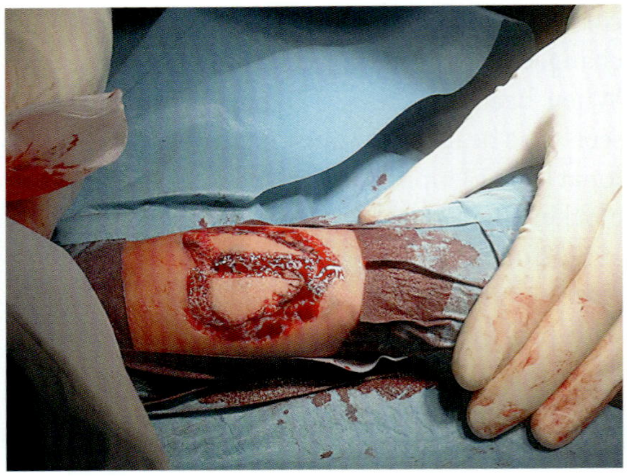

Fig. 12. Standard operation setting with sterile conditions.

tome or the Watson® dermatome is used for harvesting the split-skin transplant, if indicated. The *donor site* is often selected near the recipient site to ensure color match. A mesh graft machine is used to mesh the split-skin transplant. This gives the best result, compared to 'hand mesh' performed as needle puncture manually through the split-skin transplant.

Procedure
The tattoo area affected is excised, covered with a split-skin transplant, and meshed 1:1.5 or 1:3 by the mesh graft machine. To prevent pyogenic infection, a single-dose antibiotic can be given during or immediately before the operation.

Bandages. Recipient site: Gitter gaze, several layers of sterilized foams and compression bandage for 2–4 days. Donor site: absorbent dressing, preferably several layers of alginate, covered with semipermeable film, applied under elastic compression bandage for 7–10 days.

Postoperative Treatment
Bandages. Recipient site: after 2–4 days, change to a simple dressing and compression until healing. Donor site: after 7–10 days, application of absorbent foam and compression for some months.

When healed, the recipient and donor sites must not be exposed to the sun for at least 12 months, or alternatively treated eagerly with a sun blocker.

Outcome
The recipient site often shows hyper- or hypopigmentation along with scarring. The donor site may show similar changes.

Setting of Surgery

The setting of surgery is typically a 1-day outpatient procedure. Standard anesthesia is infiltration anesthesia with mepivacaine hydrochloride (carbocaine, 1% with no adrenaline). Patients with large tattoo areas are operated under regional anesthesia (peripheral nerve block) or general anesthesia. Often used peripheral nerve blocks are the n. axillaris, n. femoralis, and n. poplitea blocks. General anesthesia is uncommon but necessary in selected cases. If the reacting tattoo is located on a special and difficult anatomical site (the face, the neck, or the back of the patient), general anesthesia may be necessary.

Operations are conducted in a standard operation theater under sterile conditions (fig. 11,

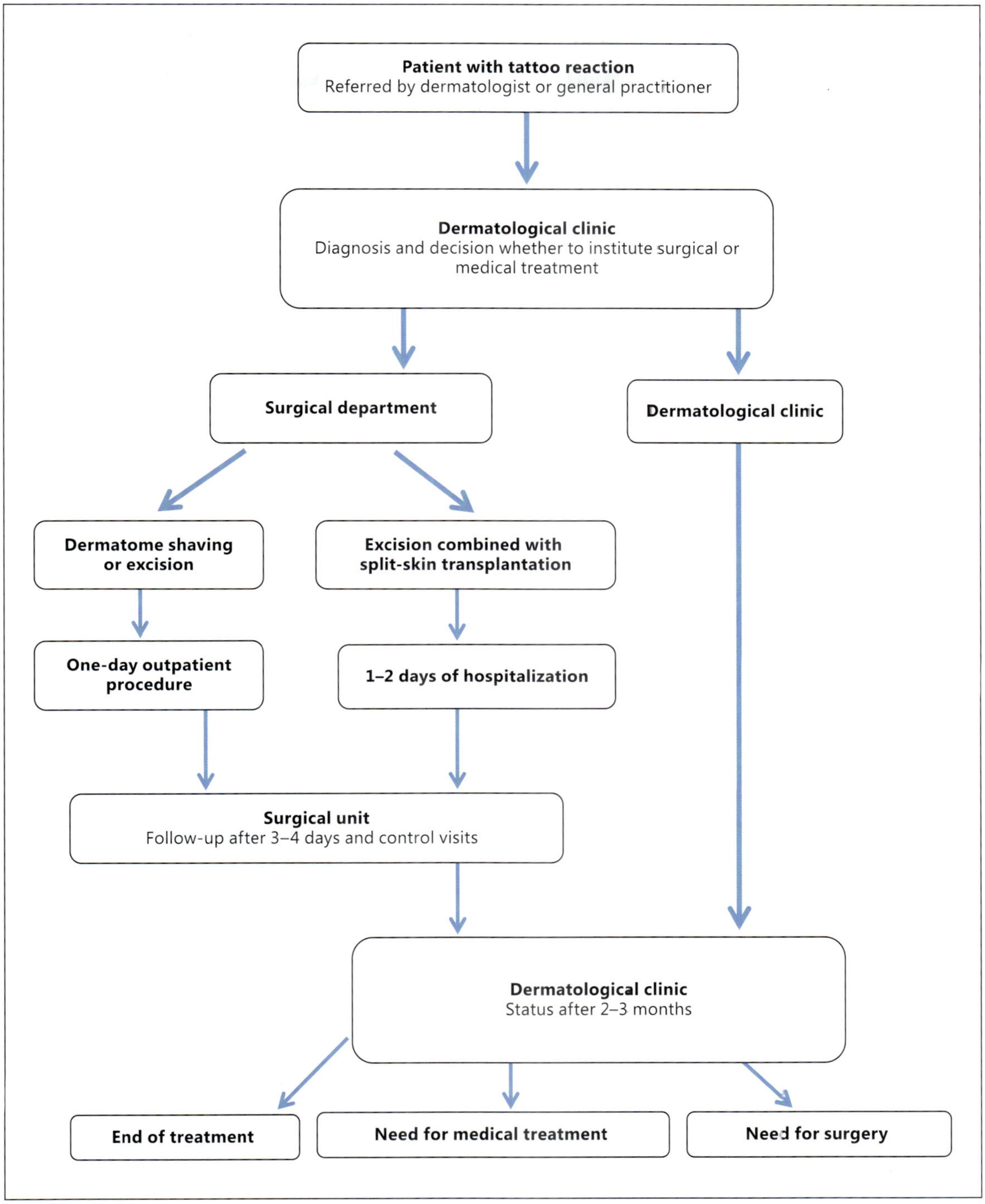

Fig. 13. Algorithm for surgical treatment and follow-up of patients with chronic tattoo reactions.

12). In general, postoperative antibiotics or sedatives are not used. In cases when the patient has an infection or is at 'high risk', such as in diabetes and when receiving immunosuppressive treatment, antibiotics are used to prevent infections.

The patient and the surgeon will both benefit of a 'pleasant environment' during the surgery. To achieve this, relatives are welcome to support the patient during the surgery. The patient is allowed to listen to music and communicate while the operation takes place, which prevents anxiety and may eliminate the need for sedatives. In our published study, the patients were directly asked if the operation was a burden to them. On a rating scale from 0 to 3 (0 = no problem, 3 = terrible, 'I would never do it again'), the average rating was 0.6 [12].

From Symptoms to Rational Treatment

With presently more than 500 tattoo reactions examined in the 'Tattoo Clinic' since 2008 and with more than 140 operations performed in the Wound Healing Center, much experience and routine has been achieved [9]. Especially the daily routine, with excisions and harvesting of split-skin for transplantation of many different ulcers, leads to familiarity with the instruments, technics, and procedures. This positions us to provide recommendations on the rational and effective treatment of tattoo reactions. The algorithm from tattoo reaction and diagnosis to rational treatment is illustrated in figure 13.

Postoperative follow-up is important. After 2–3 months the dermatologist sees the patient to conclude the healing after operation and the treatment outcome and, possibly, initiate further treatment (fig. 13). Often the treatment ends after a long-term follow-up. In our experience, 13% of patients with primary dermatome shaving underwent a secondary dermatome shaving due to persistent symptoms and remaining pigment [12]. In our opinion, recurrences due to remnants of pigment deep in the dermis shall appear at some acceptable level since too aggressive removal with the dermatome will produce more adverse reactions with scarring and disfiguring. Surgery of tattoo reactions is the delicate balance between doing just the necessary and not too much.

Instrument Suppliers

Watson® dermatome. Sterile scalpel, hand-operated dermatome. Skin graft knife without blades, 300 mm, 12″ (spare blades, sterile, sales unit: PAK = package of 10 pieces). BRAUN®, www.bbraun.com.

Miltex® blade. Bioblade, Shave Biopsy Blade, sterile. Technology by kai medical, INTEGRA®, www.integralife.com/integramiltex.

DermaBlade®. Sterile surgical blades. Personna International® UK limited. www.personna-blades.com.

(The list of instruments and suppliers refers to those instruments we use in the Wound Healing Center.)

References

1 Engel E, Vasold R, Santarelli F, et al: Tattooing of skin results in transportation and light-induced decomposition of tattoo pigments – a first quantification in vivo using a mouse model. Exp Dermatol 2009;19:54–60.

2 Vasold R, Naarmann N, Ulrich H, et al: Tattoo pigments are cleaved by laser light – the chemical analysis in vitro provide evidence for hazardous compounds. Photochem Photobiol 2004;80: 185–190.

3 Engel E, Spannberger A, Vasold R, et al: Photochemical cleavage of a tattoo pigment by UVB radiation or natural sunlight. J Dtsch Dermatol Ges 2007;5:583–589.

4 Kuperman-Beade M, Levine VJ, Ashinoff R: Laser removal of tattoos. Am J Clin Dermatol 2001;2:21–25.

5 Bernstein EF: Laser treatment of tattoos. Clin Dermatol 2006;24:43–55.
6 Prinz BM, Vavricka SR, Graf P, et al: Efficacy of laser treatment of tattoos using lasers emitting wavelengths of 532 nm, 755 nm and 1,064 nm. Br J Dermatol 2004;150:245–251.
7 Ross EV, Naseef G, Lin C, et al: Comparison of responses of tattoos to picosecond and nanosecond Q-switched neodymium: YAG lasers. Arch Dermatol 1998;134:167–171.
8 Karsai S, Raulin C: Laser treatment of tattoos and other dyschromia; in Raulin C, Karsai S (eds): Laser and IPL Technology and Dermatology and Aesthetic Medicine. Heidelberg, Springer, 2011, pp 189–210.
9 Serup J, Sepehri M, Hutton Carlsen K: Classification of tattoo complications in a hospital material of 493 adverse events. Dermatology 2017, in press. DOI 10.1159/000452315.
10 Sepehri M, Hutton Carlsen K, Serup J: Papulo-nodular reactions in black tattoos as markers of sarcoidosis: study of 92 reactions from a hospital material. Dermatology 2017, in press. DOI 10.1159/000452148.
11 Hutton CK, Serup J: Quality of life and subjective complaints of tattoo reactions measured by DLQI and the ISS score of itch. Skin Res Technol 2015;21:101–107.
12 Sepehri M, Jørgensen B, Serup J: Introduction of dermatome shaving as first line treatment of chronic tattoo reactions. J Dermatolog Treat 2015;26:451–455.

Mitra Sepehri, MD
The Wound Healing Centre, Department of Dermatology
Bispebjerg University Hospital, Bispebjerg Bakke 23
DK–2400 Copenhagen NV (Denmark)
E-Mail mitrasepehri9@hotmail.com

Serup J, Bäumler W (eds): Diagnosis and Therapy of Tattoo Complications. With Atlas of Illustrative Cases.
Curr Probl Dermatol. Basel, Karger, 2017, vol 52, pp 94–104 (DOI: 10.1159/000450809)

Laser Treatment of Tattoos: Basic Principles

Wolfgang Bäumler

Department of Dermatology, University of Regensburg, Regensburg, Germany

Abstract

Tattooing has become very popular worldwide during the past decades, and millions of people have one or many tattoos at different anatomical sites. The color of tattoos is mainly black, followed by red, green, blue, and other colors. A part of the tattooed people regret tattooing or have permanent problems with tattoos and therefore seek for tattoo removal. Tattoos consist of solid pigment particles in the skin. Thus, tattoo removal requires fragmentation of these permanently incorporated particles. The gold standard of tattoo removal is laser therapy. Short light pulses at high intensities are applied to the tattooed skin surface. The laser light penetrates the skin and is selectively absorbed in the pigment particles. The absorbed laser light leads to heat-up and fragmentation of the particles. Due to the complex chemistry of the various tattoo pigments, the efficacy of this fragmentation process is frequently unpredictable. Due to the short and intense pulses, nonlinear effects of light and thermal properties of tattoo particles may play a role, and the assumptions of selective photothermolysis may not reflect the real process of tattoo particle fragmentation as a whole. In case fragmentation occurs, the concentration of pigment particles in the skin decreases, yielding a fading of the tattoo color in the skin. Laser therapy is most effective in black tattoos and less effective for colored tattoos. The rate of side effects is low due to the selectivity of the treatment. Laser light may change the chemistry of the tattoo pigments and hence provoke toxic decomposition products.

Tattooing is an ancient procedure to stain the skin of humans, and its history goes back thousands of years. In the past, people used various colorants and devices to stain the skin permanently [1, 2]. Nowadays, the colorants are usually injected as a suspension into the skin by the use of solid needles, which are actuated by tattoo machines. A fraction of the colorant stays in the dermis as particles causing the color of the tattoo, while an unknown fraction of the injected colorant is removed from the skin via the lymphatic system. As a result, tattoo colorants can be found in the lymph nodes located next to the tattoo [3–7].

From time to time, tattooed individuals ask for tattoo removal stating various reasons, such as change of social status, dissatisfaction with the tattoo, or medical problems. A survey in German-speaking countries revealed a rate of about 5% of tattooed individuals who desire tattoo removal [8]. Several treatment procedures were applied in the past decades to remove tattoo colorants from skin. Surgical excision may remove a tattoo completely but leaves scars and is usually limited to small tattoos. Laser treatment raised hope of selective destruction of tattoo particles in the skin without leaving scars. In 1983, Rox Anderson described such a selective laser application and called it 'precise microsurgery by selective absorption of pulsed radiation' [9]. The so-called selective photothermolysis was born in laser medicine.

Prior to this, T.H. Maiman published the first report on laser emission from a ruby crystal in 1960 [10]. Five years later, one of the first laser treatments of tattoos was published by Goldman and coauthors in the *Journal of Investigative Dermatology* [11]. The report was entitled 'Radiation from a Q-switched ruby laser. Effect of repeated impacts of power output of 10 megawatts on a tattoo of man'. The authors summarized their findings as follows: 'Repeated experiments with Q-switched ruby laser impacts produced transient, edematous blanched areas in a dark tattoo of the forearm but not in the white skin. As yet, the mechanism of this change in the skin reactions of the tattoo to Q-switched ruby lasers is not known, but the differences were probably not due entirely to thermal factors'.

Since then, Q-switched lasers evolved to standard laser technology, which has been applied for many years to destroy tattoo particles in skin, yielding a lightening of the tattoo color [12–15]. Meanwhile, scientific investigations revealed the mechanisms associated with Q-switched lasers and tattoo particles in the skin. In comparison to other targets in laser medicine, like blood vessels, however, the knowledge about the processes is still incomplete with regard to the lightening of tattoo colors in the skin when using short and intense laser pulses.

Tattooed Skin

During the process of tattooing, tattooists perforate the skin surface by using solid needles and thereby place a certain amount of tattoo colorant in the skin. Part of the injected colorant is removed from the skin by the lymphatic system weeks and months after tattooing. Due to limitations of lymphatic transportation, a certain amount of injected colorant stays in the dermis which yields a long-lasting tattoo color of the skin [16, 17]. The major component of tattoo colorants are small solid state particles consisting of pigments with a complex chemistry [2]. Thus, when tattooed people undergo laser treatment of their tattoos, the targets for the laser radiation are such small solid state particles lying randomly distributed in the dermis [18, 19].

Chemistry of Tattoo Colorants

The colorants used for tattoos are frequently called ink, a term that is somewhat misleading because it usually means 'colored water'. However, such a colorant would not stain the skin permanently. The English word 'ink' descends from the old French word *enque* which means dark writing fluid. *Enque* descends from the Latin word *encaustum*, which is what was used by the Roman emperors to sign their documents.

Colorants are chemically classified as either pigments or dyes, whereas the chemical structure of pigment molecules and dye molecules are frequently the same. In contrast to dyes, pigments are practically insoluble in the medium in which they are incorporated. Pigments are inorganic or organic, colored, white, or black materials.

In the past decades, tattooists used inorganic pigments that contained heavy metals such as mercury, chromium, or cadmium. Typical colors were yellow (cadmium sulfide), red (mercury sulfide), or green (chromium oxide). Two important inorganic pigments are still in use: titanium diox-

Table 1. Selection of colored pigments, which are classified by their chemical nature and identified either by chemical index (C.I.) or pigment shortcut (Px.y)

Trade name	Color	Pigment number
Canary Yellow	yellow	PY.14
I7	reddish yellow	PY.55
Zitronengelb	greenish yellow	PY.74
Golden Luv, Dunkelgelb	reddish yellow	PY.83
Sunset Yellow	reddish yellow	PY.87
Orange, Navel Orange, Melon, I3, P7	yellowish orange	PO.13
Dunkelrot	carmine	PR.5
I8	yellowish red	PR.9
Cardinal Red, Dragon Red, Spanish Red, P8	yellowish red	PR.22
Ruby Red, Red Velvet	red	PR.112
P1	red	PR.170
Burgandy, I5	bluish red	PR.122
I6, Pur Purple, True Purple, P3	bluish violet	PV.23
Permanent Blue, Permanent Blau, Navy Blue, Fezan Lt. Blue, I1	blue	PB.15
Permanentgrün, Waldgrün, Forest Green, I4, Fezan Blue Green, Permanent Green, P2	green	PG.7
Black inks	black	carbon black
White pigments	white	titanium dioxide

Black tattoo inks mainly consist of carbon black. Titanium dioxide is frequently applied to reduce the color strength of pigment solution.

ide for tempering and carbon black for black tattoos. About 60% of tattoos are either completely or partly black [8]. Nowadays, the colored tattoo colorants mainly consist of organic pigments like azo or polycyclic pigments, which are usually taken from the chemical industry [2].

In view of the variety of tattoo pigments on the market, a list of tattoo pigments, such as presented in table 1, is definitely incomplete. Pigments are tiny particles with diameters of a few tenths of nanometers (fig. 1). Tattooists usually purchase ready-to-use suspensions which contain the respective pigment, solvents, emulsifier, anti-foam agents, preservatives, and other substances. The absorption spectra provide evidence of the high color strength of the pure pigments (fig. 2). Therefore, the pigments are often mixed with titanium dioxide to change the color strength.

The Basics of Lasers

The acronym LASER is derived from the most important elements: Light Amplification by Stimulated Emission of Radiation. The process of spontaneous emission of photons describes the emission of radiation from a usual light source. After excitation, atoms or molecules can emit photons at different times, in any direction, and usually with different wavelengths. Therefore, such a radiation is incoherent, divergent, and spectrally broadband.

In contrast, a laser medium consists of identical atoms or molecules which are excited by different means. Such photon emitters are placed in a substrate like a solid state. After excitation, which is called pumping, the atoms or molecules return from the excited to the ground state and thereby

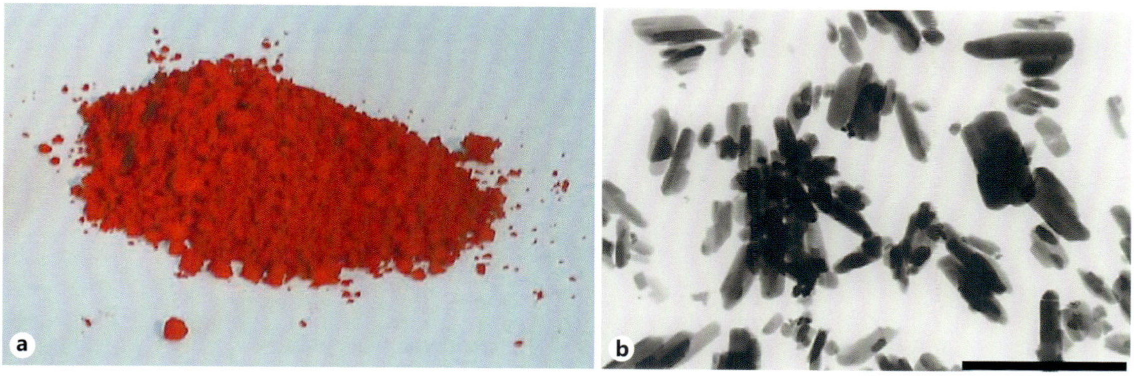

Fig. 1. a Azo pigment PR.22 powder. **b** Electron microscopy image of the disazo-diarylide pigment PY.82 powder. Scale bar, 1 µm.

emit photons with a specific wavelength λ that is determined by the energy difference ΔE of the excited and the ground state, with $\Delta E = hc/\lambda$.

The combination of such identical transitions and photons with the same wavelength λ in a confined volume called laser medium (e.g. glass rod) allows another process to come to the fore: the stimulated emission of photons, as described and published by Albert Einstein in 1917 (4). A laser medium consists of up to 10^{20} photon-emitting atoms or molecules, which provides an immense number of stimulated photons. For example, a laser pulse (energy: 1 J) in the visible spectrum contains about 10^{19} photons. Thus, the light amplification is actuated by the stimulated emission of radiation, as described by the acronym LASER. The process of light amplification does not change the energy of photons but increases their number exponentially.

To promote the stimulated emission of radiation and hence optimize the process of light amplification, the laser medium is placed in an optical resonator that consists of two or more mirrors. Due to the reflection of laser photons inside the resonator, the number of photons continues to increase until the maximum is reached. The temporal behavior of the laser emission depends on the temporal behavior of the excitation (energy supply) of the atoms or molecules. When the energy supply is limited to a certain time interval by using, e.g. a flash lamp, pulsed excitation take place and the laser emits pulses accordingly, usually in the range of milliseconds to microseconds.

Pulse durations in the nanosecond range (10^{-9} s) can be achieved by switching the quality of the resonator (Q-switch) by using an electro-optical device. The device contains an optically nonlinear crystal, which prevents photons from running back and forth inside the resonator (low quality of the resonator) as long as the crystal is connected to high voltage. When the voltage is switched off within nanoseconds, the switch abruptly becomes transparent, increasing the quality of the resonator and yielding a very intense emission peak.

The mode-locking of the longitudinal modes in the laser resonator may result in ultrashort pulse duration in the picosecond (10^{-12} s) or femtosecond (10^{-15} s) range. Active mode-locking appears when devices such as optoacoustic modulators are placed in the resonator. Also, passive mode-locking is possible by applying a saturable absorber like dye molecules.

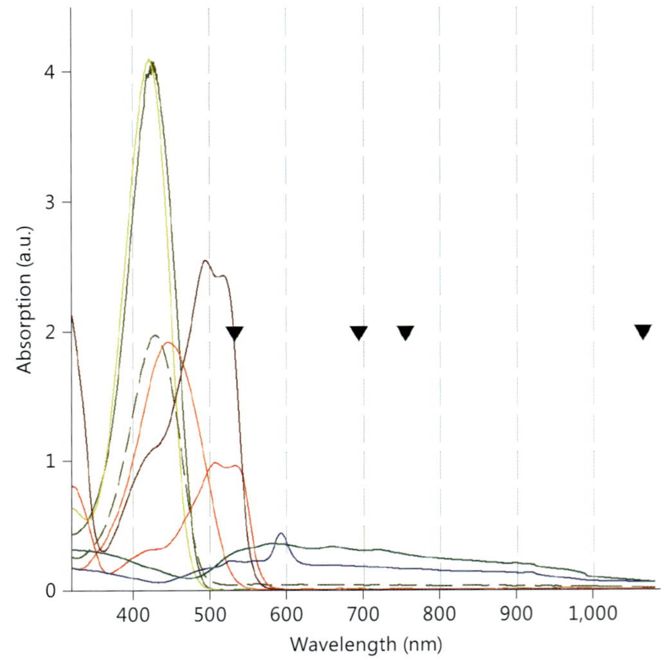

Fig. 2. The image shows the different light absorption (absorption cross-section) of some colored pigments dissolved in appropriate solvents. The four black triangles indicate the wavelengths of typical Q-switched lasers used for tattoo removal: frequency doubled Nd:YAG laser (532 nm), ruby laser (694 nm), alexandrite laser (755 nm), and Nd:YAG laser (1,064 nm).

Laser Tattoo Removal

Background

It remains unclear how many people desire the removal of their tattoos. In a survey, about 5% of people indicated that they plan tattoo removal [8]. The reasons for tattoo removal are either health problems or dissatisfaction with the tattoo. Tattoo colorants in the skin can be removed via surgical excision or laser therapy [20, 21]. When using the CO_2 laser, the tattoo pigments are removed unselectively together with the skin area treated, which leads to unwanted scar formation. Contrarily, when using Q-switched lasers, the ultrashort and intense laser pulses are suitable to destroy only the pigment particles in the skin via selective photothermolysis with harming the surrounding tissue [9]. This principle requires the proper selection of wavelength, light energy, and pulse duration of the laser pulses applied.

Selective Photothermolysis

Wavelength of Laser Pulse

The color of organic pigments is caused by light absorption in the delocalized electrons of a conjugated system in the pigment molecule. The pigment molecules strongly absorb light in a specific wavelength range. The unabsorbed light is reflected to viewers' eyes and hence represents the color of a given pigment. This provides a first indication of which wavelength could be appropriate in case of using laser light for tattoo removal. The light absorption maximum of different pigment molecules may be located anywhere in the UV and visible spectrum (200–700 nm), yielding a huge variety of colored pigments. This, however, hampers the selection of appropriate laser wavelength for tattoo removal, because neither tattooists nor patients usually know the identity of the pigment used for tattooing.

The lasers used in practice are frequency-doubled Nd:YAG laser (532 nm), ruby laser (694 nm), alexandrite laser (755 nm), and Nd:YAG laser (1,064 nm). Depending on the respective pigment, the laser light does not necessarily match the absorption spectra of tattoo pigments (fig. 2). Moreover, tattoos having similar colors may contain different pigments and therefore exhibit a different absorption behavior. Physicians, who treat tattoos with lasers, therefore apply wavelengths according to the published clinical studies and the clinical experience. However, the numerous different pigments face a small number of laser wavelengths available, which are limited due to technical and commercial reasons.

Energy of Laser Pulse

After tattooing, the pigment particles are exclusively found intracytoplasmatically, lying in membrane-bound structures, identified as secondary lysosomes. This is due to active phagocytosis into dermal cells (macrophages, fibroblasts) [6]. Then, the pigment particles show diameters up to a few micrometers being visible when using normal light microscopy in histology. Now, the goal of tattoo treatment with Q-switched lasers is the fragmentation of these tattoo particles in the skin allowing transportation of the pigment material away from skin. Consequently, the color of the tattoo in the skin should fade.

Thus, the light energy absorbed in the pigment particle must be sufficient for particle fragmentation. When treating tattoos with lasers, the first mechanism is the absorption of light in the pigment and hence the conversion of absorbed light energy to any excitation energy inside the particle (e.g. heat). Assuming a simple heat-up process, the absorbed light energy correlates to the produced heat energy. This energy must be sufficient to heat up the entire pigment particle.

Duration of Laser Pulse

The pulse duration must be in the order of nanoseconds at least for the following two reasons. Firstly, such short pulse duration allows very high laser light intensities that enable rapid heat-up of the tattoo particles, which is necessary for particle fragmentation. Secondly, the heated particle starts to transfer the heat energy to the adjacent tissue by means of thermal conductivity. This effect should be limited to a sufficiently short time to avoid heating of adjacent tissue, reducing the risk of damaging the surrounding tissue.

Laser Tattoo Removal

Penetration of Light into the Skin

After tattooing, the pigment particles are randomly distributed inside the dermis of the skin. When treating tattoos with lasers, the laser light is applied to the skin surface with different spot sizes with diameters of a few millimeters. Then, the light penetrates tissue to reach the pigment particles, which are located in different depths of the dermis.

Propagation of optical radiation through normal media such as air or glass can be described in a straightforward fashion, in particular for monochromatic and collimated laser light. Reflection, refraction, and absorption dominate the propagation. However, when optical radiation penetrates turbid media like the skin, scattering of radiation inside tissue must be considered, which hampers light propagation in a complex manner.

When optical radiation strikes the skin, part of the photons is reflected back due to the different refractive index of air and skin. Photons inside the skin do not propagate straight on but frequently and abruptly change their direction due to collision with skin constituents (scattering). The mode and the extent of scattering depend on the size of the scattering objects and the wavelength of the radiation. The size of the scattering objects ranges from a few nanometers (small cell organelles, cell membranes) to a few micrometers (large cell organelles, cells, collagen) and to hundreds of micrometers (hair follicle, sweat glands).

The extent of scattering decreases with increasing wavelength. With increasing wavelength, photons are less deflected on their path into skin. Thus, the longer the wavelength, the higher is the penetration depth of radiation in the skin. UVB radiation (around 300 nm) penetrates the skin up to a few tenths of millimeters only, whereas infrared radiation (e.g. Nd:YAG, 1,064 nm) achieves a penetration depth of up to a few millimeters. However, the increase in penetration depth with increasing wavelength reverses for wavelengths longer than about 1,100 nm because radiation is increasingly absorbed by water in the skin. Unfortunately, the scattering changes the beam geometry in the skin and thereby substantially affects the dosimetry. It is complex to determine the number of photons that reach a target (e.g. a vessel) in the skin.

The higher the number of photons reaching the target, the more heat can be produced inside the target. Thus, the deeper tattoo particles are located in skin, the less photons reach the particle and the less is the fragmentation efficacy that limits the therapeutic effect of lasers for tattoo removal.

Mechanisms of Action

The current assumption regarding the mechanisms of action is heat production in the tattoo particle by the absorbed light energy. So far, it is unclear whether and to which extent the heat-up process alone describes the entire process of tattoo particle destruction. Other processes like release of electronic bonds in the particle might also play a role.

Nonetheless, as a response to this laser impact with appropriate parameters, a multitude of mechanisms may occur at the same time. Large aggregates and agglomerates break down into smaller particles. Molecules can break up, resulting in hazardous decomposition products like hydrogen cyanide and aromatic amines [22–24]. Due to fragmentation of the tattoo particles, small pigment particles, unknown decomposition products, and newly generated chemical compounds may then be removed from the skin via the lymphatic system. This mechanism could induce a decrease of the color strength of the pigments responsible for a noticeable lightening of a colored tattoo.

The heating of the particle should be processed in a very short time yielding high temperatures. Then, the extremely hot surface of the particle may cause ultrashort heating-up of a thin shell of surrounding tissue. The following expansion of this water-containing shell may induce a negative pressure and a shock wave near to the surface of the pigment. These shock waves may help to fragment the tattoo particles mechanically. Such an anomalous photoacoustic effect was reported when a suspension of small particles in water was irradiated by a Q-switched Nd:YAG laser (532 nm), where high-temperature reactions and gas expansions induced shock waves [25].

Histological investigation of tattooed skin samples directly after laser impact showed that these shock waves occurred upon treatment with Q-switched lasers. Small vacuoles were exclusively formed in the dermis, which caused a clinically visible whitening of the skin. These vacuoles usually resolve within a few hours after laser impact [19].

Laser Tattoo Removal and Selective Photothermolysis

So far, little is known about the removal of tattoos by using Q-switched lasers. Laser treatment of many skin disorders has been performed under the terms of selective photothermolysis for decades [9]. Shortly again, the energy of laser pulses applied to the skin is selectively absorbed by a target that undergoes thermal damage, while the damage is confined to the target by choosing the appropriate pulse duration. The pulse duration correlates to the thermal relaxation time, which can be estimated when knowing the size of the target. Tattoo pigment particles show a small size requiring a pulse duration of a few nanoseconds.

However, selective photothermolysis is frequently based on simplified models assuming linear optics and linear thermodynamics. In addition, the density, the composition, as well as the optical and thermal properties of the heated target (e.g. tattoo particle) are considered homogenous. It is additionally assumed that these properties do not change during the heat-up process. This is an appropriate assumption to begin with. However, the assumption may not reflect the real and complex process of tattoo particle fragmentation as a whole.

Laser Tattoo Removal

Linear and Nonlinear Effects

At low light intensities, e.g. nonlaser sources, the properties of materials remain independent of the light intensity. Light waves can pass through materials or be reflected from boundaries and interfaces without interacting with each other.

However, laser sources can provide sufficiently high light intensities to modify the optical properties of materials. Then, light waves can interact with each other causing nonlinear optical effects. This interaction of light waves can result in the generation of optical fields at new frequencies (wavelengths) including optical harmonics of incident radiation or frequency mixing (e.g. frequency-doubling effects, two-photon absorption). Nonlinear optics is the area where the response of the material system to the applied electromagnetic field is nonlinear in the amplitude of this field.

With regard to the short laser pulses (10^{-9}–10^{-12} s) used in tattoo removal, the intensity of such laser pulses should be high enough (up to hundreds of MW/cm^2) to allow nonlinear processes such as frequency doubling and two-photon absorption. Numerous dye molecules show light absorption at half of the wavelength that is applied for excitation [26, 27].

Regarding tattoo removal, so far, the assumptions of the selective photothermolysis are based on the linear absorption of laser photons in a pigment molecule. The extent of photon absorption (A) is described by the Beer-Lambert law: $A = 1 - exp(-\mu_a d)$, where μ_a is the linear absorption coefficient and d the thickness of the light absorbing sample. Due to the high intensities of Q-switched lasers, the simultaneous absorption of two photons might occur. That is, two photons of a ruby laser (694 nm) can absorb like one photon at 347 nm. At present, however, it has not been investigated whether and to which extent such a nonlinear process of two-photon absorption might contribute to the effect of light absorption in tattoo pigments.

Complex Properties of Tattoo Particles

As mentioned above, tattoo pigments are usually industrial pigments consisting of inorganic or organic molecules. Inorganic pigments such as carbon black (black tattoos) show numerous and complex morphologies. Commonly, the carbon black particles can be divided into four different types of morphologies, spheroidal, ellipsoidal, linear, or branched, which are caused by different production and finishing processes [28]. Organic pigments such as azo or polycyclic pigments (colored tattoos) are closer to the amorphous state than to the idealized crystal. However, pigments are frequently treated with different methods to enhance crystallinity [29, 30]. When used for tattoos, it is usually unknown which pigment particles in which crystallinity state were applied. In addition, the small particles may agglomerate after tattooing into the skin by different mechanisms of phagocytosis. Thus, the particles of black and colored tattoos in the skin may show various particle structures and sizes that clearly influence any interaction with light. In particular when heated up by laser radiation, such variations may lead to different fragmentation mechanisms and efficacies.

Ho et al. [31] investigated whether the mechanism of the breakup process can be identified via computer simulations and proposed a treatment strategy that can potentially minimize the collateral damage to the surrounding tissues. The authors calculated the magnitude of the tensile stress generated inside graphite tattoo particles as functions of laser pulse length and particle size. The authors concluded that the breakup of tattoo particles is photoacoustic and the optimal pulse length is approximately 10–100 ps to minimize the laser fluence and the collateral damage. However, these calculations are based on homogenous graphite particle keeping the respective values for density, specific heat, and thermal conductivity constant.

In contrast to that, it has recently been shown that the values for density and thermal conductivity of carbon black decrease and the value of specific heat increases with increasing temperature [32]. That is, these values of carbon black might also change when heated up by intense laser pulses during tattoo removal. As mentioned above, tattooists usually apply black pigments that contain no graphite particles but carbon black with various morphologies and hence various optical and thermal properties. In addition, the interaction of intense laser pulses with carbon black and carbon-based material may produce nonlinear effects. Lim et al. [33] have recently reported that under intense laser excitation, thin films and suspensions of graphite and its nanostructure, including carbon black, nanotubes, few-layer graphenes and graphene oxides, exhibit multi-photon absorption and induced transparency due to saturable absorption. When using nanosecond pulses, the authors reported the detection of microbubbles and microplasmas that causes nonlinear light scattering.

Another computer-assisted model (finite element method) was applied to simulate the fragmentation of tattoo pigment particles. Interestingly, the authors concluded that an increased spot diameter and beam fluence improve the lightening response of tattoos. This correlated to the authors' observations from the simulation. Conversely, variations in the pulse width are shown to have little influence on the fragmentation response [34].

The situation should be even more complex when laser light interacts with the various morphologies of colored pigment particles based on azo or polycyclic compounds. On one hand such modeling work is important, but the results might not reflect the reality when a laser pulse hits a tattoo particle of unknown origin and morphology in skin.

An animal study was published in 1999 showing better clearance of black tattoos when using pulse duration of 500 ps (titanium:sapphire laser, 795 nm) as compared to 50 nanoseconds (alexandrite laser, 752 nm) [35]. The question remains whether and to which extent the different wavelengths possibly affected the results. In 1998, a preliminary clinical study showed that picosecond laser pulses yielded better results than nanosecond pulses [36]. The authors used a Nd:YAG laser with a pulse duration of 35 ps, which was considerably shorter than that used in the few recent studies (350–900 ps) [37–40].

Conclusion

At first view, the treatment of tattoos appears to be a rather simple process that has been well understood in the past decades. However, on closer inspection, the fragmentation of complex morphological structures such as tattoo pigment particles, consisting of various molecules, is a rather complex process that involves known and many unknown facts. This includes nonlinear optical effects as well as unknown thermal properties of various pigment particles with different morphologies. This might hamper the application of the usual theory of selective photothermolysis or lead to the conclusion that this theory might not be appropriate in its current form. In view of all these unknown facts, the simple change of a single laser parameter such as shortening of the pulse duration – as frequently recommended – might be a premature and oversimplified recommendation.

References

1 Laux P, Tralau T, Tentschert J, Blume A, Al Dahouk S, Baumler W, Bernstein E, Bocca B, Alimonti A, Colebrook H, de Cuyper C, Dahne L, Hauri U, Howard PC, Janssen P, Katz L, Klitzman B, Kluger N, Krutak L, Platzek T, Scott-Lang V, Serup J, Teubner W, Schreiver I, Wilkniss E, Luch A: A medical-toxicological view of tattooing. Lancet 2016; 387:395–402.

2 Baumler W, Eibler ET, Hohenleutner U, Sens B, Sauer J, Landthaler M: Q-switch laser and tattoo pigments: first results of the chemical and photophysical analysis of 41 compounds. Lasers Surg Med 2000;26:13–21.

3 Lehner K, Santarelli F, Vasold R, Penning R, Sidoroff A, Konig B, Landthaler M, Baumler W: Black tattoos entail substantial uptake of genotoxicpolycyclic aromatic hydrocarbons (PAH) in human skin and regional lymph nodes. PLoS One 2014;9:e92787.

4 Sokolovskaya E, Shariff Y: Calcifications in axillary lymph nodes on negative mammograms: tattoo pigment mimicking axillary lymph node calcifications. Breast J 2015;21:678–679.

5 Pinto A, Wieshmann H, Triantafyllou A, Shaw R: Tattoo-pigmented cervical lymph node that masqueraded as the sentinel lymph node in oral squamous cell carcinoma. Br J Oral Maxillofac Surg 2015;53:886–887.

6 Manganoni AM, Sereni E, Pata G, Ungari M, Pavoni L, Farisoglio C, Calzavara-Pinton PG, Farfaglia R: Pigmentation of axillary sentinel nodes from extensive skin tattoo mimics metastatic melanoma: case report. Int J Dermatol 2014;53:773–776.

7 Kluger N, Koljonen V: The surgeon, the tattoo and the black lymph node. J Plast Reconstr Aesthet Surg 2013;66:561–562.

8 Klugl I, Hiller KA, Landthaler M, Baumler W: Incidence of health problems associated with tattooed skin: a nationwide survey in German-speaking countries. Dermatology 2010;221:43–50.

9 Anderson RR, Parrish JA: Selective photothermolysis: precise microsurgery by selective absorption of pulsed radiation. Science 1983;220:524–527.

10 Maiman TH: Stimulated optical radiation in ruby. Nature 1960;187:493–494.

11 Goldman L, Wilson RG, Hornby P, Meyer RG: Radiation from a q-switched ruby laser. Effect of repeated impacts of power output of 10 megawatts on a tattoo of man. J Investig Dermatol 1965;44:69–71.

12 Pohl L, Kaiser K, Raulin C: Pitfalls and recommendations in cases of laser removal of decorative tattoos with pigmented lesions: case report and review of the literature. JAMA Dermatol 2013; 149:1087–1089.

13 Hsu VM, Aldahan AS, Mlacker S, Shah VV, Nouri K: The picosecond laser for tattoo removal. Lasers Med Sci 2016;31: 1733–1737.

14 Choudhary S, Elsaie ML, Leiva A, Nouri K: Lasers for tattoo removal: a review. Lasers Med Sci 2010;25:619–627.

15 Kilmer SL, Anderson RR: Clinical use of the Q-switched ruby and the Q-switched nd:Yag (1,064 nm and 532 nm) lasers for treatment of tattoos. J Dermatol Surg Oncol 1993;19:330–338.

16 Engel E, Santarelli F, Vasold R, Maisch T, Ulrich H, Prantl L, Konig B, Landthaler M, Baumler W: Modern tattoos cause high concentrations of hazardous pigments in skin. Contact Dermatitis 2008; 58:228–233.

17 Engel E, Santarelli F, Vasold R, Ulrich H, Maisch T, Konig B, Landthaler M, Gopee NV, Howard PC, Baumler W: Establishment of an extraction method for the recovery of tattoo pigments from human skin using HPLC diode array detector technology. Anal Chem 2006; 78:6440–6447.

18 Izikson L, Farinelli W, Sakamoto F, Tannous Z, Anderson RR: Safety and effectiveness of black tattoo clearance in a pig model after a single treatment with a novel 758 nm 500 picosecond laser: a pilot study. Lasers Surg Med 2010;42: 640–646.

19 Ferguson JE, Andrew SM, Jones CJ, August PJ: The Q-switched neodymium:Yag laser and tattoos: a microscopic analysis of laser-tattoo interactions. Br J Dermatol 1997;137:405–410.

20 Reid R, Muller S: Tattoo removal by CO laser dermabrasion. Plast Reconstr Surg 1980;65:717–728.

21 Kaur RR, Kirby W, Maibach H: Cutaneous allergic reactions to tattoo ink. J Cosmet Dermatol 2009;8:295–300.

22 Vasold R, Engel E, Konig B, Landthaler M, Baumler W: Health risks of tattoo colors. Anal bioanal chem 2008;391: 9–13.

23 Schreiver I, Hutzler C, Andree S, Laux P, Luch A: Identification and hazard prediction of tattoo pigments by means of pyrolysis-gas chromatography/mass spectrometry. Arch Toxicol 2016;90: 1639–1650.

24 Schreiver I, Hutzler C, Laux P, Berlien HP, Luch A: Formation of highly toxic hydrogen cyanide upon ruby laser irradiation of the tattoo pigment phthalocyanine blue. Sci Rep 2015;5:12915.

25 Chen HX, Diebold G: Chemical generation of acoustic-waves – a giant photoacoustic effect. Science 1995;270:963–966.

26 Albota M, Beljonne D, Bredas JL, Ehrlich JE, Fu JY, Heikal AA, Hess SE, Kogej T, Levin MD, Marder SR, McCord-Maughon D, Perry JW, Rockel H, Rumi M, Subramaniam G, Webb WW, Wu XL, Xu C: Design of organic molecules with large two-photon absorption cross sections. Science 1998;281:1653–1656.

27 Pawlicki M, Collins HA, Denning RG, Anderson HL: Two-photon absorption and the design of two-photon dyes. Angew Chem Int Ed Engl 2009;48:3244–3266.

28 de Uralde JL, Ruiz I, Santos I, Zubillaga A, Bringas PG, Okariz A: Automatic morphological categorisation of carbon black nano-aggregates; in Lecture Notes in Computer Science, vol 6262. Berlin, Springer, 2010, p 185.

29 Schmidt MU, Dinnebier RE, Kalkhof H: Crystal engineering on industrial diaryl pigments using lattice energy minimizations and X-ray powder diffraction. J Phys Chem B 2007;111:9722–9732.

30 Herbst W, Hunger K: Industrial Organic Pigments. Weinheim, Wiley-VCH, 2006, p 44.

31 Ho DD, London R, Zimmerman GB, Young DA: Laser-tattoo removal – a study of the mechanism and the optimal treatment strategy via computer simulations. Lasers Surg Med 2002;30:389–397.

32 Humphries A, Lister TS, Wright PA, Hughes MP: Determination of the thermal and physical properties of black tattoo ink using compound analysis. Lasers Med Sci 2013;28:1107–1112.
33 Lim GK, Chen ZL, Clark J, Goh RGS, Ng WH, Tan HW, Friend RH, Ho PKH, Chua LL: Giant broadband nonlinear optical absorption response in dispersed graphene single sheets. Nat Photonics 2011;5:554–560.
34 Humphries A, Lister TS, Wright PA, Hughes MP: Finite element analysis of thermal and acoustic processes during laser tattoo removal. Lasers Surg Med 2013;45:108–115.
35 Herd RM, Alora MB, Smoller B, Arndt KA, Dover JS: A clinical and histologic prospective controlled comparative study of the picosecond titanium:sapphire (795 nm) laser versus the Q-switched alexandrite (752 nm) laser for removing tattoo pigment. J Am Acad Dermatol 1999;40:603–606.
36 Ross V, Naseef G, Lin G, Kelly M, Michaud N, Flotte TJ, Raythen J, Anderson RR: Comparison of responses of tattoos to picosecond and nanosecond Q-switched neodymium: YAG lasers. Arch Dermatol 1998;134:167–171.
37 Bernstein EF, Schomacker KT, Basilavecchio LD, Plugis JM, Bhawalkar JD: A novel dual-wavelength, Nd:YAG, picosecond-domain laser safely and effectively removes multicolor tattoos. Lasers Surg Med 2015, Epub ahead of print.
38 Alabdulrazzaq H, Brauer JA, Bae YS, Geronemus RG: Clearance of yellow tattoo ink with a novel 532-nm picosecond laser. Lasers Surg Med 2015;47:285–288.
39 Saedi N, Metelitsa A, Petrell K, Arndt KA, Dover JS: Treatment of tattoos with a picosecond alexandrite laser: a prospective trial. Arch Dermatol 2012;148:1360–1363.
40 Brauer JA, Reddy KK, Anolik R, Weiss ET, Karen JK, Hale EK, Brightman LA, Bernstein L, Geronemus RG: Successful and rapid treatment of blue and green tattoo pigment with a novel picosecond laser. Arch Dermatol 2012;148:820–823.

Prof. Dr. Wolfgang Bäumler
Department of Dermatology, University of Regensburg
DE–93042 Regensburg (Germany)
E-Mail baeumler.wolfgang@klinik.uni-regensburg.de

Serup J, Bäumler W (eds): Diagnosis and Therapy of Tattoo Complications. With Atlas of Illustrative Cases.
Curr Probl Dermatol. Basel, Karger, 2017, vol 52, pp 105–112 (DOI: 10.1159/000450811)

Removal of Tattoos by Q-Switched Nanosecond Lasers

Syrus Karsai

Department of Dermatology, Klinikum Darmstadt, Darmstadt, and Department of Dermatology, University Hospital Greifswald, Greifswald, Germany

Abstract

Tattoo removal by Q-switched nanosecond laser devices is generally a safe and effective method, albeit a time-consuming one. Despite the newest developments in laser treatment, it is still not possible to remove every tattoo completely and without complications. Incomplete removal remains one of the most common challenges. As a consequence, particular restraint should be exercised when treating multicoloured tattoos, and patients need to be thoroughly informed about remaining pigment. Other frequent adverse effects include hyper- and hypopigmentation as well as ink darkening; the latter is particularly frequent in permanent make-up. Scarring is also possible, although it is rare when treatment is performed correctly. It is becoming more widespread for laser operators to encounter allergic reactions and even malignant tumours in tattoos, and treating these conditions requires a nuanced approach.

General Thoughts about Plain Tattoo Removal Using a Q-Switched Nanosecond Laser

Clinical experience has demonstrated that in about one third of all cases, even months of treatment are not enough to adequately remove a tattoo using a laser. In these cases, it may make more sense not to treat a tattoo at all than to attempt an effort that will likely prove unsatisfactory, especially when multicoloured tattoos with many blended shades are involved. In ideal cases, the laser operator will need 4–6 treatment sessions for amateur tattoos and 15–20 sessions for professional tattoos, if not more. The most frequently used laser systems in tattoo removal are the Q-switched ruby (694 nm), Nd:YAG (532 and 1,064 nm), and alexandrite (755 nm) lasers. An overview of how different tattoo inks may respond to laser treatment is summarized in table 1. It must be noted that an individual's response is hardly foreseeable [1]. Consequently, trial sessions on a small and inconspicuous area are strongly recommended.

Table 1. Overview of Q-switched laser systems and the response to commonly used colours

Colour	Ruby (694 nm)	Alexandrite (755 nm)	Nd:YAG (532 nm)	Nd:YAG (1,064 nm)
Black	+++	+++	–	+++
Blue	+++	+++	–	+++
Brown	+	+	+	+
Violet	+	–	–	–
Red	–	–	+++	–
Orange	–	–	++	–
Yellow	–	–	+	–
Green	+++	+++	–	–

– = No response; + = moderate response; ++ = good response; +++ = very good response.

We can only speculate as to which tattoos will respond well to treatment and which ones will respond poorly, if at all. A recently published retrospective study identified factors which may be relevant to the lightening process and need to be taken into account in the informed-consent discussion [2]. Coloured tattoos, especially those with green and yellow, respond more poorly (red is an exception, however), and so do larger tattoos (>30 cm^2) and those with a greater pigment density. Compared with tattoos at other sites, the lower extremities do not respond as well; tattoos which are over 36 months old or treated at shorter intervals (≤8 weeks) yield similarly poor responses. Interestingly, smoking cigarettes appears to have a negative impact on the lightening process. The probability of successfully removing a tattoo from a smoker's skin after 10 treatment sessions was nearly 70% lower in the aforementioned study. If we reflect upon the context of how tattoo pigments break down after laser treatment, this observation may be surprising, but it is fully logical. It is a well-known fact that nicotine has a negative effect on numerous immunological processes such as the phagocytic activity of macrophages, which means it indirectly affects the process of clearing tattoo particles.

Practical Approach to Plain Tattoo Removal via Q-Switched Nanosecond Laser

Prior to Treatment

Prior to treatment, an anaesthetic cream can be applied to the appropriate area if the tattoo is very large or the patient is anxious. Please note, however, that if the fluence is inadvertently set too high, pain is no longer present as a 'red flag', and the risk of burning the skin thus increases. Proper eye protection is essential for everyone involved (patient, laser surgeon and operating room personnel): each person must wear optically coated goggles that specifically match the emission spectrum of the laser being used. Of note, the patient is given special protective goggles which do not permit laser light to pass through the gap along the lower edge where it rests on the cheek.

During Treatment

During treatment, the hand piece is held perpendicular to the skin to ensure that the tattoo is evenly covered. If adequate fluences are available, select the largest spot size possible to achieve the greatest possible penetration depth while also minimizing epidermal debris. Here, the primary therapeutic endpoints are a transient whitening of the tattoo that occurs immediately after treatment as well as pinpoint bleeding in individual spots. Depending on these reactions, 1–2 passes are to be conducted with minimal overlapping of the laser pulses. Dermal urticarial response in the treated skin is also frequently observed; it is not to be equated with an allergic reaction. It is due to traumatic histamine release in the skin causing wheal and flare. It fades in a few hours. Furthermore, blisters and crusting may develop but resolve within 1–2 weeks.

After Treatment

After the session, the treated area is covered with an antiseptic ointment and bandaged to prevent infection. Although several patients want to have as many sessions as possible within a short time, treatment should take place with long intervals between sessions (≥8 weeks), since the immunological breakdown process means that tattoos continue to lighten several weeks after treatment.

Laser-Induced Complications and Their Management

This chapter focuses on *laser-induced* complications and how to manage them. Please refer to the appropriate chapters to read about potential complications which can occur even years after a tattoo is applied and do not have any correlation to laser treatment [see the chapters by Serup, this vol., pp. 58–73, and Hutton Carlsen et al., this vol., pp. 124–131]. A distinction must be made here between complications and the concomitant reactions described above; the latter may be observed during treatment as a therapeutic endpoint (whitening, pinpoint bleeding), or shortly after treatment (blistering or crusting) without malpractice having occurred.

Hypopigmentation
The most prevalent laser-induced complications include (transient) hypopigmentation (fig. 1), which is especially common with the ruby or 532-nm Nd:YAG laser and can last up to 6 months [3]. This adverse event is observed far less frequently when the 1,064-nm Nd:YAG laser is used, since the light at this wavelength is not absorbed as well by melanin. The number of treatment sessions and fluence settings has a positive correlation with the risk of hypopigmentation. The greatest risk factor, however, is suntanned skin. In cases of persistent hypopigmentation, an attempt can be made to induce re-pigmentation with an excimer laser, but it should be noted that multiple laser sessions are required. In one case study, stable re-pigmentation was only possible after 40 sessions [4].

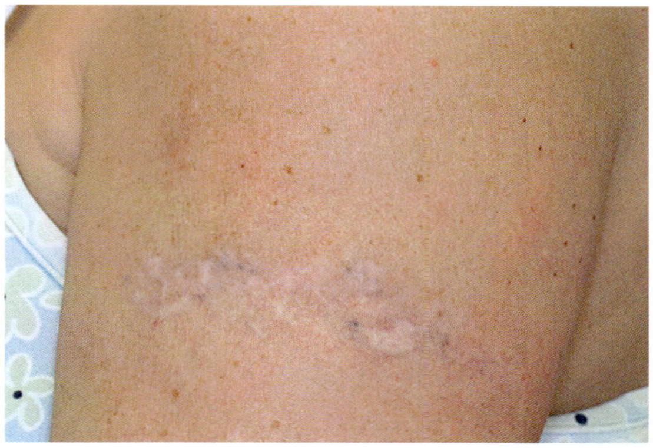

Fig. 1. Near-complete removal of a professional tattoo with persistent hypopigmentation. Courtesy of Springer [29].

Hyperpigmentation
This symptom manifests most commonly amongst darker skin types and if there was inadequate UV protection immediately following laser treatment; as a rule, it is transient. In some cases, nonablative fractional photothermolysis can be used to treat (postinflammatory) hyperpigmentation successfully [5].

Ink Darkening
The chemical compounds iron oxide and titanium dioxide are responsible for the laser-induced change from red to green or black observed in permanent make-up. Both substances are chemically reduced by high-energy laser pulses; the result is the so-called ink darkening (fig. 2). Experience shows that this reaction is most common in white or skin-coloured tattoos, which may contain titanium dioxide almost exclusively. When removing such tattoos, it is advisable to thoroughly inform the patient about this potential complication. Importantly, several trial sessions should be conducted at one and the same test site to assess the therapeutic response. Contrary to the widely held doctrine that ink darkening means a worse response to laser treatment [6], our experience in the past several years has been very dif-

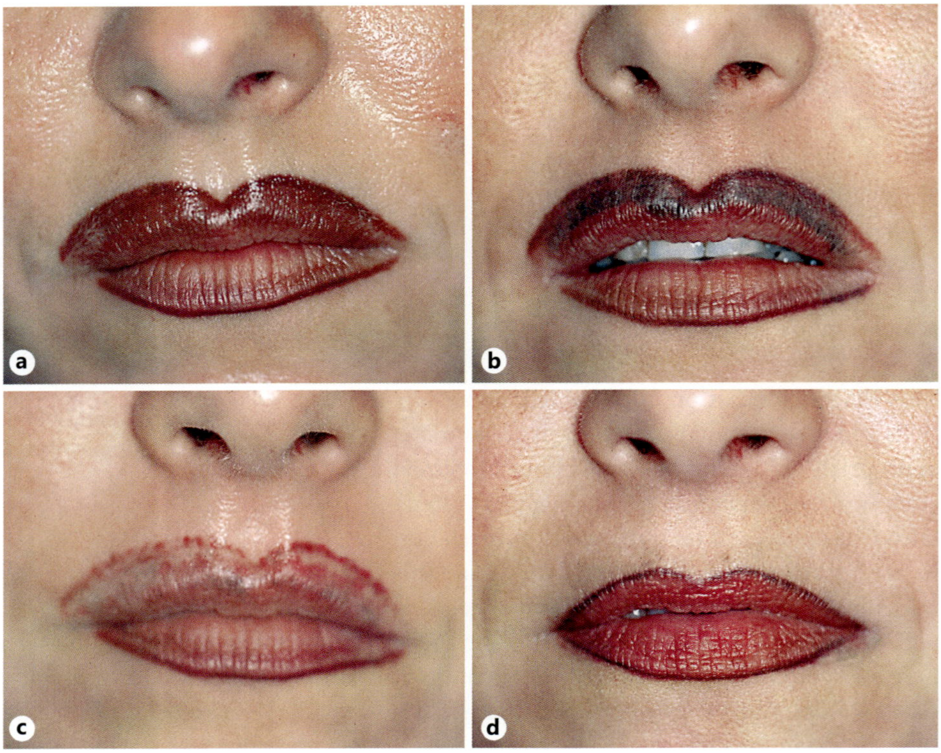

Fig. 2. a Female patient whose permanent make-up had been corrected several times by a cosmetician. **b** One month after the first treatment, the colour shifted from red to black. **c** One month after the seventh treatment with a Q-switched ruby laser. **d** Six months after five further treatments with a Q-switched 532-nm Nd:YAG laser. Courtesy of Springer [29].

ferent. If treatment is consistently continued despite the colour change, even permanent make-up may respond well to laser treatment. This is also the case with faded permanent make-up. Please note that the wavelength may need to be adapted in the course of treatment. If the permanent make-up does not respond further after a colour change, one alternative is to very cautiously attempt a (fractional) ablative laser treatment.

Patients who take or have taken gold salts (e.g. for rheumatoid arthritis) pose a special challenge. Treatment with a Q-switched laser system can cause uneven hyperpigmentation (chrysiasis). Interestingly, these cases respond especially well to treatment with a long-pulsed ruby laser (3 ms) [7].

Scarring

Fundamentally speaking, scarring can occur after any laser treatment, although it is rare when lasers are used correctly. To prevent scars, please make very certain that the fluences selected at the beginning of treatment are not set too high, especially when treating very densely inked tattoos. By contrast, larger spot sizes have a lower risk of scarring. One problem which is not to be underestimated is the scars which formed in the course of applying the tattoo and is not visible to the patient until the pigments have been removed (fig. 3). A (fractional) Er:YAG or CO_2 laser can contribute to cosmetic and functional improvement [8].

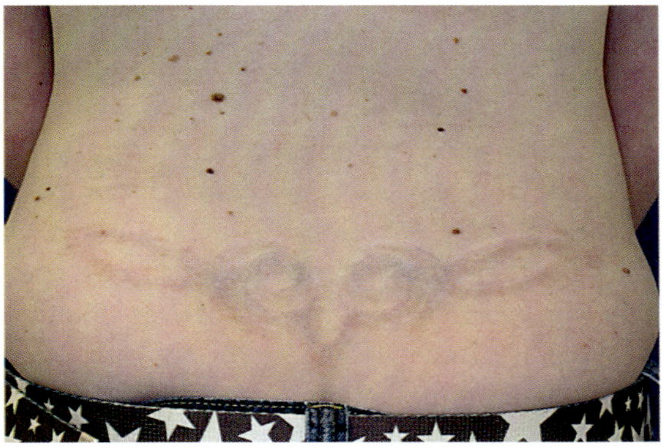

Fig. 3. Complete removal of a lower-back tattoo using a Q-switched laser. There is evidence of scarring that resulted from the tattooing per se. In cases such as these, the initial findings should be meticulously photographed for forensic reasons. Courtesy of Springer [29].

Partial Removal

For a variety of reasons, tattoo pigments may linger in the skin even after many labour- and time-consuming as well as expensive treatment sessions. This issue is currently the largest challenge facing laser tattoo removal. The most common causes of incomplete removal include scarring (caused by the tattooing process itself), which makes it more difficult for the laser light to penetrate the dermis due to scattering processes. This in turn reduces the light absorption in the ink particles.

The following therapeutic strategies should be taken into account or at least discussed as a means of optimizing the outcome of treatment:

1 The penetration depth of the laser light can be optimized by using a spot size that is as large as possible (at least 4 mm) [9]; this approach also makes it possible to reach pigment particles deep in the dermis.

2 Fractional photothermolysis can be used in conjunction with a Q-switched laser to destroy the dermoepidermal junction and thus increase the transepidermal elimination of colour pigments [10, 11].

3 One innovative approach is known as the R20 method. The idea here is for multiple rounds of treatment to occur in a single session at intervals of 20 min each [12]. The rationale for selecting this interval is biophysical: within a few minutes after treatment, vacuoles can clearly be seen forming in the dermis, a phenomenon which can be clinically confirmed by the whitening effect, i.e. the lasered area turning white. Since the vacuoles are reabsorbed within 20 min, the R20 method means that treatment can be resumed after this interval. As a result, tattoos may be removed more effectively in fewer sessions. Positive case studies notwithstanding, treatment with the R20 method is not without challenges. For example, the procedure is very time consuming: a treatment session can take several hours and must be scheduled accordingly. To sidestep this problem, colleagues in the US recommend the use of perfluorodecalin as a gel, since it can absorb gases and thus dramatically reduce the intervals between treatments [13]. Please note, however, that perfluorodecalin contributes considerably to global warming. A more environmentally friendly option with comparable effects is simply applying a damp compress after each pass. Furthermore, experience tells us that in pigmented skin there is a considerable risk of blistering, scarring, and pigmentary alteration.

4 Other approaches for simpler and more effective tattoo removal include the development of new inks ('permanent but easily removable ink') as well as individual determination of the absorption characteristics of the pigments. This makes it possible to select the optimal laser wavelengths before treatment begins [14]. Both of these approaches are currently undergoing clinical trials.

5 At present, we are studying whether the number of treatment sessions can be reduced by using lasers with pulse durations in the picosecond (or rather sub-nanosecond) range; this is-

sue is currently a matter of speculation. The findings from the only randomized controlled trial to date showed no clinical or statistical difference in treating black tattoos compared to a conventional Q-switched 1064-nm Nd:YAG laser [15]. Whether the use of a picosecond laser offers any advantages in treating coloured tattoos must be analyzed in investigator-initiated studies (ideally in a split-side study design).

Allergic Reactions

In terms of differential diagnostics, a distinction must be made between allergic reactions to tattoo pigments (whether immediate or delayed onset) and reactions to local anaesthetics or other substances which may be used in the course of laser treatment (e.g. antiseptic ointments). In rare cases, there have been reports of local allergic reactions to the metal salts once commonly used, e.g. mercury (red), cadmium (yellow), chrome (green), cobalt (blue), and above all, nickel. These reactions take place in the form of lichenoid or granulomatous skin lesions. Decades ago there was a shift away from the metal salts listed above and towards industrially manufactured organic pigments (e.g. the azo compounds in red pigments) [16]. A description of the tattoo inks currently used and their composition is listed in the chapter by Serup [this vol., pp. 1–17], which also reviews the biokinetics and toxicology of tattoo inks and ingredients.

Since the extent of allergic reactions cannot be anticipated in advance [17, 18], there is a fundamental need to ensure that laser treatments are conducted solely by physicians [19]. If an allergic reaction within the tattoo has occurred or the patient has an allergic reaction following laser treatment, further laser treatments must not be performed so as to prevent allergens from being distributed within the body and avoid a systemic reaction [17, 18]. Since tattoo pigments always absorb light and thus are subject to photochemical breakdown when exposed to powerful laser light, an existing allergy may be triggered or a new allergy induced through a primary sensitization acquired with the laser treatment [see the chapter by Bäumler, this vol., pp. 94–104]. Individual case studies on allergies after laser tattoo removal have described continuing treatment with a Q-switched laser; however, this approach cannot be unconditionally recommended. Ashinoff et al. [17] report about a patient with an allergic reaction who experienced lightening of over 75% after two laser treatments. Conceivably, the inflammatory and immunological reaction which manifests after laser treatment contributed to the lightening [17]. Nevertheless, if there is an allergic reaction, treatment should be seriously reconsidered and only take place or be continued with the greatest of care, since there is no way to rule out the risk of allergenic ink particles distributing throughout the body due to the continued laser treatment; the consequence can be hematogenous contact dermatitis, urticarial reactions or even anaphylactic shock. Prophylactic treatment with oral antihistamines and corticosteroids has been discussed, but to date there has not been any widespread clinical experience with this indication, which potentially may have a fatal outcome.

Unless there is unequivocal clinical evidence (which indeed is often the case), it is advisable to take a skin biopsy, although histology cannot distinguish a common unspecific inflammatory reaction (fig. 4) from a genuine allergic reaction as discussed in detail in the chapter by Serup [this vol., pp. 42–57]. As a second phase, other diagnostic steps can be taken, such as allergy tests. In many patients with allergic reactions to tattoo pigments, however, no reaction is evident in patch testing even if the culprit ink is used. It is likely that the antigens were not present in the tattoo ink bottle; instead, the pigment needs to be haptenized in the dermis over an extended period of months or years in order to become immunogenic, as described in a previous study [20]. As a word of caution, we must emphasize here that a delayed-onset allergic reaction may take place months or even years afterwards. In the time that has elapsed since the tattoo was applied, the tattoo

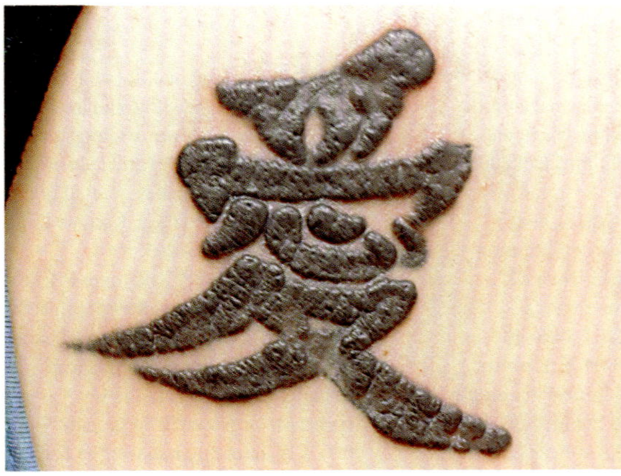

Fig. 4. Delayed-onset reaction in a black tattoo 13 years (!) after applying the tattoo. This reaction was granulomatous and of the papulonodular type, which is nonallergic and related to pigment agglomeration in the dermis with slow formation of large pigment clusters causing the reaction. This type of reaction is associated with sarcoidosis.

ink product originally used is often unknown or no longer available, and adequate information about product characteristics can be hard to obtain in the tattoo world of often short-lived commercial products and businesses.

The first-line approach to treating allergic reactions to tattoo inks is locally and/or intralesionally applied corticosteroids, although they are not effective enough in severe granulomatous reactions. One new alternative frequently cited in the medical literature is ablative fractional laser treatment to eliminate the allergic ink portion of a multicoloured tattoo [21]. Dermatome shaving of the outer skin layers, a process that was introduced many years ago, can be considered a permanent solution with radical removal of the pigment, which has spontaneously concentrated in the outer dermis. The procedure is primarily applicable to chronic inflammatory tattoo reactions and causes no new sensitization. A recent study documented the method to be effective with a high score of patient satisfaction [22]. The method is discussed in detail in the chapter by Sepehri and Jørgensen [this vol., pp. 82–93] and calls for critical deliberation about whether the allergens deep in the dermis can indeed be eliminated this way without creating disfiguring scars.

Malignant Skin Tumours

A variety of tattoo pigments may break down into toxic and/or carcinogenic compounds after laser treatment. For example, the deep-blue copper phthalocyanine (photo-)thermally breaks down into benzonitrile, benzene, and hydrocyanic acid [23]. To date, however, the correlation between tattoo inks (or their breakdown products) and local/systemic carcinogenic effects is an issue of great speculation and is supported primarily by case reports which were collected over the course of a century. These findings were recently summarized in the highly esteemed journal *The Lancet Oncology* [24]. The majority of the 50 cases reported in the world literature involved tumours of epidermal origin, such as pseudoepitheliomatous hyperplasia, keratoacanthoma, squamous cell carcinoma, and basal cell carcinoma. Pathogenetically speaking, a number of carcinogenic compounds (e.g. polycyclic aromatic hydrocarbons) were thought to play a role, and they are detected especially often in black tattoo inks [25]. However, the Lancet review concluded that any correlation between tattoos and cancer are pure coincidence, since reports of cancers in tattoos are very few, and the incidence of spontaneous skin cancer is about 2 million new cases in the world per year. Independently of that, keratoacanthoma in particular often can manifest after laser treatments or dermatosurgical interventions per se [26]. No matter the aetiology of the tumours found in tattoos, all carcinomas need to be biopsied, histologically classified, and treated appropriately. Another factor which is not to be underestimated is the fact that tattoo-pigment deposits in locoregional lymph nodes may make it more difficult to diagnose metastases of malignant melanoma [27]; correspondingly, the presence of tattoos may complicate the ability to diagnose malignoma correctly [28].

References

1 Bäumler W, Eibler E, Hohenleutner U: Q-switched laser and tattoo pigments: first results of the chemical and photophysical analysis of 41 compounds. Lasers Surg Med 2000;26:13–21.
2 Bencini PL, Cazzaniga S, Tourlaki A, et al: Removal of tattoos by q-switched laser: variables influencing outcome and sequelae in a large cohort of treated patients. Arch Dermatol 2012;148:1364–1369.
3 Leuenberger ML, Mulas MW, Hata TR, et al: Comparison of the Q-switched alexandrite, Nd:YAG, and ruby lasers in treating blue-black tattoos. Dermatol Surg 1999;25:10–14.
4 Gündogan C, Greve B, Hausser I, et al: Repigmentierung persistierender laserinduzierter Hypopigmentierungen nach Tätowierungsentfernung mit dem Excimerlaser. Hautarzt 2004;55:549–552.
5 Schmitt L, Raulin C, Karsai S: Fraktionierte Photothermolyse. Behandlung der postinflammatorischen Hyperpigmentierung nach Wiesengräserdermatitis. Hautarzt 2009;60:573–577.
6 Anderson RR, Geronemus R, Kilmer SL, et al: Cosmetic tattoo ink darkening. A complication of Q-switched and pulsed-laser treatment. Arch Dermatol 1993;129:1010–1014.
7 Yun PL, Arndt KA, Anderson RR: Q-switched laser-induced chrysiasis treated with long-pulsed laser. Arch Dermatol 2002;138:1012–1014.
8 Glaich AS, Rahman Z, Goldberg LH, et al: Fractional resurfacing for the treatment of hypopigmented scars: a pilot study. Dermatol Surg 2007;33:289–294.
9 Karsai S, Pfirrmann G, Hammes S: Treatment of resistant tattoos using a new generation Q-switched Nd:YAG laser: influence of beam profile and spot size on clearance success. Lasers Surg Med 2008;40:139–145.
10 Hantash BM, Bedi VP, Sudireddy V: Laser-induced transepidermal elimination of dermal content by fractional photothermolysis. J Biomed Opt 2006;11:041115.
11 Marini L, Kozarev J, Grad L, et al: Fractional Er:YAG skin conditioning for enhanced efficacy for Nd:YAG Q-switched laser tattoo removal. J Laser Health Acad 2012;1:35–40.
12 Kossida T, Rigopoulos D, Katsambas A, et al: Optimal tattoo removal in a single laser session based on the method of repeated exposures. J Am Acad Dermatol 2012;66:271–277.
13 Zawar V, Sarda A, De A: Bindi tattoo on forehead: Success with modified R-20 technique using low fluence Q-switched Nd Yag laser: a case report. J Cutan Aesthet Surg 2014;7:54–55.
14 Haedersdal M, Bech-Thomson N, Wulf HC: Skin-reflectance – guided laser selections for the treatment of decorative tattoos. Arch Dermatol 1996;132:403–407.
15 Pinto F, Große-Büning S, Karsai S, et al: Nd:YAG (1064-nm) picosecond laser versus Nd:YAG (1,064-nm) nanosecond laser in tattoo removal: a randomized controlled single-blind clinical trial. Br J Dermatol 2016, Epub ahead of print.
16 Laux P, Tralau T, Tentschert J, et al: A medical-toxicological view of tattooing. Lancet 2016;386–402.
17 Ashinoff R, Levine VJ, Soter NA: Allergic reactions to tattoo pigment after laser treatment. Dermatol Surg 1995;21:291–294.
18 Zemtsov A, Wilson L: CO_2 laser treatment causes local tattoo allergic reaction to become generalized. Acta Derm Venereol 1997;77:497.
19 Karsai S, Krieger G, Raulin C: Tattoo removal by non-professionals – medical and forensic considerations. J Eur Acad Dermatol Venereol 2010;24:756–762.
20 Serup J, Hutton Carlsen K: Patch test study of 90 patients with tattoo reactions: negative outcome of allergy patch test to baseline batteries and culprit inks suggests allergen(s) are generated in the skin through haptenation. Contact Dermatitis 2014;71:255–263.
21 Ibrahimi OA, Syed Z, Sakamoto FH, et al: Treatment of tattoo allergy with ablative fractional resurfacing: a novel paradigm for tattoo removal. J Am Acad Dermatol 2011;64:1111–1114.
22 Sepehri M, Jørgensen B, Serup J: Introduction of dermatome shaving as first line treatment of chronic tattoo reactions. J Dermatolog Treat 2015;26:451–455.
23 Schreiver I, Hutzler C, Laux P, et al: Formation of highly toxic hydrogen cyanide upon ruby laser irradiation of the tattoo pigment phthalocyanine blue. Sci Rep 2015;5:12915.
24 Kluger N, Koljonen V: Tattoos, inks and cancer. Lancet Oncol 2012;13:e161–e168.
25 Wiener DA, Scher RR: Basal cell carcinoma arising in a tattoo. Cutis 1987;39:125–126.
26 Kwiek B, Schwartz RA: Keratoacanthoma: an update and review. J Am Acad Dermatol 2015;74:1220–1233.
27 Pinto A, Wieshmann H, Triantafyllou A, et al: Tattoo-pigmented cervical lymph node that masqueraded as the sentinel lymph node in oral squamous cell carcinoma. Br J Oral Maxillofac Surg 2015;53:886–887.
28 Pohl L, Kaiser K, Raulin C: Pitfalls and recommendations in cases of laser removal of decorative tattoos with pigmented lesions: case report and review of the literature. JAMA Dermatol 2013;149:1087–1089.
29 Raulin C, Karsai S (eds): Laser and IPL Technology in Dermatology and Aesthetic Medicine. Heidelberg, Springer, 2011.

Syrus Karsai
Department of Dermatology, Klinikum Darmstadt
Heidelberger Landstrasse 379
DE–64297 Darmstadt (Germany)
E-Mail syrus.karsai@mail.klinikum-darmstadt.de

Serup J, Bäumler W (eds): Diagnosis and Therapy of Tattoo Complications. With Atlas of Illustrative Cases.
Curr Probl Dermatol. Basel, Karger, 2017, vol 52, pp 113–123 (DOI: 10.1159/000450812)

New and Advanced Picosecond Lasers for Tattoo Removal

Maurice A. Adatto[a, b] • Ruthie Amir[c] • Jayant Bhawalkar[d] • Rafael Sierra[e] • Richard Bankowski[e] • Doran Rozen[c] • Christine Dierickx[f] • Moshe Lapidoth[g]

[a]Skinpulse Dermatology, Laser and Beauty Centers, Geneva, and [b]Department of Dermatology, Bern University Hospital, Bern, Switzerland; [c]Syneron Medical Ltd., Yokneam, Israel; [d]Syneron Candela Co., Wayland, Mass., and [e]Cynosure Inc., Westford, Mass., USA; [f]Skinperium, Boom, Belgium; [g]Laser Unit, Department of Dermatology, Rabin Medical Center, Petah Tiqwa, Israel

Abstract

Early methods of tattoo removal ultimately resulted in unacceptable cosmetic outcomes. While the introduction of laser technology was an improvement over the existing chemical, mechanical, and surgical procedures, the use of nonselective tattoo removal with carbon dioxide and argon lasers led to scarring. Q-switched lasers with nanosecond (10^{-9}) pulse domains were considered to have revolutionized tattoo treatment, by selectively heating the tattoo particles, while reducing the adverse sequelae to adjacent normal skin. Theoretical considerations of restricting pulse duration, to heat tattoo particles to higher temperatures, proposed the use of subnanosecond pulses to target particles with thermal relaxation times lower than the nanosecond pulses in Q-switched lasers. Initial studies demonstrated that picosecond (10^{-12}) pulses were more effective than nanosecond pulses in clearing black tattoos. Advances in picosecond technology led to the development of commercially available lasers, incorporating several different wavelengths, to further refine pigment targeting.

The removal of unwanted tattoos has been practiced for as long as the art of tattooing has existed. The first evidence of tattoo removal attempts was found in Egyptian mummies, dated to have lived 4,000 years BC [1]. Early methods included chemical, mechanical, and surgical procedures, which almost inevitably resulted in unacceptable cosmetic outcomes. With the introduction of lasers in the 1960s, specifically CO_2 lasers in the millisecond domain, cosmetic outcomes improved but continued to result in adverse sequelae (scarring), as the thermal damage in the surrounding tissue was far too extensive. The first major improvement in treatment outcome was ushered in by the advent of Q-switched lasers in the 1990s. These lasers provide nanosecond (10^{-9}) duration pulses that can disrupt cells containing tattoo ink particles, resulting in effective clearance and greatly reduced collateral skin damage [2]. The use of Q-switched lasers was rapidly accepted, and numerous commercial products became available. Despite this improvement, many drawbacks exist with the use of Q-switched lasers, such as residual and/or resistant pigments, hypopigmentation, and scarring. In the 20 years that followed, there was essentially no advancement in tattoo removal technology to address these limitations. The need for safer and more effective treatment led to the consideration of using shorter pulse durations to target tattoos more effectively.

Why Shorter Pulse Durations?

Even as Q-switched lasers were being adopted, the possibility of even shorter picosecond duration lasers was being considered. In 1993, Jacques [3] and others analyzed laser tissue interaction over a broad range of pulse durations and concluded that tattoo removal would benefit greatly from the introduction of sub-nanosecond lasers. Based on work by Dingus and Scammon [4], Jacques argued that pulse durations in the order of the acoustic transit time of the target particle would result in the buildup of mechanical stresses within the target. He also identified the acoustic transit time as the time required for an acoustic wave to traverse the target. Sierra [5] solved the heat diffusion and acoustic wave equations, for the case of realistic laser pulses with rise times of several acoustic transit times. His results showed that the peak tensile stress σ, obtained at the center of the tattoo target, is given by the equation:

$$\sigma = -3\gamma\mu F(\tau\_a/\tau)\text{^}2, \qquad (1)$$

where F is the laser irradiance (fluence), τ_a and τ are the acoustic transit time and laser pulse duration, respectively, μ is the absorption coefficient of the target material at the laser wavelength, and γ is a constant that depends only on the properties of the target. If the tensile stress exceeds the tensile strength of the target material, there is a high probability of not only releasing but also breaking down the target particles.

Equation 1 clearly demonstrates why picosecond laser pulses can be expected to outperform nanosecond laser pulses. At equal laser irradiance, a 600-ps laser pulse will result in 100 times greater tensile stress at the tattoo target than obtained using a 6-ns Q-switched laser pulse. This greater mechanical stress significantly improves the probability of fragmenting the tattoo particle and suggests that it may be possible to use pulses with lesser irradiance, without degradation in the outcome and possibly greater safety.

It should be noted that absorption of light by the tattoo particle is still a primary requirement even at sub-nanosecond pulse durations. Therefore, the wavelength of these lasers still needs to be matched to the absorption spectrum of the tattoo particle. Interestingly, yellow tattoos, which were very resistant to nanosecond pulses at 532 nm, react very well to picosecond pulses at the same wavelength, as described below. For a multicolor tattoo, this requirement implies the need for a multi-wavelength laser source.

Methods of Generation of Picosecond Laser Pulses

Q-switching is a well-known technique for the generation of short pulses and forms the basis for a majority of tattoo removal lasers [6]. In most of these lasers, Q-switching is done by an electro-optic switch called a Pockel's cell. The shortest pulse generated by Pockel's cell Q-switching is limited by the laser gain medium selected and the practical constraints on the laser resonator length. Pulse durations achieved from these lasers are typically 5–10 ns for a Q-switched Nd:YAG laser to about 50–100 ns for a Q-switched alexandrite laser. This technique does not lend itself to generate pulses shorter than about 1 ns.

The earliest methods of generation of picosecond pulses included a technique called mode-locking. This technique has since demonstrated pulse durations down to several femtoseconds [7]. One of the earliest demonstrations of tattoo removal, using picosecond laser pulses, was re-

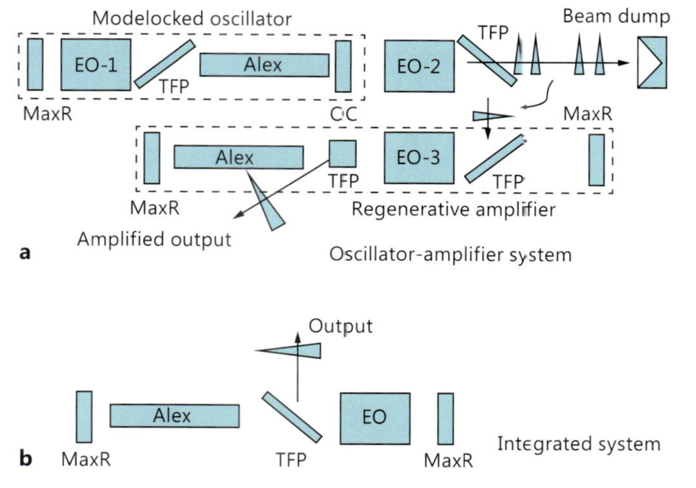

Fig. 1. Two picosecond laser systems. **a** A typical large complex system as commonly seen in laboratories. Two laser stages are shown. The oscillator generates a string of pulses, one of which is redirected into the amplifier stage. Three electro-optic switches (EO-1, 2, 3) route the pulse through the system. Not shown are isolation and beam management optics. **b** A commercially available picosecond laser with a much simpler configuration uses a sophisticated control system and re-programmable electro-optic switch to achieve the same results.

ported by Kilmer et al. [8], using a large complex mode-locked Ti:Sapphire laser system at the Lawrence Livermore National Lab. Figure 1a shows a system with a simplified diagram. Harter et al. [9] demonstrated an alexandrite laser system of this type with picosecond pulses of energy up to 10 mJ. However, to provide higher energy with hundreds of millijoules, as necessary for tattoo treatments, additional amplification stages would need to be added. In short, such cumbersome systems are simply not commercially viable.

Commercially Available Picosecond Lasers

The first commercially available tattoo laser that offered picosecond duration pulses was a 755-nm alexandrite laser (PicoSure; Cynosure, Westford, Mass., USA). It replaced the complex architecture of earlier systems with a much simpler design (fig. 1b). Here, a single-gain medium replaced the multiple stages used above, greatly reducing the number of components and size requirements. The new system was designed to produce a consistent and repeatable performance in tattoo removal.

Sub-nanosecond pulses can also be generated using a technique called passive Q-switching that can result in very compact and robust systems. Unlike Pockel's cell Q-switched lasers, passive Q-switching is achieved without the need for any high voltage or high-speed electronics, enabling very compact lasers [10].

The first commercial Nd:YAG-based 1,064/532-nm picosecond tattoo removal laser (PicoWay; Syneron Candela Corp., Wayland, Mass., USA) was based on passive Q-switching, followed by an amplification stage. The pulse characteristics, such as pulse duration and beam quality, are determined by the passively Q-switched laser, which acts as a seed laser generating a very low energy pulse. A subsequent amplification stage increases the energy to the desired level, while maintaining the other characteristics of the seed laser pulse. These 2-stage systems are often referred to as Master Oscillator Power Amplifier (MOPA) systems. The simplicity of the passively Q-switched MOPA configuration allows for robust systems that are scalable to high powers.

There has been a proliferation of sub-nanosecond lasers in the tattoo removal market in recent

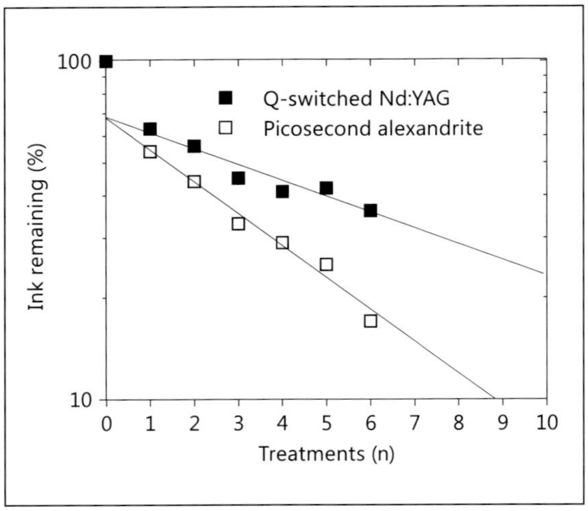

Fig. 2. Tattoo response to irradiation with nanosecond (Nd:YAG) and picosecond (alexandrite) lasers. YAG laser parameters were set in accordance with manufacturer's recommendation. Picosecond alexandrite was fixed at 3 J/cm^2. The use of picosecond pulses achieves equivalent clearance in half the number of treatments.

years. These have been based on some of the technologies described in this section. With improvements to technology, pulse durations below 100 ps could be commercially available in the future. Theory predicts that this is the range of pulse duration where near complete thermal and acoustic confinement of the laser energy is possible, which should result in better efficacy of tattoo clearance.

Clinical Studies

The use of shorter pulse durations was already published as far back as 1998, when Ross et al. [11] described a study in which 16 patients with black tattoos were treated with 10 ns pulses compared to 35 ps pulses from a 1,064-nm YAG laser. Patients received a total of 4 treatments at 4-week intervals. All laser pulse parameters were held constant except pulse duration. Radiation exposure was 0.65 J/cm^2 at the skin surface. In 12 of the 16 tattoos, there was significant lightening in the picosecond-treated areas compared with those treated with nanosecond pulses. This was the first published study concluding that picosecond pulses are more efficient than nanosecond pulses in clearing black tattoos. A second study was published in 1999 by Herd et al. [12] that compared treatments to black tattoos on porcine skin with a 795-nm, 500-ps titanium:sapphire laser and a Q-switched alexandrite 752-nm, 50-ns laser. Results were similar to those of the first study, showing better clearance of pigment in the picosecond-treated areas. It should be noted that the picosecond lasers used at that time for both studies were lab prototypes and not commercially available.

One of the earliest demonstrations of tattoo removal, using a new commercially available picosecond laser (PicoSure, Cynosure), was reported by Sierra and Mirkov [13] in Innsbruck in 2012. A picosecond alexandrite laser was used to compare the efficacy of this new laser with that of nanosecond lasers on split tattoos. Commercially available nanosecond lasers, an alexandrite laser (Accolade, Cynosure) and Nd:YAG 1,064/532-nm laser (RevLite, Cynosure), were used for comparison of black and multicolor tattoos. The tattoos were split, with 1 side treated using the picosecond laser at a fixed 3 J/cm^2 irradiance and 3 mm spot size, and the other half treated using one of the nanosecond lasers with parameters set in accordance with the manufacturer's recommendations. The picosecond alexandrite laser was found to achieve clearance equivalent to that obtained with the nanosecond lasers (fig. 2) but required half the number of treatments and one half to one third the irradiance as compared with the nanosecond lasers. As shown in figure 2, there was a rapid initial drop in the fraction of ink remaining after each treatment, followed by an exponential decrease of 10% per treatment for the picosecond laser and 5% per treatment for the Q-switched YAG laser. Although the study was limited with only 5 tattoos included in the Nd:YAG comparison and 10 in the nanosecond alexandrite comparison, the data clearly support expected outcomes.

Table 1. Benefits of picosecond lasers over nanosecond lasers in tattoo removal

Benefits	Reference
Fewer number of treatment sessions	14, 15, 21, 23, 24
Less time required for complete removal	As less sessions are required, less time is needed (pers. experience)
Better clearance of colors, especially blue, green, and yellow	15, 19–24
Removing ghost of tattoo remaining after multiple sessions with nanosecond	25, pers. experience

Geronemus and colleagues [14] demonstrated, at a 1-month follow-up, that 92% of the subjects treated had >75% clearance of the 12 tattoos containing blue and green pigment after 1 or 2 treatments with a picosecond, 755-nm alexandrite laser. Another study demonstrated that 75% of all subjects had >75% clearance in 2–4 treatments of black and blue tattoo inks [15]. While there was no nanosecond control group in this study, the authors used historical controls to assess the comparative efficacy of the picosecond laser device. Previous publications by Fitzpatrick and Goldman [16] and Alster [17] reported that using a Q-switched alexandrite laser required 8.9 treatments and 8.5 treatments, respectively, on average to achieve clearance similar to that observed with the 755-nm picosecond alexandrite laser with 4.3 treatments, thereby reducing the number of treatments by approximately 50%.

In a recent publication, a Nd:YAG 1,064-nm picosecond laser (PicoWay, Syneron Candela) was compared to a Nd:YAG 1,064-nm nanosecond laser (ConBio Medlite C6, Cynosure) for tattoo removal [18]. The authors concluded that there was no statistically significant and no clinical relevant difference between picosecond and nanosecond technologies using 1,064-nm lasers. This study was limited to 2 treatments and the conclusion that additional subsequent treatment sessions would result in no statistical difference between 2 lasers was based on a mathematic model.

This is contrary to the examples in figure 3, which clearly demonstrates that 2 different split tattoos had more efficacious clearing of black and colored ink with 755-nm picosecond technology compared to both 755-nm nanosecond (Accolade, Cynosure) and 1,064/532-nm nanosecond (Revlite, Cynosure) technologies. Figure 4 also demonstrates the same result in favor of picosecond, showing a black tattoo treated with 1,064 nm; one side was done with picosecond (Picoway, Syneron-Candela Corporation) and the other with nanosecond (Alex TriVantage, Candela Corporation), at same fluences. After 4 sessions, the picosecond side showed better pigment clearance than the one treated with nanosecond. Also, in the published review article from Torbec et al. [20], a specific PubMed search yielded 10 articles on picosecond technology that met the search criteria. The authors concluded from the review of the relevant published information that picosecond lasers are most effective requiring less treatments and lower fluences compared to nanosecond lasers [20].

The Challenge of Removing Various Tattoo Colors

As described previously, the choice of wavelength is still important for targeting different pigment colors. Therefore, the first wavelength commercially available, 755 nm, was successful to remove

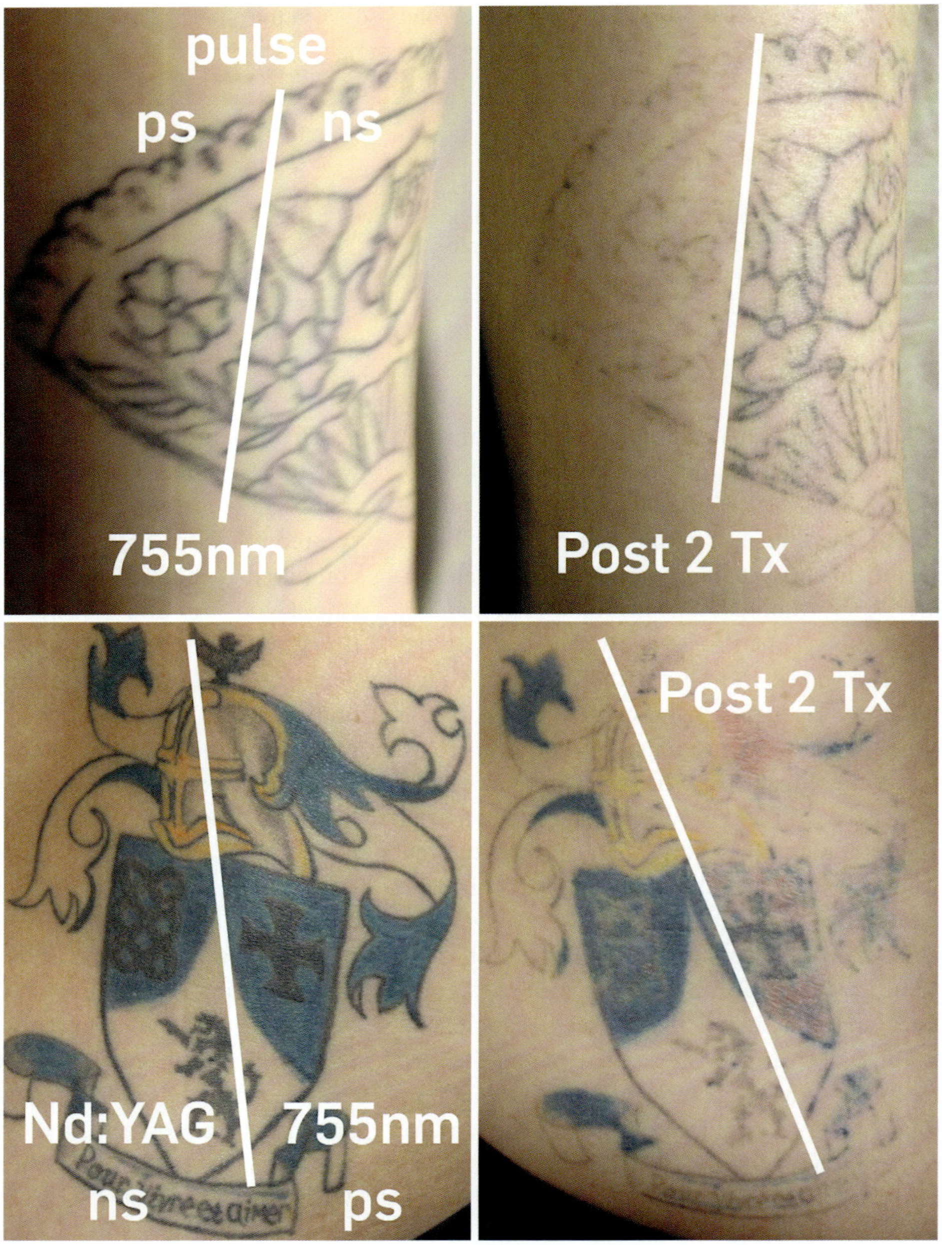

Fig. 3. Comparison of 755 nm picosecond (ps) pulse exposure with existing nanosecond (ns) technologies after 2 treatments. Upper photos: 755-nm picosecond 4.9 J/cm^2 vs. 755-nm nanosecond 10 J/cm^2. Lower photos: 755-nm picosecond 3 J/cm^2 vs. Nd:YAG (1,064/532 nm) up to 6 J/cm^2. The use of picosecond duration pulses leads to faster clearance even at lower fluence. Tx, treatment.

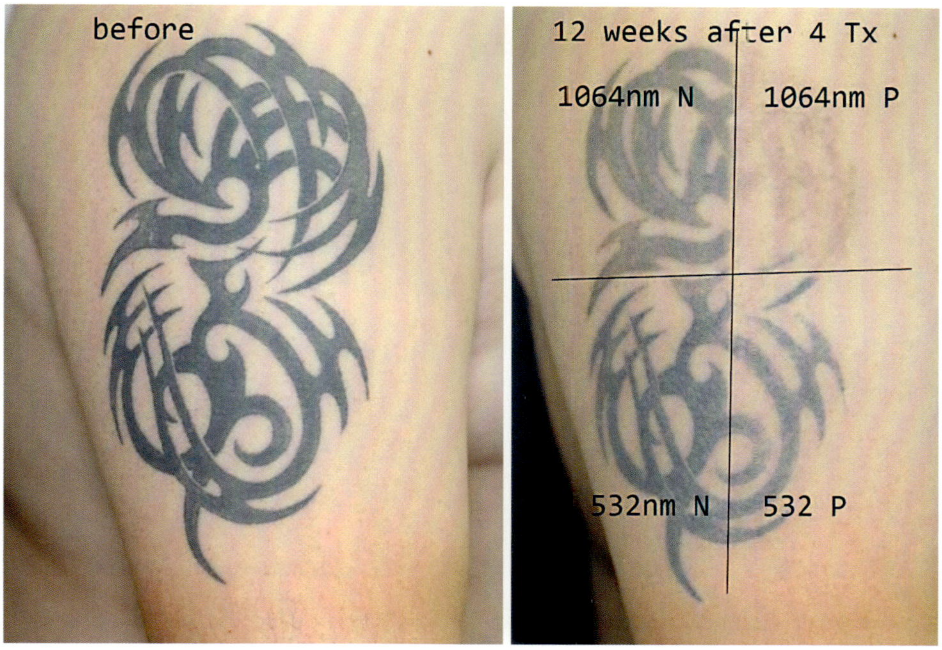

Fig. 4. Comparison of 1,064- and 532-nm picosecond pulse treatment with nanosecond pulse treatment after 4 treatments. The top left quadrant was treated with a 50-ns 1,064-nm laser (Alex TriVantage, Candela Corporation) while the top right quadrant was treated with 450-ps 1,064-nm (PicoWay, Syneron Candela Corporation) at equal fluence. The lower quadrants compare 532-nm 50-ns on the left side with 532-nm 450-ps on the right side. Substantially greater lightening of the tattoo is seen on the 1,064-nm 450-ps side. Tx, treatment. Photo courtesy of Taro Kono, MD.

black, blue, and green colors [14, 15], but was less efficient on colors like red, yellow, and orange. Another approach to treating this wide range of tattoo ink colors is a new dual-wavelength Nd:YAG 1,064/532-nm picosecond laser (PicoWay, Syneron Candela). A study was conducted comparing the efficacy of this dual-wavelength picosecond laser with a Q-switched 50-ns 532/1,064-nm laser (Alex Trivantage, Syneron Candela) on 11 multicolor and 12 black tattoos in Asian patients [19, 20]. The efficacy of the picosecond laser was shown to be significantly better than the efficacy of the nanosecond laser in both wavelength choices for both black and multicolor tattoos. Clearance of red, yellow, and orange tattoos was further demonstrated in a multicenter study by Bernstein et al. [21], in which 75 tattoos in 60 subjects, of all Fitzpatrick skin types I–VI, were safely treated. Blinder reviewer evaluation showed an average of 79% clearance score after an average of 6.5 treatments in multicolored tattoos. Using the 1,064-nm wavelength, after 7 treatments black ink showed the greatest clearing at 92%, followed by purple at 78%, green at 65%, and blue at 43%. Using the 532-nm wavelength, after 7 treatments, yellow ink showed 85% clearance and red ink 80%.

The need for multiple wavelengths in tattoo removal led to the development of 2 additional wavelengths for the 755-nm PicoSure, with 532 nm and 1,064 nm, and 1 additional for Picoway, 785 nm. Most of the new picosecond laser systems coming out now on the market offer at least 3 wavelengths (1,064 nm, 532 nm, and a third wavelength between 670 and 785 nm).

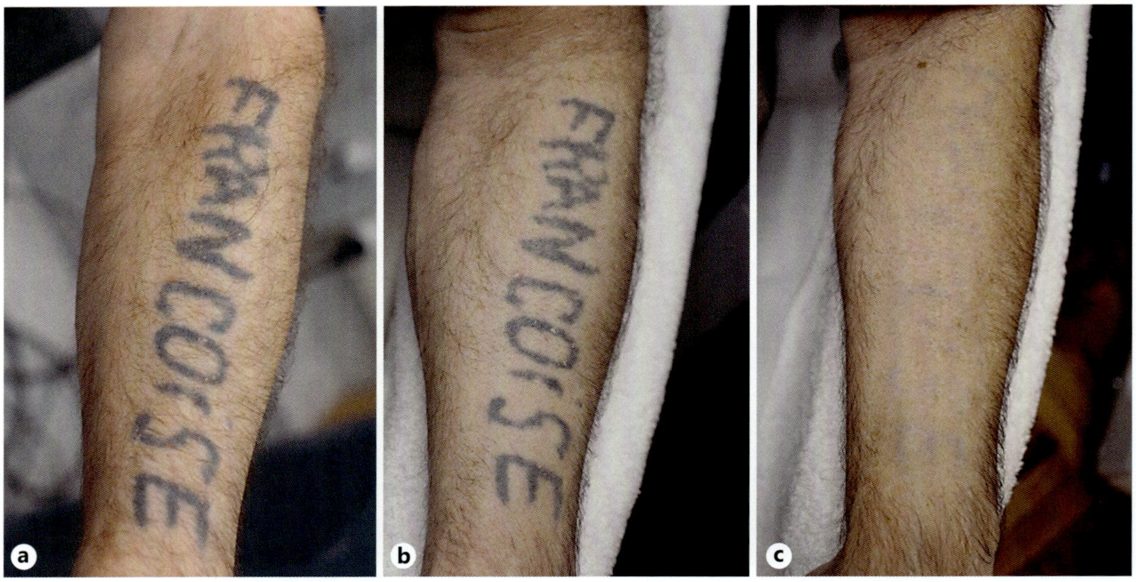

Fig. 5. a Dark amateur black tattoo on the left forearm of a male patient. **b** Six sessions were performed over 1 year with a Q-switched laser at 1,064 nm, with very little improvement. **c** Four additional sessions with a 755-nm picosecond laser improved the situation dramatically. Photo courtesy of M.A. Adatto, MD.

Geronemus and colleagues [22] demonstrated that most tattoo ink colors are effectively treated with 755 and 532 nm. Red, orange, and yellow inks showed >75% improvement with an average of 2 treatments using the 532-nm wavelength. The 755- and 1,064-nm wavelengths produced comparable results in treating black ink; however, greater caution should be exercised when using 755 nm in the darkest of skin types for tattoo removal. This was also the first documentation of the clearing of yellow ink with a picosecond laser [23]. In a second study with picosecond 755, 1,064, and 532 nm from Dover and Arndt and colleagues [24], multicolored tattoos were improved on average by 50% 2 two treatments and by 75% after 4 treatments using 532-, 755-, and 1,064-nm wavelengths. Blue and green ink responded best to 755 nm, while black ink responded slightly better to 755 nm compared to 1,064 nm in this particular study.

Practical Considerations

In most cases, picosecond lasers have shown to remove tattoos in a much more efficient way than nanosecond lasers, with fewer sessions, reduced time, and less risks of side effects, especially residual scarring and incomplete removal, as sometimes seen after nanosecond laser treatment [25]. Another benefit is that picosecond lasers are able to clear very stubborn colors: the 755-nm picosecond laser was shown to efficiently remove bright blue and green colors, while the 532-nm picosecond laser can remove purple, orange, and yellow colors. These colors were very difficult to remove with nanosecond technology. However, tattoos come in many different compositions due to the differences in the quality and the quantity of the tattoo particles, the depth of placement, and the mixing of different tattoo colors. This unknown factor means that we have to set realistic expectations with our patients and

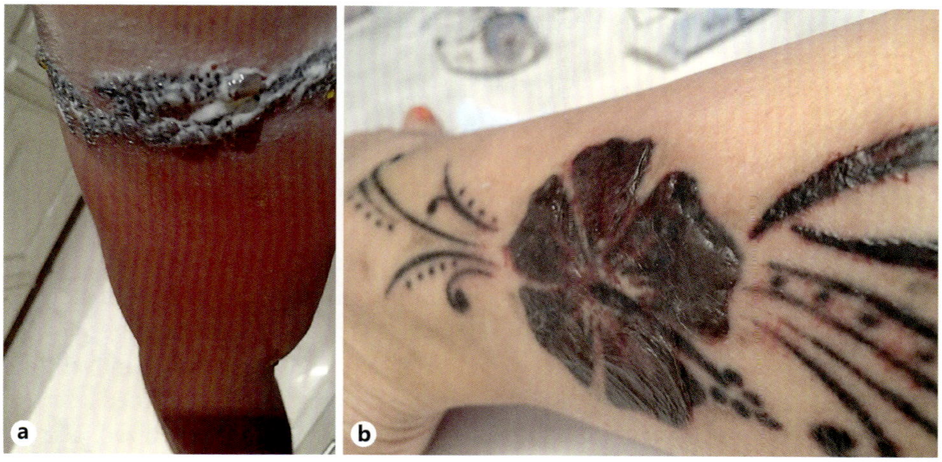

Fig. 6. a Bullae after 755-nm picosecond. **b** Bullae after 1,064-nm picosecond. Photos courtesy of M.A. Adatto, MD.

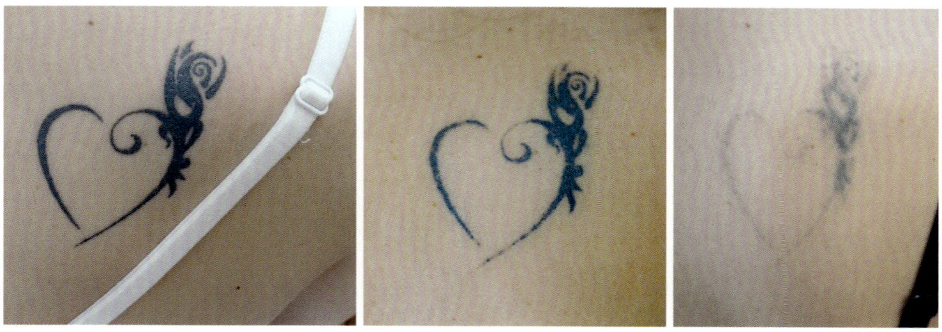

Fig. 7. Difficult tattoo to remove, even with picosecond at 755 and 1,064 nm. The resistant area is a re-tattooing, requiring more sessions as the density of pigment is higher. Photos courtesy of M.A. Adatto, MD.

explain that the exact number of treatments to remove a tattoo is always unknown, but that, in general, the clearance is expected to be faster with the picosecond lasers, due to the more efficient way of fracturing and consequently removing the very small ruptured tattoo particles. Tattoo colors resistant to treatment do exist, even with picosecond technology, but such cases are rare. With tattoos that have been redone or covered up, more treatments are still required to remove the double-ink load. However, theoretically, the picosecond laser could potentially produce faster clearance than nanosecond lasers. A comparative study with nano- and picosecond lasers for this subtype of tattoos is therefore warranted.

After a session, we typically see a higher incidence of bulla formation (fig. 5) after the use of picosecond lasers (up to 50% during first sessions when the targeted pigment is located superficially and especially on lower extremities) The exact mechanism remains unclear, and the question remains as to the mechanical effect on epidermis from back-scattered fragmented tattoo particles. The fact is that these bullae heal very quickly (within 4–5 days), without any sequelae, if managed properly. One way to diminish the incidence of these bullae could be to use the picosecond laser in combination with a fractional ablative CO_2 laser [26]. Another approach is to use either fractional picosecond laser immediately after treating with the flat beam or to apply a silicone gel (Strataderm®; Stratapharma, Basel, Switzerland) prior to the laser session (unpubl. results, M. Adatto, pers. experience). The endpoint of treatment should remain the same, with an immediate crisp whitening of the tattoo pigment, right after the laser impact.

Another indication where picosecond lasers are beneficial is to remove old, darkened pigment, composed of iron or zinc oxide [27]. Due to its already described characteristics, picosecond lasers remove quicker and more efficiently previously darkened and recalcitrant pigments. However, it should be stated that picosecond lasers do not prevent this darkening.

Conclusions

Picosecond lasers are a significant improvement in the management of tattoo removal. Usually, fewer sessions are needed and, therefore, the overall treatment removal time is reduced compared with Q-switched lasers. The benefit for the patient is then realized. Use of picosecond technology also allows the physician to treat difficult conditions (resistant colors, darkened or residual pigment after nanosecond treatment) in a much easier way. Understandably, as a new technology, not all the optimal treatment parameters and mechanisms of action are fully understood, and further studies are warranted to elucidate some of them (i.e. bulla formation).

References

1 Adatto MA, Halachmi S, Lapidoth M: Tattoo removal; in Bogdan Allemann I, Goldberg DJ (eds): Basics in Dermatological Laser Applications. Curr Probl Dermatol. Basel, Karger, 2011, vol 42, pp 97–110.
2 Adatto MA: Laser tattoo removal: benefits and caveats. Med Laser Appl 2004; 19:175–185.
3 Jacques SL: Role of tissue optics and pulse duration on tissue effects during high-power laser irradiation. Appl Opt 1993;32:2447–2454.
4 Dingus RS, Scammon RJ: Grüneisen-stress-induced ablation of biological tissue. Proc SPIE Int Soc Opt Eng 1991: 1427;45–54.
5 Sierra R: Impact of pulse duration from nanoseconds to picoseconds on the thermal and mechanical effects during laser interaction with tattoo targets. Lasers Surg Med 2013;45(S25):29–30.
6 Kent KM, Graber EM: Laser tattoo removal – a review. Dermatol Surg 2011; 38:1–13.
7 Morgner U, Kärtner FX, Cho SH, Chen Y, Haus HA, Fujimoto JG, Ippen EP, Scheuer V, Angelow G, Tschudi T: Sub-two-cycle pulses from a Kerr-lens mode-locked Ti:sapphire laser: addenda. Opt Lett 1999;24:920.
8 Kilmer SL, Fitzpatrick RE, DaSilva LB, Marshall R, Ghiselli R: Picosecond and femtosecond laser treatment of tattoo ink (abstract). Lasers Surg Med 1996;19: 36.
9 Harter DJ, Pessot MA, Squier JA, Nees JA, Bado P, Mourou GA: Short pulse amplification in tunable solid state materials. Proc SPIE Int Soc Opt Eng 1990; 1229:19–28.
10 Miller IJ, Alcock AJ, Bernard JE: Experimental Investigation of Cr4+ in YAG as a Passive Q-switch Advanced Solid State Lasers OSA Proceedings Series 1992, Paper LM13.
11 Ross V, Naseef G, Lin G, Kelly M, Michaud N, Flotte TJ, Raythen J, Anderson RR: Comparison of responses of tattoos to picosecond and nanosecond Q-switched neodymium:YAG lasers. Arch Dermatol 1998;134:167–171.
12 Herd RM, Alora MB, Smoller B, Arndt KA, Dover JS: A clinical and histologic prospective controlled comparative study of the picosecond titanium:sapphire (795 nm) laser versus the Q-switched alexandrite (752 nm) laser for removing tattoo pigment. J Am Acad Dermatol 1999;40:603–606.
13 Sierra R, Mirkov M: Tattoo Treatment: A new technology for an old problem (abstract). Laser Innsbruck Conference 2012, Innsbruck Austria, September 2012.
14 Brauer JA, Reddy KK, Anolik R, Weiss ET, Karen JK, Hale EK, Brightman LA, Bernstein L, Geronemus, RG: Successful and rapid treatment of blue and green tattoo pigment with a novel picosecond Laser. Arch Dermatol 2012;148:820–823.

15 Saedi N, Metelitsa A, Petrell K, Arndt KA, Dover JS: Treatment of tattoos with a picosecond alexandrite laser: a prospective trial. Arch Dermatol 2012;148:1360–1363.
16 Fitzpatrick RE, Goldman MP: Tattoo removal using the alexandrite laser. Arch Dermatol 1994;130:1508–1514.
17 Alster TS: Q-switched alexandrite laser treatment (755 nm) of professional and amateur tattoos: J Am Acad Dermatol 1995;33:69–73.
18 Pinto F, Grosse-Büning S, Karsai S, Weiss C, Bäumler W, Hammes S, Felcht M, Raulin C: Nd:YAG (1,064-nm) picosecond laser vs Nd:YAG (1,064-nm) nanosecond laser in tattoo removal: a randomized controlled single-blind clinical trial. Br J Dermatol 2016, DOI: 10.1111/bjd.14962.
19 Kono T, Shek S, Chan H, Groff W, Imagawa K, Miyasaka M: Comparison study of a 532/1,064 nm picosecond laser vs a 532/1,064 nm nanosecond laser in the treatment of multi-color tattoos in Asians (abstract). Lasers Surg Med 2016;S27.
20 Torbeck R, Bankowski R, Henize S, Saedi N: Lasers in tattoo and pigmentation control: role of the PicoSure® laser system. Med Devices (Auckl) 2016;9:63–67.
21 Bernstein EF, Schomacker KT, Basilavecchio LD, Plugis JM, Bhawalkar JD: A novel dual-wavelength, Nd:YAG, picosecond-domain laser safely and effectively removes multicolor tattoos. Lasers Surg Med 2015, Epub ahead of print.
22 Bloom B, Alabdulrazzaq H, Bae YS, Brauer JA, Neckman J, Bernstein L, Weiss E, Anolik R, Geronemus, RG: A 1,064, 532 and 755 nm laser system for the treatment of unwanted tattoos (abstract). Lasers Surg Med 2016;S37:13.
23 Alabdulrazzaq H, Brauer JA, Bae YS, Geronemus RG: Clearance of yellow tattoo ink with a novel 532-nm picosecond laser. Lasers Surg Med 2015;47:285–288.
24 Prather H, Desai S, Kruter L, Depina J, Doherty S, Arndt K, Dover J: Clinical Evaluation of the picosecond 532, 755, and 1,064 nm wavelengths for the removal of tattoos (abstract). Lasers Surg Med 2015;S58:20.
25 Alabdulrazzaq H, Bae YS, Bloom B, Brauer JA, Anolik R, Bernstein L, Weiss E, Geronemus RG: A new paradigm for optimal tattoo removal using three picosecond laser wavelengths (abstract). Lasers Surg Med 2015;S54:19.
26 Au S, Liolios AM, Goldman MP: Analysis of incidence of bulla formation after tattoo treatment using the combination of the picosecond alexandrite laser and fractionated CO_2 ablation. Dermatol Surg 2015;41:242–245.
27 Bae YC, Alabdulrazzaq H, Brauer J, Geronemus R: Successful treatment of paradoxical darkening. Lasers Surg Med 2016;48:471–473.

Dr. Maurice A. Adatto
Skinpulse Dermatology, Laser and Beauty Centers
5 Rond-Point de Plainpalais
CH–1205 Geneva (Switzerland)
E-Mail madatto@skinpulse.ch

Serup J, Bäumler W (eds): Diagnosis and Therapy of Tattoo Complications. With Atlas of Illustrative Cases.
Curr Probl Dermatol. Basel, Karger, 2017, vol 52, pp 124–131 (DOI: 10.1159/000450813)

Laser Surgeon, Client Education, and Satisfaction with Tattoo Removal

Katrina Hutton Carlsen[a] · Jørgen Esmann[b] · Jørgen Serup[a]

[a]The 'Tattoo Clinic', Department of Dermatology, Bispebjerg University Hospital, Copenhagen, and [b]Centre for Laser Surgery, Hellerup, Denmark

Abstract

Studies of satisfaction with tattoo removal outcomes by laser, rated by clients themselves, including qualitative aspects, are sparse. We studied long-term results and client satisfaction with tattoo removal by Q-switched YAG laser. Client satisfaction is influenced by numerous factors: pretreatment expectations, objective observations, pretreatment information, laser treatment procedures, and outcome, including subjective experiences such as pain. Client-surgeon interaction during the full laser treatment course is a major determinant of client satisfaction. The client is in a dynamic state of mind and undergoes a change of opinion during a laser treatment course as a result of his/her experiences. In this continuous process of learning, expectations are changed from a state of high expectation before treatment to a more realistic state with acceptance of outcome. The laser surgeon shall be aware of his/her role as a tutor and prepare the client for a situation, where outcomes can be acceptable albeit not ideal.

Tattoo removal by laser has increased due to the rising number of tattoo acquirements and thereby regrets. Laser tattoo removal involves many aspects besides selecting the appropriate laser equipment with efficient settings. Published studies on outcome of tattoo removal by lasers are often evaluated by the treating laser surgeons and not by clients themselves [1–10].

Acquiring tattoos and having them removed is comprised of many aspects, e.g. health risks and culture; therefore, the laser surgeon is encouraged to see tattoo laser removal in a broad perspective [11, 12]. There are essentially two scenarios, e.g. removal of tattoos due to regret and removal of tattoos with inflammatory complications such as allergic and nonallergic reactions [11, 12]. This chapter will primarily address tattoo removal by laser due to regret.

At the 'Centre for Laser Surgery', a private clinic in Copenhagen, Denmark, a questionnaire study of 154 persons was recently conducted concerning client satisfaction with tattoo removal by Q-switched laser performed by a dermatologist specialised in laser techniques [13]. Clients, who had completed a laser treatment course, were invited to participate by completing a questionnaire with predefined and open questions. The laser surgeon and his team were blinded from data handling, which was conducted by the 'Tattoo Clinic', Bispebjerg University Hospital.

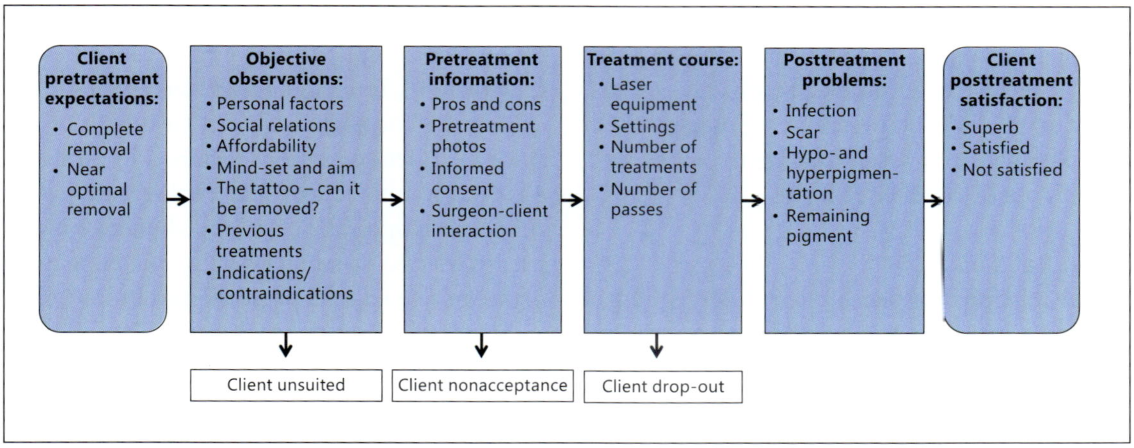

Fig. 1. Tattoo removal by laser: flow chart of the treatment course.

A laser treatment course has different phases, as illustrated in figure 1, influencing client satisfaction. These will be described in the following and summarized with suggestions to laser surgeons on how to conduct a situation with hopefully high client satisfaction.

In many fields of dermatology, the physician-client interaction influences adherence to therapy, and thereby treatment result, and is therefore of uttermost importance [14]. These findings can be transferred to the practice of tattoo removal.

The data behind the guidance is provided in an original publication, supplemented with our experiences from the clinic [13]. The essence of the guidance is that client satisfaction ranges beyond objective outcome of the full laser treatment course. Client satisfaction is a learning process with the laser surgeon having the role as a tutor.

Client Pretreatment Expectations

It is important to clarify clients' pretreatment expectations before offering laser surgery. In our recently published study, pretreatment expectations were rated as follows: complete removal without a blemish, near optimal removal, partial removal, no effect but took the chance, or other expectations. Most clients (66%) expected complete removal of their tattoos without a blemish.

A full laser treatment course can take up to 2–3 years to complete, and in some cases entire clearance is impossible [9]. Especially multicoloured tattoos can be very difficult or impossible to remove, which the client should understand and accept before treatment starts. Fortunately, during the process of treatments most clients adjust their expectations and adapt a more realistic view of outcomes.

Objective Observations

Before the start of treatment, the laser surgeon must understand the individual client and his/her personality. Different individual factors can influence the laser treatment course and thereby the result and satisfaction rate. In the following, the different factors will be outlined: personal factors, social relations, affordability, mind-set and aim of treatment, the tattoo (can it be removed?), previous treatments, and indications/contraindications.

Personal Factors

Personal factors, e.g. low motivation, health problems, psychiatric disorders, pregnancy, or distance to the clinic, may result in some patients not completing a full laser treatment course and, thereby, an incomplete removal.

Social Relations

Social relations influence clients' perception of treatment satisfaction more than we realise, and treatment dropout or change of clinic can be due to friends' positive or negative comments or experiences.

Affordability

Removal of a tattoo by laser can become very expensive, as some tattoos require multiple treatments. Not all clients can afford a full laser treatment course and may drop out, choose intermittent treatment, or proceed at another laser clinic that is cheaper, and therefore, client satisfaction will be nominal.

Mind-Set and Aim of Treatment

Some clients may from the start decide on a partial tattoo removal simply to fade the existing motif to acquire a cover-up tattoo thereafter. A cover-up tattoo is a newly applied tattoo covering the original tattoo. Clients should be informed about the vulnerable condition of the skin after laser treatments. A new cover-up tattoo can be associated with prevalent complications, and the healing of the cover-up tattoo may be delayed.

The Tattoo – Can It Be Removed?

Tattoo colour, anatomical site, status of tattooists (professional/amateur), and length of time with the tattoo can influence treatment result and clients' rating of satisfaction. Effectiveness relative to tattoo colour was rated on a visual analogue scale from 0 (no effect) to 10 (complete removal), and clients scored a mean of 9.5 (blue), 9.3 (black), 8.8 (red), 8.5 (yellow), and 6.5 (green). Clients with green colour rated their overall satisfaction rather low, even though all other colours in the tattoo were completely removed, because they felt the green ink remnants resembled a bruise. The anatomical site may also affect treatment results since treatment on tattoos localised in thin skin, e.g. the lower inner arm, may easily result in scarring. The skin on the chest and shoulders is also predisposed to scarring. Usually, amateurs install pigments deeper than professional tattooists, and amateur tattoos are therefore more difficult to remove.

Previous Treatments

Some clients may have had previous laser treatments on their tattoos at other clinics. In the above-mentioned study, 18% had received laser treatments at other clinics prior to treatments at the 'Centre for Laser Surgery'. Reasons for changing clinic were low effectiveness of treatments, advice from friends and family, lower price of treatment, and neighbouring vicinity to the Centre.

Indications and Contraindications

Health problems and pregnancy are factors that the laser surgeon cannot alter. Pregnant and lactating women should never receive laser treatment because of the potential risk of fragmented ink particles and formation of photochemical breakdown products after laser treatment [15, 16]. Patients with health conditions, e.g. diabetes, heart problem, epilepsy, relevant skin disease, pathological scar formation, photosensitivity, and allergic reaction, may also not be treated due to health risks. Clients with a low pain threshold may be unable to fulfil a treatment course.

Laser removal of inflammatory tattoo complications is a field of special concern. Allergic reactions in red tattoos are a relative contraindication, as laser treatment can boost the allergic reaction [17–20]. Figure 2 shows an allergic reaction in a red tattoo. Complications worsened after laser treatments.

Abnormal personality and psychiatric disorders may also contraindicate tattoo removal.

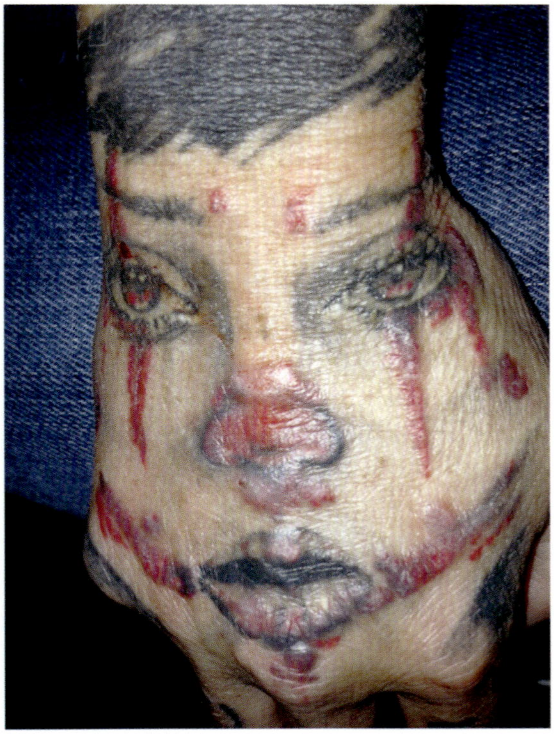

Fig. 2. A patient with an allergic reaction in a red tattoo on the right hand, treated with laser, which resulted in relapse of allergy and posttreatment scarring. Laser treatment was performed by a provider who was not a medical doctor. The patient was afterwards treated with dermatome shaving and intralesional corticoid at Bispebjerg University Hospital. Photo provided by Bispebjerg University Hospital.

Client Suited or Unsuited?

The decision on whether a client is suited for laser treatment should be taken after objective observations and determining the client's pretreatment expectations, but it should also be influenced by the quality of the interaction between the client and surgeon. The interaction should be built on mutual confidence and trust. Suitable clients must be presented with pretreatment information before their acceptance for enrolment.

Pretreatment Information

Pretreatment information is essential for the client to accept laser treatment and also legally important. Apart from general information on laser treatment, more detailed information should be conveyed concerning advantages and disadvantages for each specific tattoo to be removed. It is normal routine that laser surgeons provide the following basic information to clients before the first treatment:

1 Treatment: immediately after laser treatment, the treated area will appear white. This is normally a sign of good laser light absorption by the ink [21]. The skin will be sore, with oedema and peeling, but within 7 days the skin will heal.

2 After treatment: the tattoo will begin to fade after the process of wound healing. This process may take weeks until the skin has recovered, whereby an interval of at least 6 weeks between treatment sessions is recommended.

In the original article, 84% experienced moderate to extreme pain during treatment [13]. Thus, information to the client about pain is necessary before treatment. Applying ice as a routine procedure can relieve pain during and after treatments.

The primary objective is to remove the tattoo without a blemish. Adverse effects may occur, e.g. scarring, hypo- and hyperpigmentation (fig. 3). The risk of scarring is low when lasers are used up to professional standard, but clients may have scarring from the tattoo procedure, which becomes visible during the course of treatment [21].

Surgeon-Client Interactions

The surgeon-client interaction is important and will most likely influence the clients' acceptance of treatment, experiences during treatments, and satisfaction afterwards.

The level of trust is essential. It is of course important that laser surgeons are well educated and experienced. The use of laser equipment by an in-

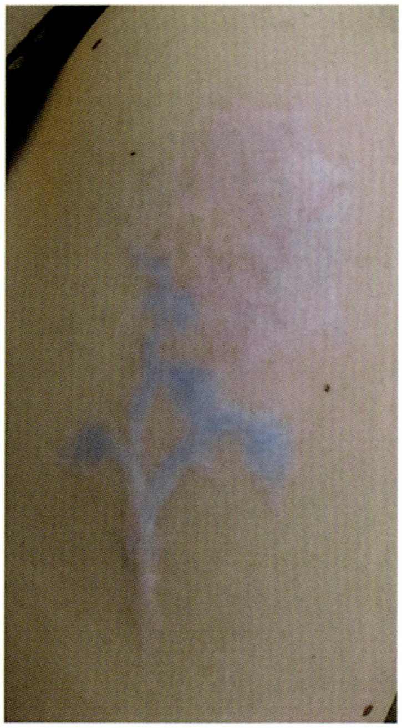

Fig. 3. The shoulder of a woman who had received laser treatments by an operator who was not a medical doctor. The treatment resulted in scarring and hypopigmentation. She was afterwards treated with dermatome shaving at Bispebjerg University Hospital. During shaving, a previous tattoo with pigments deep in the dermis became visible. The final treatment outcome was not satisfactory. Photo provided by Bispebjerg University Hospital.

experienced layperson (cosmetologist, tattooist, private nurse) can result in numerous complications [22]. Competence and professional style from start to end of treatment course should be provided.

Suggestions:

- Provide both oral and written information. Information on tattoo removal by laser should consist of personal letter format information.
- Clients appreciate being listened to, understood, and treated in a polite and friendly atmosphere. Be aware of the mind-set of the client who can be nervous, unrealistic, critical, neglectant, or very sensitive to pain.
- Motivate clients prior to laser treatments, e.g. acquaint clients with images of positive and poor outcomes from other clients.
- Older and faded tattoos are easier to remove. Knowledge of tattoos' age can be helpful in estimating required laser treatments. The professional laser surgeon should have the personal ability to inform and instruct clients in a manner where expectations are met on both sides. Unrealistic expectations and goals concerning tattoo removal will result in a dissatisfied and frustrated clientele.
- Tattoos can be very difficult to remove completely; therefore, do not exaggerate forthcoming treatment results. Note that multicoloured tattoos, hereby green, require numerous treatments and may be impossible to remove with a satisfactory outcome. If possible, avoid laser treatment on white-coloured tattoos. Paradoxical ink darkening may occur due to colour change (titanium dioxide) [15].
- Always enquire as to whether a tattoo is a cover-up tattoo before initiating removal, since other colours may be concealed underneath.
- Align the burden and side effects of treatment, e.g. short-term complications such as infections, and long-term complications such as dyspigmentation, scarring, and ink retention [15].
- Gain information on previous treatments: at which clinic, number of treatments, reason for changing clinic, and colours responding to or not responding to treatment. This information will give an indication of the difficulty in removing the tattoo, level and depth of ink pigment, and whether the client has too high expectations.
- In certain cases, when estimating the number of treatments required for removing a tattoo, it can be beneficial to give an estimate a little higher than expected. The client will be more content when treatment is completed with fewer treatments and thereby save both time and money.

- Tattoo laser removal can be very expensive. Sometimes discounts can be granted depending on the surgeons' opinion and policy.
- Information on the price of treatments should have second priority. It is often preferable that results and price of treatment be discussed after initial examination, but some clients may wish to have the price issue clarified up-front. It is important to give the client a precise and realistic price from the start. Some tattoos may require more laser treatments than others, making a precise price estimate difficult. The price per laser treatment may be preferred instead of a total price for a complete treatment course.
- Take photos prior to the first and after the last laser treatment session to avoid misunderstandings and disputes. Photos prior to treatment should be of high quality and taken under standardised conditions, including close-up images. Photos after the last treatment are useful both to document results and for the laser surgeon's own production control.

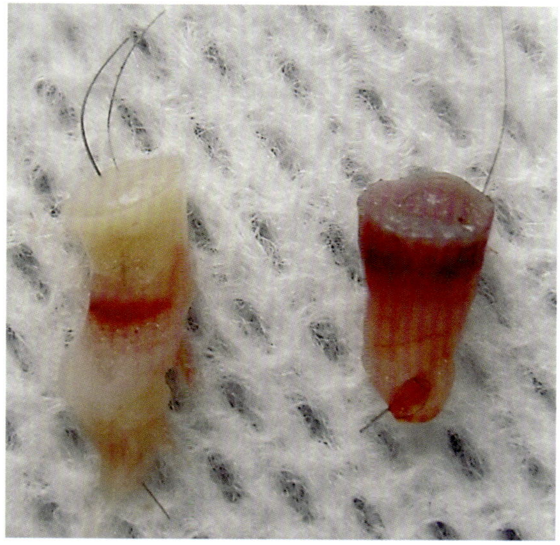

Fig. 4. Raw punch biopsies from 2 tattoos. Left: after laser treatment; pigment in lower dermis not bleached. Right: before laser treatment; pigment is concentrated in the outer dermis. Photo provided by Bispebjerg University Hospital.

Client Acceptance or Nonacceptance?

By following the suggested steps in figure 1, the client is now prepared to decide whether he/she accepts the terms and receives laser treatments on the tattoo. Gain formal signed consent from the client before treatment start. Nonacceptance should be respected and persuasion to change of mind discouraged.

Treatment Course

Obviously, treatment results affect the clients' degree of satisfaction and will benefit with state of the art technology and relevant settings. The precise number of treatments and passes influence the degree of client satisfaction. It is the laser surgeon's decision, as a specialist, to select equipment and settings.

The effect of laser treatment is dependent on the amount of ink deposited, the depth of ink in the dermis, and skin thickness (fig. 4). Pigments deep in the dermis may be beyond the bounds for lasers. In allergic tattoo reactions, these pigments will cause relapse.

Old amateur tattoos and tattoos containing little ink are easier to remove and require fewer laser treatments compared to tattoos heavily packed with ink, e.g. over-tattooed skin [9]. Fortunately, tattoo pigments often relocate in the dermis and concentrate in the outer dermis, where laser light is effective.

Some clients will discontinue their tattoo removal course due to pain, disappointing effect, complications, economic reasons, or distance to the clinic.

Suggestions:

The laser surgeon has two important roles; one is mastering the technique and the operation, the other one is being a tutor and educating the client.

- Follow what is 'state of art' and considered good practice. Respect contraindications.
- Use optimal equipment and settings, and cool skin to reduce pain. It is imperative that the surgeon has experience with the equipment being used.
- Time spent with the client, during the entire treatment course, is an opportunity for continuing education of the client. Respect individual needs of the client and respond to upcoming issues during the process. The client comes from pretreatment expectations and thoughts, and through direct experience in dialogue with the surgeon, the client will during the course of treatment gain much more insight in the process of treatment and the logic outcomes.

Posttreatment Problems

Posttreatment problems, e.g. early and long-term problems, may occur. Infections are only seen as early problems compared to scarring, hypo- and hyperpigmentation, and remaining pigment, which may be visible, both at early and long-term stages [6, 7, 11]. These problems are well known to laser surgeons.

Suggestions:

- Misunderstandings concerning complications and less acceptable results can be helped by showing photos taken prior to treatment as a reference.
- Handling dissatisfied clients: be empathic, careful, and polite, and offer a follow-up consultation or refer the client to an independent dermatologist for a second opinion.

Client Posttreatment Satisfaction

In the original article, clients rated their overall assessment from 'superb', very good, fairly well, acceptable, inferior, and rather poor to unacceptable [13]. 85% of clients rated their treatment and results to be acceptable to superb, while 15% rated their treatment and results to be inferior to unacceptable due to ink retention or complications.

Only 1/3 of the clients (30%) rated their satisfaction to be 'superb', contrasting 2/3 of clients (66%) who expected complete removal without a blemish before treatment. Overall, the majority of clients were satisfied with treatment. This illustrates that clients had adapted a more realistic view during the treatment course.

Discussion

The laser surgeon has many roles. The main role is to provide technically high-standard treatment with selection of optimal equipment and settings and thereby remove the tattoo as efficiently as possible. The other role is to master the interaction with the client at a personal level in a positive, respectful, and mutual manner during the full laser treatment course. The laser treatment course is a learning process for the client with the laser surgeon as the tutor. Likewise, it is also a learning process for the laser surgeon who should be aware of relevant personal details of the persons being treated. The client should generally have a positive experience from the treatment course, and by observing the attempt to remove the tattoo, most clients will learn, respect, and accept if their tattoo could not be removed successfully despite having a qualified laser surgeon. They will hopefully see this as an inferiority of methodology relative to the tattoo and finally achieve acceptance with the result, albeit at a lower level than expected.

References

1 Haedersdal M, Bech-Thomsen N, Wulf HC: Skin reflectance-guided laser selections for treatment of decorative tattoos. Arch Dermatol 1996;132:403–407.

2 Biesman BS, O'Neil MP, Costner C: Rapid, high-fluence multi-pass q-switched laser treatment of tattoos with a transparent perfluorodecalin-infused patch: a pilot study. Lasers Surg Med 2015;47:613–618.

3 Reddy KK, Brauer JA, Anolik R, Bernstein L, Brightman L, Hale E, Karen J, Weiss E, Geronemus RG: Topical perfluorodecalin resolves immediate whitening reactions and allows rapid effective multiple pass treatment of tattoos. Lasers Surg Med 2013;45:76–80.

4 Kossida T, Rigopoulos D, Katsambas A, Anderson RR: Optimal tattoo removal in a single laser session based on the method of repeated exposures. J Am Acad Dermatol 2012;66:271–277.

5 Sardana K, Ranjan R, Chakravarty P, Goel K, Tenani A, Madan A: Pigmented lesions and tattoos; in Sardana K, Garg VK (eds): Lasers in Dermatological Practice, ed 1. New Delhi, Jaypee Brothers Medical Publishers (P) Ltd, 2014, pp 101–171.

6 Barua S: Laser-tissue interaction in tattoo removal by q-switched lasers. J Cutan Aesthet Surg 2015;8:5–8.

7 Weiss ET, Geronemus RG: Combining fractional resurfacing and Q-switched ruby laser for tattoo removal. Dermatol Surg 2011;37:97–99.

8 Aurangabadkar SJ: Shifting paradigm in laser tattoo removal. J Cutan Aesthet Surg 2015;8:3–4.

9 Mankowska A, Kasprzak W, Adamski Z: Long-term evaluation of ink clearance in tattoos with different color intensity using the 1,064-nm Q-switched Nd:YAG laser. J Cosmet Dermatol 2015;14:302–309.

10 Sardana K, Ranjan R, Ghunawat S: Optimising laser tattoo removal. J Cutan Aesthet Surg 2015;8:16–24.

11 Serup J, Harrit N, Linnet JT, Møhl B, Olsen O, Westh H: Tattoos – Health, Risks and Culture. The Council on Health and Disease Prevention, Copenhagen, 2015. www.vidensraad.dk

12 Serup J, Kluger N, Bäumler W (eds): Tattooed Skin and Health. Curr Probl Dermatol. Karger, Basel, 2015, vol 48.

13 Hutton Carlsen K, Esmann J, Serup J: Tattoo removal by Q-switched YAG laser: client satisfaction. Questionnaire follow-up assessment of 154 clients. J Eur Acad Derm 2017, in print.

14 Davis SA (ed): Adherence in Dermatology. Switzerland, Springer International Publishing, 2016, pp 3–178.

15 Eklund Y, Rubin AT: Laser tattoo removal, precautions, and unwanted effects; in Serup J, Kluger N, Bäumler W (eds): Tattooed Skin and Health. Curr Probl Dermatol. Basel, Karger, 2015, vol 48, pp 88–96.

16 Vasold R, Naarmann N, Ulrich H, Fischer D, König B, Landthaler M, Bäumler W: Tattoo pigments are cleaved by laser light-the chemical analysis in vitro provide evidence for hazardous compounds. Photochem Photobiol 2004;80:185–190.

17 Ashinoff R, Levine VJ, Soter NA: Allergic reactions to tattoo pigment after laser treatment. Dermatol Surg 1995;21:291–294.

18 Izikson L, Avram M, Anderson RR: Transient immunoreactivity after laser tattoo removal: report of two cases. Lasers Surg Med 2008;40:231–232.

19 Ibrahimi OA, Syed Z, Sakamoto FH, Avram MM, Anderson RR: Treatment of tattoo allergy with ablative fractional resurfacing: a novel paradigm for tattoo removal. J Am Acad Dermatol 2011;64:111–114.

20 Harper J, Losch AE, Otto SG, Zirwas M, Delaney KO, Wakelin JK: New insight into the pathophysiology of tattoo reactions following laser tattoo removal. Plast Reconstr Surg 2010;126:313–314.

21 Karsai S, Raulin C: Laser treatment of tattoos and other dyschromia; in Raulin C, Karsai S (eds): Laser and IPL Technology in Dermatology and Aesthetic Medicine. Springer, Berlin, Heidelberg, 2011, pp 189–202.

22 Karsai S, Krieger G, Raulin C: Tattoo removal by non-professionals – medical and forensic considerations. J Eur Acad Dermatol Venereol 2010;24:756–762.

Katrina Hutton Carlsen
The 'Tattoo Clinic', Department of Dermatology, Bispebjerg University Hospital
Bispebjerg Bakke 23
DK–2400 Copenhagen (Denmark)
E-Mail Katrinahuttoncarlsen@hotmail.com

Serup J, Bäumler W (eds): Diagnosis and Therapy of Tattoo Complications. With Atlas of Illustrative Cases.
Curr Probl Dermatol. Basel, Karger, 2017, vol 52, pp 132–138 (DOI: 10.1159/000452966)

Guide to Treatment of Tattoo Complications and Tattoo Removal

Jørgen Serup[a] • Wolfgang Bäumler[b]

[a]The 'Tattoo Clinic', Department of Dermatology, Bispebjerg University Hospital, Copenhagen, Denmark;
[b]Department of Dermatology, University of Regensburg, Regensburg, Germany

Abstract

Clinicians in the fields of general medicine, dermatology, and plastic surgery are in their work now and then confronted with tattoo complications. Recognizing the rather few important diagnostic groups and urgencies, the medical 'decision tree' of treatment becomes quite simple. Acute conditions are dominated by bacterial infections needing antibiotic treatment. Systemic infection is a matter of urgency and requires intravenous treatment in a hospital without delay to prevent septic shock. Inflammatory reactions are a real challenge. Chronic allergic reactions in red tattoos are mostly nonresponsive to topical corticoid and best treated with dermatome shaving with complete removal of the hapten concentrated in the outer dermis. Laser treatment of allergic reactions can boost the allergy with worsening and a potential risk of anaphylaxis and is thus *not* recommended in tattoo allergy. Chronic papulonodular reactions in black tattoos with pigment agglomeration can respond to local corticoid or be treated with dermatome shaving or lasers depending on availability. It is important to recognize sarcoidosis, which is strongly associated with reactions in black tattoos. Tattoo complications also include many rare but specific entities, which require individual treatment depending on the case and the disease mechanism. Removal of tattoos in individuals regretting their tattoo is performed using Q-switched nanosecond lasers and the recently introduced picosecond lasers. In view of the various tattoo pigments with different absorption spectra and the limited number of laser wavelengths, it is difficult to predict treatment outcome, and it is recommended to pretreat small test spots. Black and red colors are removed best, while other colors are difficult. Removal of large tattoos, especially when multicolored, is hardly achievable and not recommended. Clients often have unrealistic expectations, and informed consent and dialogue between the client and the laser surgeon before and during a treatment course is important since the client shall know the risk that removal can be unsuccessful, with complications and even disfiguring leading to regret at the end.

The treatment of tattoos in clinics and hospitals is grouped into 2 major categories, namely treatment of medical complications and treatment of patients who regret their tattoo due to change of mind and fashion. The following guide to treatment follows this main distinction.

Treatment of Medical Complications

Proper diagnosis is a paramount need behind choice of rational treatment, which in this field is widely empiric due to the paucity of systematic studies. An armamentarium of diagnostic approaches and methods is described in the chapter by Serup [this vol., pp. 42–57]. In the chapter by Serup [this vol., pp. 58–73] a modern concept of diagnostic classification of the broad spectrum of tattoo complications is presented with definitions and clues to diagnosis. There are many entities of very different causes and mechanisms.

In the clinic a major distinction is made between complications, which are acute, chronic, local in the tattoo, regional, generalized in the skin, or systemic, the latter possibly with impairment of the general condition and, ultimately, life threatening.

Acute Complications
Acute complications happen during and immediately after tattooing or during the phase of healing. There are a number of conditions, which can make the person faint during tattooing, with pain, exhaustion, dehydration, and hypoglycemia as the commonest reasons. *Syncope* due to cordial disease or epilepsy can happen as casualties needing hospital treatment. *Bacterial infections*, local, regional, and systemic, are by far the largest group and require treatment with oral or intravenous antibiotics [see chapter by Serup, this vol., pp. 30–41]. In systemic infection institution of treatment is urgent and critically needed. *Allergic reactions* with severe generalized rash within a day after tattooing in persons with a known strong allergy to nickel, and after a few weeks in primary sensitization against preservatives and other new contact allergens, may require oral prednisone followed by other immunosuppressant. *Allergy to latex* provoked by tattooists' gloves is exceptional but dangerous with risk of anaphylactic collapse. Urticarial reactions to tattoos are discussed under Chronic Complications. *Photosensitivity reactions* of dark-colored tattoos are rather common as a mild and sometimes acute complaint [see chapter by Serup, this vol., pp. 18–29], but reactions can be chronically intermittent and reach the burden of disease. Treatment is standard physical and chemical photo protection as recommended for photosensitive skin. *Burning sensation during magnetic resonance scanning* is acute and may interrupt scanning. Often it is followed by inflammation for a few hours, but it is not a thermal burn, thus ulceration has not been reported. Burning sensation is predominantly seen in cosmetic tattoos in the sensitive periorbital skin.

Chronic Complications
Chronic complications are mostly local in the tattoo but sometimes there are manifestations of systemic disease.

Inflammatory tattoo reaction is by far the largest group. The separation of inflammatory reactions into allergic and nonallergic cases is essential and critical in the choice of proper treatment and, thus, must be sharp. The distinction is guided by the color of the tattoo and by the specific clinical pattern [see chapter by Serup, this vol., pp. 58–73]. *Allergic reactions* are very often seen in red tattoos or in nuances of red affecting every part of the tattoo of that particular color at the same time, with 'plaque elevation' (in the past given the imprecise label 'lichenoid reaction'), with 'excessive hyperkeratosis', and with ulcerating affections with dermal necrosis if allergy is strong. Therapeutic response to local corticoids very often is poor, and reactions remain cumbersome. Some dermatologists may favor intralesional corticoid; however, such treatment is symptomatic, needs repeated injections, and may easily cause skin atrophy. As in other cutaneous allergies, the fundamental treatment is elimination of the allergen, in this case a hapten formed in the dermis over time. Pigment and hapten are located in the outer part of the dermis, and therefore surgery with dermatome shaving is rational and positioned as the first-line treatment [see chapter by Sepehri and Jørgensen, this vol., pp. 82–93]. Dermatome shaving is documented in recent research. Surgical excision is only feasible in some cases and may require coverage with a transplant. Surgical excision often leaves ugly scars that cannot be fixed contrasting acceptable scarring after dermatome shaving with the option to have a cover-up tattoo. In *allergic cross-reaction* with accompanying reactions of old tattoos triggered by a fresh allergic reaction in a red tattoo, the reacting tattoo(s) normally need no treatment. Spontaneous regression occurs once the trigger tattoo has undergone full removal of the pigment hapten from the skin by surgery. *Laser removal of allergic tattoo reactions should be seen as contraindicated* due to the risk of laser light-induced photochemical breakdown of pigment boosting the allergy, with worsening and the reported potential risk of anaphylaxis. Pretreatments such as antihistamine and oral corticoid cannot eliminate this risk. Laser clinics are not equipped for, not staffed for, and not experienced in treating severe allergy with acute cardiovascular collapse. Furthermore, lasers are an incoherent multiple-spot treatment of uncertain depth control, thus as a method not able to produce the consequent, supervised, and clean-cut removal of pigment obtained with a dermatome, which slice by slice removes the outer skin to a desired level under the pigment. Red pigment can absorb laser light of YAG laser systems, but blue, green, and yellow are mostly poor absorbers. Allergic reactions seldom may occur in blue, green, violet, purple, and yellow tattoos. *Nonallergic reactions* are predominant in black tattoos with only some parts of the tattoo being affected with variably sized papules and nodules, i.e. with the 'papulonodular' pattern [see chapter by Serup, this vol., pp. 58–73]. The severity of the reaction depends on the dose of black pigment in the dermis and the pigment's tendency to spontaneous aggregation and formation of pigment foreign bodies in the skin causing the inflammation. Sometimes reactions respond to local corticoids, which should be tried as first-line treatment.

Cumbersome reactions of high pigment density are best treated with dermatome shaving or with Q-switched nanosecond lasers and picosecond lasers depending on what methods are available and feasible also considering the anatomical site and tattooed area [see chapters in this vol. by Sepehri and Jørgensen, pp. 82–93; Karsai, pp. 105–112; Adatto et al., pp. 113–123]. With black tattoos there is no concern regarding use of lasers and potential risk of provoking allergy. Black pigment is a strong absorber of light and the favorite color of laser surgeons.

Tattooing is directly accompanied by obligatory traumatic urticarial reactions due to the multiple needle pricks of tattooing, a condition not needing any treatment or any special precaution [see chapter by Serup, this vol., pp. 18–29]. *Chronic urticaria* after tattooing can be active for several months, very cumbersome, and require treatment with antihistamines in normal, double, or triple dose, which nevertheless often are of limited benefit. Oral prednisone dosed individually is often efficient and can be supplemented with cyclosporine or another immunosuppressant for long-term control. There is no experience with the biologic omalizumab on this indication.

A simplified 'decision tree' with suggested therapies of inflammatory tattoo reactions is presented in table 1. The table summarizes experiences from the 'Tattoo Clinic' obtained in more than 500 patients.

Tattoo reactions representing *uncommon and specific entities* [see chapter by Serup, this vol., pp. 58–73] are treated depending on the suggested cause of the problem and the mechanism behind the manifestation. For example, an abnormal scar after traumatic tattooing with hazardous needle damage to the skin and sensory hypersensitivity with chronic hyperalgesia and invalidating pain in a tattoo require very different approaches, depending on the specific case. *Keratoacanthoma* is

Table 1. Therapy of inflammatory tattoo reactions: simplified 'decision tree' and hypothetical pathology

Local in the tattoo	
Allergic reaction[a] (mainly red color*), chronic	
Local corticoid (occlusive, intralesional)	1
Dermatome shaving	1
Surgical excision	2
Prednisone/immunosuppressant	3
No laser	
Cross-reactions[a] in other red tattoos, allergic[1]	
Eliminate trigger tattoo, no treatment observation of reacting tattoos	1
Local corticoid*	2
Nonallergic inflammation[b] (mainly black color), chronic	
Local corticoid	1
Dermatome shaving	2
Laser removal	2
Photosensitivity (dark colors), intermittent	
Sun screen (chemical and physical)	1
Local corticoid	2
Generalized in the skin or systemic	
Allergic rash (any color**), acute	
Prednisone	1
Immunosuppressant	2
Urticaria (any color***), chronic	
Antihistamine	1
Prednisone	2
Immunosuppressant	3
Sarcoidosis[c] (black color****), chronic	
Prednisone	1
Local corticoid	1
Immunosuppressant	2
Dermatome shaving	3
Laser removal	3
'Rush phenomenon' in other black tattoos, autoimmune[2]	
Prednisone	1
Local corticoid	2

The numbers in the second column indicate treatment priority 1, 2, and 3. Priority may depend on local availability of treatment.

[a] Manifested as plaque elevation (lichenoid) pattern or excessive hyperkeratosis. Ulceronecrotic allergy shall be observed, surgery contraindicated. [b] Manifested as papulonodular reaction pattern. [c] Manifested as a papulonodular reaction (a special subgroup with granulomatous reaction or sarcoid granuloma in the tattoo by histology).

* Caused by pigment-related hapten made in the skin over time; allergic reactions are widely resistant to local corticoid given as open application. ** Suggested to be caused by nonpigment ingredients of ink (preservatives, etc.), contaminants (nickel, etc.), or soluble pigment breakdown products. *** Cause of allergy unknown; self-limiting and thus unlikely to be due to insoluble pigment. **** Caused by large pigment aggregates with suggested adjuvant effect resulting in autoimmunity, systemic activation, and sometimes manifest sarcoidosis.

[1] Local tattoo reaction (trigger) in a recent tattoo followed by widespread allergic reactions in older tattooos of red color (reacting tattoos) hitherto tolerated. [2] Local tattoo reaction (trigger) in a recent tattoo followed by abrupt and widespread autoimmune reactions in older tattooos of black color (reacting tattoos) hitherto tolerated; may be paralleled by other signs of active sarcoidosis in skin and internal organs.

clinically benign and is best observed until spontaneous regression occurs, which typically happens after a few months. *Skin cancers in tattoos* are considered coincidental and not related to the tattoo pigment and thus treated following common standards in skin oncology. There is no indication that radiotherapy and tattoo pigment interact. Photodynamic therapy can be influenced by the light-absorbing tattoo pigment and contribute to the already quite strong tissue response and the pain associated with this treatment. Furthermore, tattoo pigment may screen the light and in cancers invading the dermis reduce the effect of the treatment. Such screen may be significant in the perilesional skin of the cancer when the cancer is progressing subclinically and horizontally in the outer dermis. The tattoo shall not be considered a premalignant lesion, and the local site of the treated tumor shall be followed according to normal skin cancer checkup standard. Incidentally tattooed benign nevi in a larger tattoo later in life transformed into malignant melanoma shall be treated following general standards. Over-tattooed and thus camouflaged nevi carry the risk that malignant transformation and development of malignant melanoma later in life become diagnosed too late. Sentinel lymph nodes can be dark-colored due to tattoo pigment, thereby simulating regional metastasis of melanoma and complicating radical surgery.

Chronic complications also may include *hepatitis B and C*, which may need up-to-date medical treatment used in infectious medicine [see chapter by Serup, this vol., pp. 30–41]. *HIV infection* introduced by a tattoo is rare. In some countries inoculation of endemic infections by tattooing is an issue requiring treatment according to local expertise. Chronic infection of the tattoo with environmental mycobacteria, especially *Mycobacterium chelonae*, is a very uncommon infection highlighted in the literature but nevertheless rare. Infection may occur as local outbreaks. Relevant antimycobacterial treatment for a period of several months with a combination of drugs according to local microbiologists' recommendation is required.

Tattoo reaction and systemic disease are dominated by the *association between papulonodular reactions of black tattoos and sarcoidosis* affecting the tattoo, internal organs, and other parts of the skin with scar sarcoidosis and erythema nodosum sometimes occurring at the same time [see chapter by Serup, this vol., pp. 58–73]. The association is strong and with autoimmunity as the suggested linkage. The treatment of the local tattoo reactions showing granulomatous reaction or sarcoid granuloma by histology is primarily local corticoid, which may ameliorate symptoms without clearing reactions. In associated systemic disease the preferred treatment is oral prednisone, methotrexate, and another immunosuppressant. Internists should be involved. In the 'rush phenomenon', with abrupt reaction in any black tattoo all over the skin following the onset in a recent black tattoo, oral prednisone is the drug of choice and efficient. The *Koebner phenomenon* in patients with psoriasis with a psoriasis replica overlapping a fresh tattoo is treated with local corticoid or left for spontaneous healing over a few months. The association of psoriasis and tattoo is limited to newly acquired tattoos, and there is no real evidence that a tattoo can provoke psoriasis in other parts of the skin. In general worsening of psoriasis, a tattoo of course can be affected by coincidence, and treatment is then directed toward relieving psoriasis by appropriate routine treatment.

Laser Removal in Tattoo Regret

The use of lasers to treat abnormal tattoo reactions is discussed in the previous section. The following guide is directed towards treatment of normal tattoos that the person wishes to be removed due to plain regret or due to social incompetence experienced by the person in his/her private life or professional career necessitating the removal if technically achievable. Historical methods, such as chemical caustics and dermabrasion, have been replaced by modern lasers of the nonablative type, which may selectively eradicate the pigment in the skin without causing significant harm to the normal tissue. The basic principles of laser therapy are explained in the chapter by Bäumler [this vol., pp. 94–104]. Laser surgeons shall master their device and based on their skills and experience from the start make the best possible prediction of benefit and risk by treating the particular case [see chapter by Hutton Carlsen et al., this vol., pp. 124–131]. Clients request laser removal with intuitively high expectations, but about 1/3 of clients will not reach acceptable removal of the tattoo, despite the surgeons having done their very best. The surgeon shall continuously educate and challenge the client during the progress of the treatment course in the direction of realistic expectations adjusted relative to treatment experience obtained in the client, aiming at satisfaction or acceptance by the client at the end of a completed or interrupted treatment course [see chapter by Hutton Carlsen et al., this vol., pp. 124–131]. Some people with tattoo regret will regret laser removal and end up with a disfigured tattoo with some colors removed and others disturbed, blurred, or unaffected. While most of the black tattoos fade upon laser treatment, the reaction of colored tattoos is frequently unpredictable. *It is always good advice to pretreat small test spots and read lightening effect of the laser before the entire tattoo is approached.* Some individuals having smaller black tattoos can obtain a visibly complete removal with perfectly intact skin texture. In some tattoos, changes of skin texture and pigmentation may appear when the tattoo ink disappears. These changes are usually caused by the tattooing needles and not by laser treatment. The *informed consent* of the client is very important. Clients shall from the start understand and engage in shared risk taking, together with the laser surgeon. Some clients shall be denied treatment.

Today, the *Q-switched nanosecond YAG laser* is the gold standard method for tattoo removal [see chapter by Karsai, this vol., pp. 105–112]. It operates with very short pulses and thus can spare the normal tissue with less risk of scarring and dyspigmentation. This laser is primarily applicable to black and red tattoos. Blue, green, and yellow tattoos are more difficult to remove, or they cannot be removed. Laser irradiation of some tattoo pigments can cause photochemical changes of these pigments, white tattoos can turn into black color and so can tattoos made with iron pigments. Since iron pigments are commonly used in cosmetic tattoo inks, laser removal of tattoos in the orbital region can be especially unpredictable with the laser worsening the problem. The new *picosecond lasers* working with even shorter pulse durations have the potential to be more efficient with less harm to normal tissue and thus may have a better risk-to-benefit ratio [see chapter by Adatto et al., this vol., pp. 113–123]. This also implicates that this type of laser can do the job with fewer treatment sessions. The 2 types of lasers are comparable regarding wavelength versus absorbance of tattoo pigments, and benefits are mainly related to the delivery and dosing of the laser light into the skin. The preference of equipment is presently much dependent on local availability and the economy involved.

There are other types of lasers applied to tattoo removal, and such lasers may expand the range of tattoo colors, which can be treated. However, this is not a promising field and a field for laser specialists. The CO_2 laser, which is ablative and unlimited burns all tissues and pigments irrespective of color, can be used to ultimately remove any tattoo but it always leaves scars, which easily can be advanced and hypertrophic. This laser is only used for critical tattoo removal on very special indications with the client fully accepting scarring as the foreseeable outcome. Fractional CO_2 lasers, which treat the skin with narrow vertical tunnels and practically leave no scar, are sometimes used on special indications supplementary to the Q-switched nanosecond laser. This recent type of laser system has not found a defined indication in relation to laser removal. Argon lasers used in the past are today considered obsolete for tattoo removal.

Intense pulsed light (IPL) is a high-power broad-band nonlaser light that with limited control burns any tissue and thus very easily causes scarring. The treatment of small tattoo pigment particles in the skin requires pulse durations of nanoseconds or picoseconds. Being no laser, the IPL technology provides a pulse duration in the range of a few milliseconds only. Thus, the pigment particle would be heated way too long and the excessive heat would cause collateral damage in the adjacent tissue yielding a high rate of severe side effects. The IPL method, which may be offered by nonprofessional clinics in the tattoo removal business, should not be practiced on this indication.

Commentary

The tattoo removal market which, besides lasers, offers a broad spectrum of claimed treatments, including various topical remedies and injectables, such as lactic acid and other caustics, is generally poorly regulated or not regulated at all. There is no formal quality of care standard a customer can refer to or rely on. The removal marked is price sensitive, and lasers are positioned expensive. The business is a mix of many amateurs and fewer professionals. The legal position of a client making a wrong choice of provider and method of removal, laser, or other method, with a bad result and sometimes severe and disfiguring sequel is very poor. The generalist doctor on request and in the guiding of his/her patient should be aware of this situation and encourage the patient, or client, to be critical and go for professionalism, recognized method, technical skill, and ethical standard of the provider rather than a low price of the delivery.

Prof. Jørgen Serup, DMSc
Department of Dermatology D41, Bispebjerg University Hospital
Bispebjerg Bakke 23
DK–2400 Copenhagen NV (Denmark)
E-Mail joergen.vedelskov.serup@regionh.dk

Serup J, Bäumler W (eds): Diagnosis and Therapy of Tattoo Complications. With Atlas of Illustrative Cases.
Curr Probl Dermatol. Basel, Karger, 2017, vol 52, pp 139–229 (DOI: 10.1159/000453379)

Atlas of Illustrative Cases of Tattoo Complications

Jørgen Serup

The 'Tattoo Clinic', Department of Dermatology, Bispebjerg University Hospital, Copenhagen, Denmark

Abstract

Tattoos, and tattoo complications as well, are colorful and visually flashy. A clinical outlook provides important clues to diagnosis by pattern recognition. This atlas, which is a report of 79 case illustrations, is made as a practical tool and vade mecum for the clinician. The atlas can be used in the office and as a bedside tool. It includes characteristic photos, and each case is accompanied with a brief medical history, a comment with learning points, the final diagnosis, and a review of therapeutic options. This spectrum of cases illustrates the different diagnostic entities according to the newly proposed Bispebjerg University Hospital ('Tattoo Clinic') diagnostic system of tattoo complications, a system reported to the 11th revision of the WHO disease classification system. Cases include allergies predominantly seen in red tattoos manifesting the characteristic patterns of plaque elevation, excessive hyperkeratosis, ulcerating reactions, urticaria, and generalized skin rash. Each type of reaction has typical clues to diagnosis and a typical disease course. 'Cross-sensitivity' allergic reactions in old tattoos of the same color as the trigger tattoo are also illustrated. Reactions in black tattoos are dominated by a pattern with papulonodular reactions, which are nonallergic and due to pigment agglomeration in the skin. Reactions may be granulomatous and a marker of systemic sarcoidosis, sometimes associated with a general outbreak in the skin in black tattoos, e.g. 'rush phenomenon'. Bacterial infections are also illustrated. The technical hazards of tattooing and sequels as well as unwanted effects of tattoo removal by lasers are shown along with severe scarring following tattoo removal by caustics. This atlas is a tutorial in modern medical and surgical treatments of tattoo complications.

Prof. Jørgen Serup, DMSc
Department of Dermatology D41, Bispebjerg University Hospital
Bispebjerg Bakke 23
DK–2400 Copenhagen NV (Denmark)
E-Mail joergen.vedelskov.serup@regionh.dk

The Bispebjerg University Hospital ('Tattoo Clinic') diagnostic system of tattoo complications used throughout the atlas is described in a separate chapter of this book [this vol., pp. 58–73]. Definitions and delineations of the different distinctive patterns illustrated in the atlas are presented in that chapter. Therapeutic options are reviewed in other chapters of the book and summarized with a guide to treatment of tattoo complications and removal [this vol., pp. 132–138].

The original research publications behind the diagnostic classification system are:

Serup J, Sepehri M, Hutton Carlsen K: Classification of tattoo complications in a hospital material of 493 adverse events. Dermatology 2017, DOI 10.1159/000452148.

Sepehri M, Hutton Carlsen K, Serup J: Papulo-nodular reactions in black tattoos as markers of sarcoidosis: study of 92 tattoo reactions from a hospital material. Dermatology 2017, DOI 10.1159/000453315.

Serup J, Hutton Carlsen K: Patch test study of 90 patients with tattoo reactions: negative outcome of allergy patch test to baseline batteries of and culprit inks suggests allergen(s) are generated in the skin through haptenization. Contact Dermatitis 2014;71:255–263.

Index of Cases

223 Laser Removal of a Tattoo in an Amateur Setting Causing Laser Burn and a Chronic Papulonodular Reaction

224 Laser Removal of a Tattoo with Poor Outcome and Followed by Scarring and Urticaria Factitia in the Treated Field

225 Tattoo Removal by Laser with Yellow, Green, and Blue Pigment Resistance to Treatment

226 Tattoo Removal by a Caustic Product Causing a Scar

227 Caustic Tattoo Removal with Lactic Acid Causing a Scar and Psychological Complications

228 Caustic Tattoo Removal with Lactic Acid Followed by a Disfiguring Scar

229 Caustic Tattoo Removal with Lactic Acid in a Person Predisposed to Abnormal Scarring

Bacterial Tattoo Infection with Staphylococci on the Patient's Own Skin

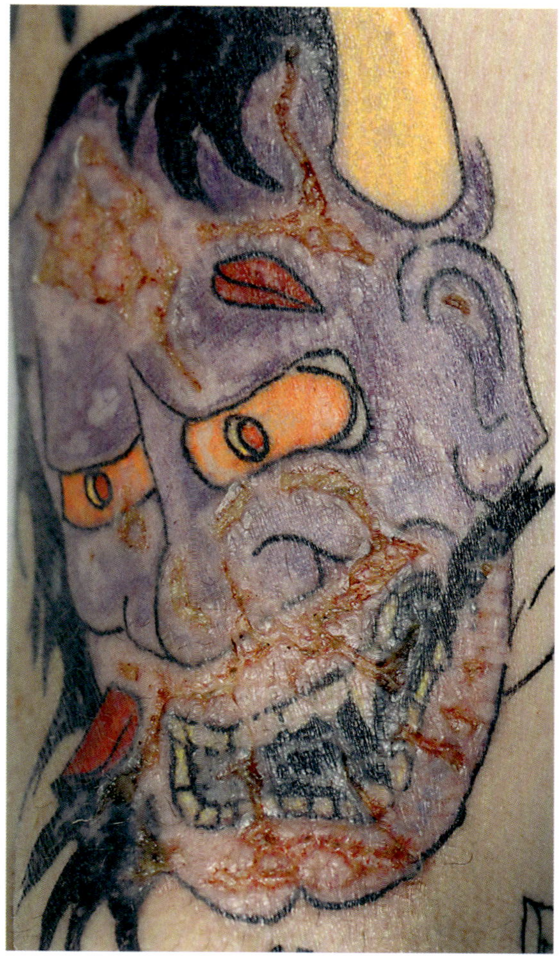

History

After 1 day, a new tattoo on the arm started to develop painful swelling and oozing involving most of the tattoo. The tattoo parlor was professional and gloves as well as single-use needles were used; the disinfection routine was unknown. The general practitioner started treatment with penicillin and fusidic acid cream. The patient had a history of abscess, paronychia, and other cutaneous infections on 3 occasions with documented staphylococci as the causative microorganism. His history also included a previous tattoo with bacterial infection of the surrounding skin.

Comment

The photo shows the tattoo infection in the state of healing, with crusts and oozing in the sites of the tattoo where the infection was severe. The sites of the tattoo that already healed, i.e. lilac parts, show pigment loss, which will also happen in additional sites presently covered with crusts. It is common that pyogenic infections destroy the color of tattoos, with massive pigment escape to the surface during infection while the skin barrier is temporarily open. Infection may also induce color change, for example from blue to greenish.

Treatment

Treatment was oral antibiotics with a combination including penicillinase-resistant penicillin. The patient was screened for staphylococci including MRSA in sites of predilection.

Bacterial Tattoo Infection with Staphylococci from the Tattoo Ink Bottle

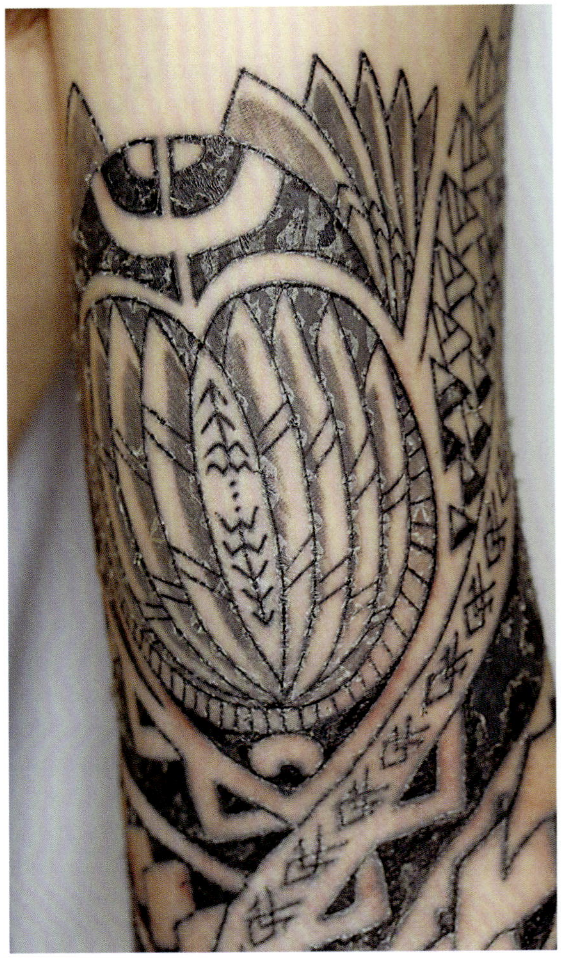

History

A newly acquired black tattoo on the upper arm started to react after a day, with swelling of the entire arm and some redness of the surrounding skin. Sites of the tattoo started to ooze. The infection was present in any part of the tattoo where the black ink was injected. Tattooing had been performed in a professional setting in a Danish parlor by a visiting star tattooist from Ireland. Needles and utensils were single use, and gloves were worn. The ink bottle was obscure and seemingly brought by the tattooist and used on different occasions.

Comment

Culture of bacteria from a black ink sample supposed to be the culprit ink showed staphylococci, which were resistant to penicillin but not to other antibiotics. The infection was concluded to be caused by the infected ink. The patient felt malaise but had no signs of blood infection.

Treatment

Treatment was a combination of oral antibiotics including penicillinase-resistant penicillin, started by the general practitioner, combined with fusidic acid cream locally. The patient recovered within 10 days, without sequels.

Bacterial Tattoo Infection with a Reused Tattoo Ink Bottle as the Suggested Source of Infection

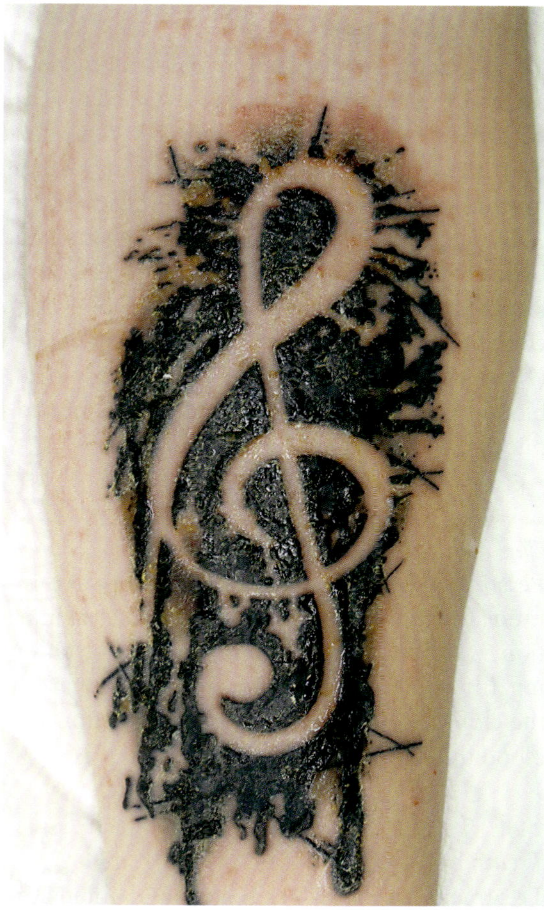

History
Two days after tattooing was performed on the arm, the patient developed redness, tenderness, and oozing of his new tattoo with redness of the surrounding skin and some tenderness of the regional lymph nodes in the armpit. His general condition was good, and apparently there had been no fever. The situation was stabilized after his practitioner had prescribed oral penicillin. The tattoo parlor was organized, and normal precautions to prevent infection had been taken. The tattoo was performed using a large bottle of black ink that had been used for a number of other customers.

Comment
Clinically it was a pyogenic infection caused by staphylococci or streptococci. Culture showed massive growth of *Enterobacter*, a marker of poor hygiene. Negative culture of cocci may be explained by ongoing penicillin treatment. The likely cause of infection was the tattoo ink bottle, which the tattooist was informed to destroy.

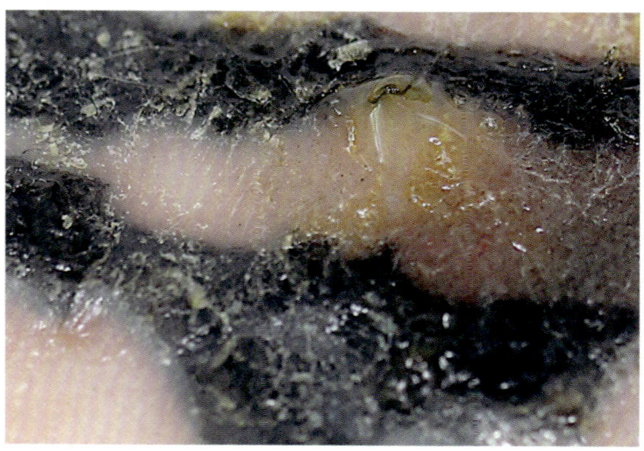

Treatment
The patient was treated with oral antibiotics, a combination of penicillin and penicillinase-resistant penicillin, combined with local treatment including sodium permanganate bath. The patient recovered perfectly.

Bacterial Tattoo Infection in a Patient with Type 1 Diabetes

History
Two days after a black tattoo had been made on the hand, the tattoo and the hand started to swell, with redness of the entire hand. The tattoo had been performed in a professional parlor taking normal hygienic precautions to prevent infection. A casualty unit diagnosed bacterial infection and instituted oral ciprofloxacin, which improved the symptoms. The patient had diabetes type 1 treated with 2 insulin products; HbA_{1c} was increased (76 mmol/mol, normal value <48). Culture from blood showed no bacteria. Healing was uncomplicated except for spotty pigment loss.

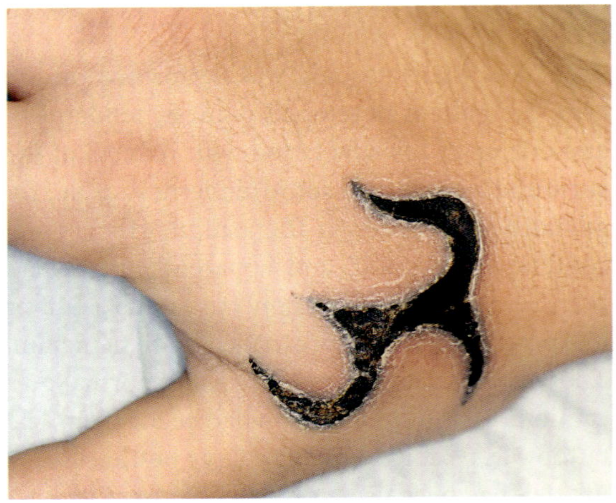

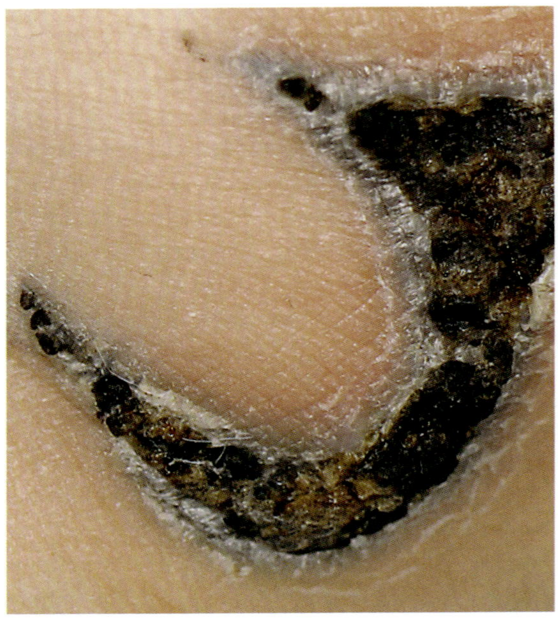

Comment
Persons with medical diseases and impaired immune function are predisposed to bacterial infection, which starts within a few days after tattooing. Infections are rather unpredictable regarding the clinical course. Progression of infection with blood infection is always a concern.

Treatment
Treatment was with antibiotics and intensified control of the patient's diabetes.

Allergic Reaction in a Red Tattoo: Type Plaque Elevation

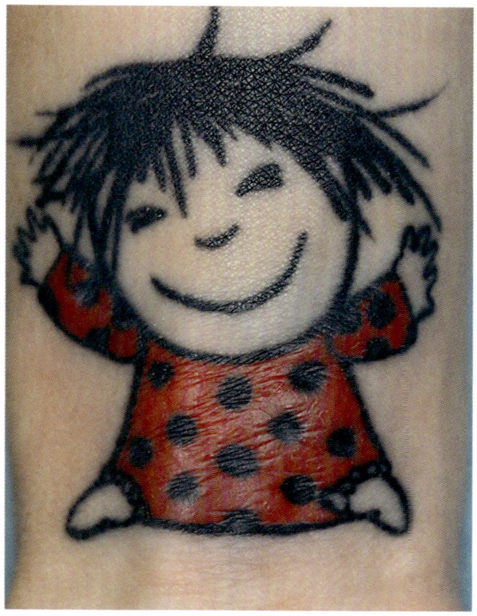

History

Eight months after tattooing with uncomplicated healing, the patient experienced thickening of the tattoo accompanied by itch. Local corticoid had minimal effect.

Comment

The patient represents a prototype of an allergic reaction of the type plaque elevation in a red tattoo. In this case, there was no significant scaling or hyperkeratosis, thus no 'lichenification' by clinical examination. Histology showed lymphocytic infiltration in the outer dermis and no special epidermal reaction; nevertheless, pathologists labelled the reaction 'what is apparent as lichenoid reaction'. Lichen and lichenoid are historical dermatological terms with several meanings and no clear definition. Dating centuries back, these terms should be considered obsolete in relation to tattoos.

Treatment

Treatment was dermatome shaving for radical elimination of the allergen. Laser removal may burst acute and delayed allergic reactions and cannot produce radical pigment removal with removal of the pigment-associated allergen. Local corticoid may help ease the itch.

Allergic Reaction in a Red Tattoo: Type Plaque Elevation

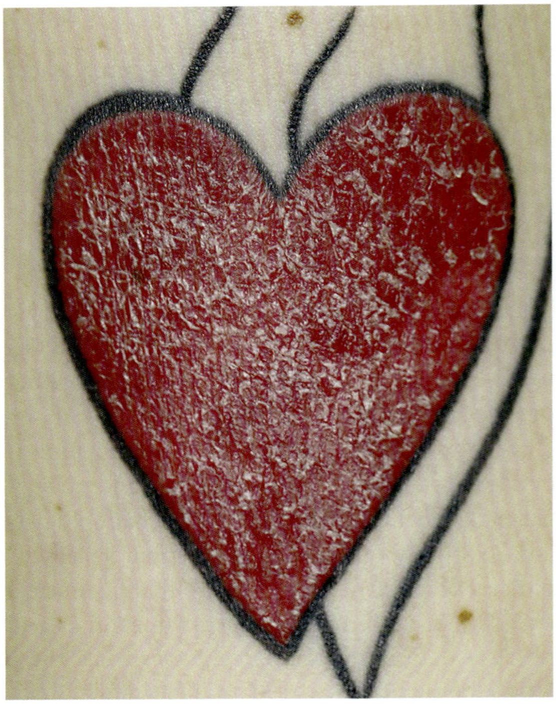

History
About 8 weeks after the patient had gotten a red tattoo and after normal initial healing, the tattoo started to thicken and itch. This was constant over months, and there was some scaling. Old tattoos including red tattoos did not react.

Comment
The patient represents a prototype case of allergy of the type plaque elevation to red pigment, with uniform thickening all over the red tattoo, rough scaling on the top of the lesion, and itch. This case represents what was called a 'lichenoid tattoo reaction' in the past, with lichenoid possibly referring to the flat and scaly look. However, 'lichenoid' coming from 'lichen' and the plant kingdom is a historical term with several meanings and diffuse delineation, thus imprecise and in relation to pathologic tattoos obsolete. In early dermatology two centuries ago, 'lichen' meant 'associated with internal disease', the historical root of the term.

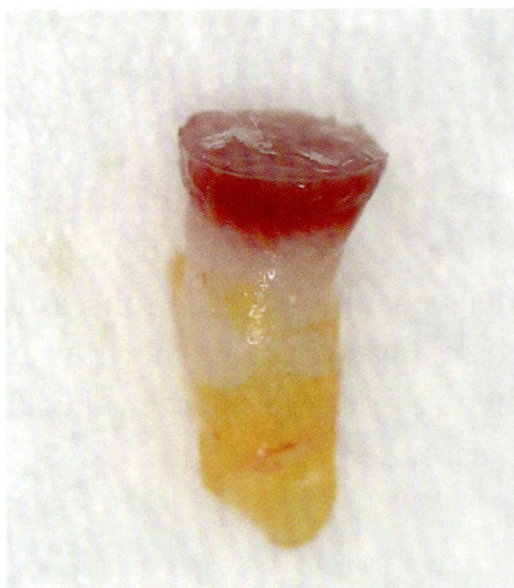

Treatment
Treatment was dermatome shaving. Raw punch biopsy showed pigment in the outer dermis only and a large scale.

Allergic Reaction in a Red Tattoo: Type Plaque Elevation

History
A Danish soldier on mission in the Middle East had the emblem of his battery tattooed on his arm. After 2 years, the tattoo suddenly started to thicken and itch 'like hell' in red parts showing an armadillo. The armadillo is a small mammal encapsulated in a hard leathery shell and with sharp claws, a symbol of military tanks and first worn as a tattoo by a military chief who was killed in the Afghan war. His company became named 'Armadillo'.

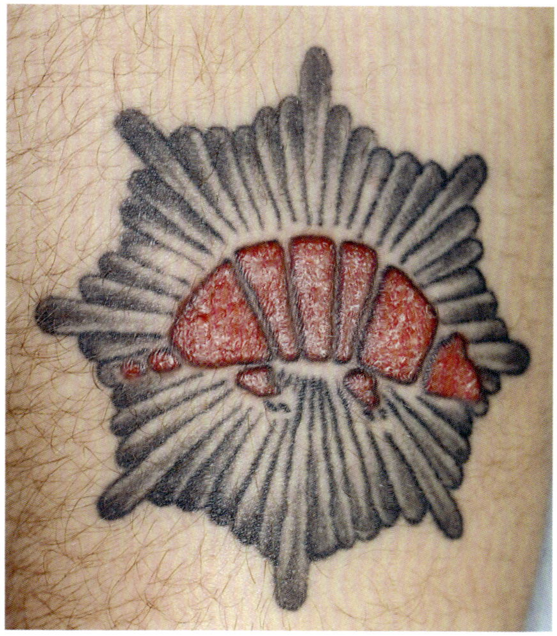

Comment
This tattoo reaction is a prototype tattoo allergy of the type plaque elevation. Biopsy showed interphase dermatitis with lymphocytic infiltration. The epidermis showed parakeratosis and minor hyperkeratosis, which was clinically seen as scaling. Raw punch showed pigment in the outer dermis.

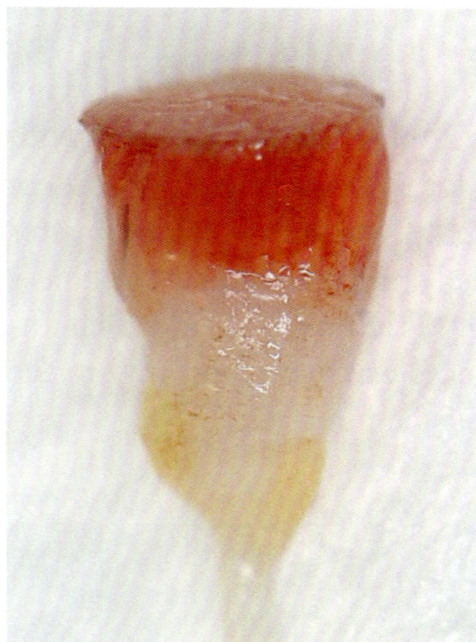

Treatment
Treatment was dermatome shaving to the middermal level. Local corticoid had no effect.

Allergic Reaction in a Red Tattoo: Type Plaque Elevation

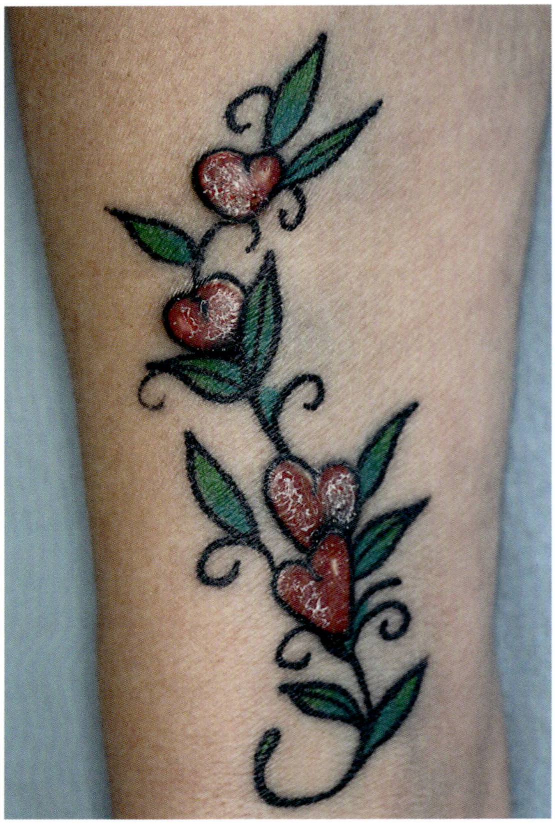

History
A red tattoo on the forearm started to itch 4 months after normal healing, and after about 6 months the tattoo started to swell with itching present day and night. Local corticoid was tried with no effect. The reaction was exclusively in the red parts of the tattoo.

Comment
The reaction was clearly allergic. There was flat elevation and lichenoid scaling all over the red parts of the tattoo, while other colors were spared. Raw punch biopsy showed red pigment distributed towards the very deep dermis nearby the interface to fat, thus, much too deep in the skin for YAG laser treatment.

Treatment
Treatment was provided as dermatome shaving performed to a level under the mid-dermis, with a second shave of local sites in the tattoo, where remnant pigment still caused a reaction after some months. Finally, the patient had no subjective symptoms but was left with a scar, which under the circumstances was acceptable and to the patient's overall satisfaction.

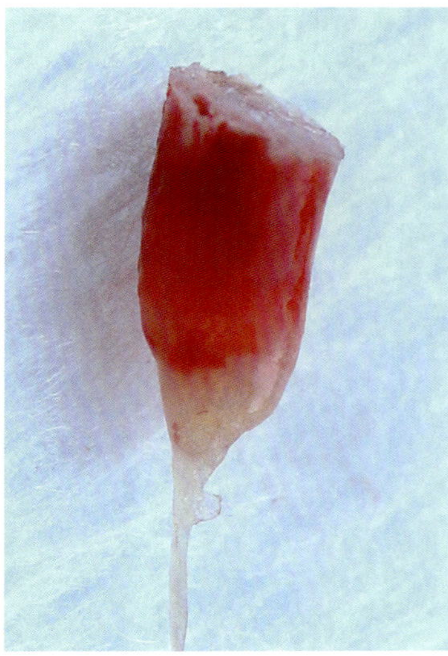

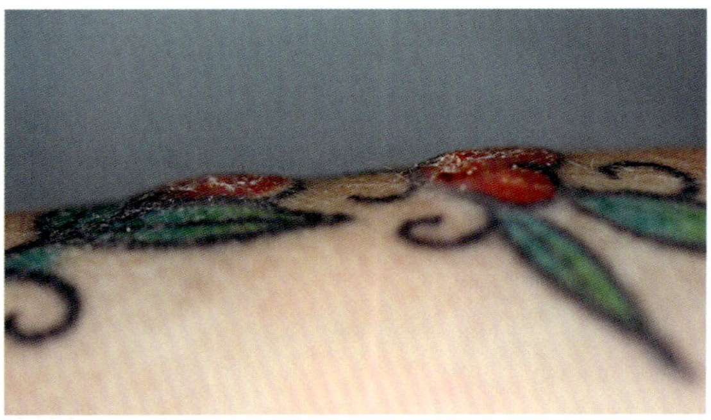

Allergic Reaction in a Red Tattoo: Type Plaque Elevation

History
The patient's only tattoo was a bracelet tattoo decorated with red hearts. About 6 months after tattooing, the red parts of the tattoo started to swell and itch. Local corticoid was without any effect.

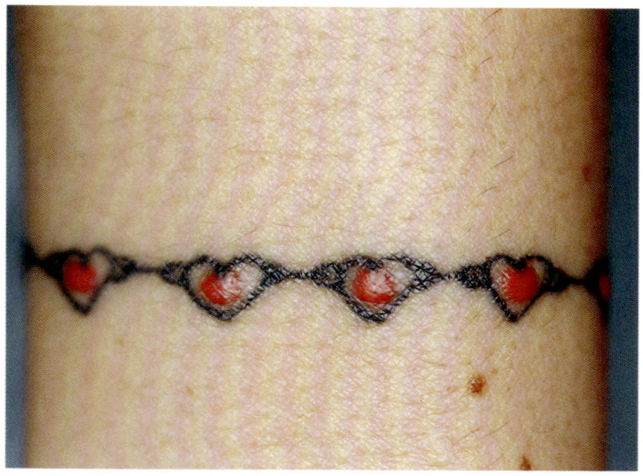

Comment
The reaction was allergic and confined to the red parts of the tattoo, supposedly caused by a red pigment hapten formed in the dermis over time.

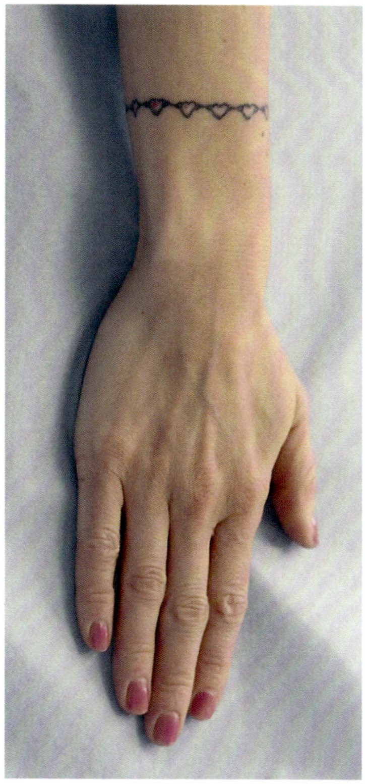

Treatment
Efficient treatment requires eradication of the culprit hapten in the dermis. Treatment was performed as dermatome shaving using shave biopsy handheld blades, which allow a precise removal of very small tattoos. Laser removal was not an option because of the risk of boosting the allergy and since pigment deep in the dermis cannot be reached by the laser; thus, complete eradiation of the pigment cannot be offered. Photography of her hand taken as follow-up showed a cosmetically favourable outcome of shaving.

Allergic Reaction in a Red Tattoo: Type Plaque Elevation

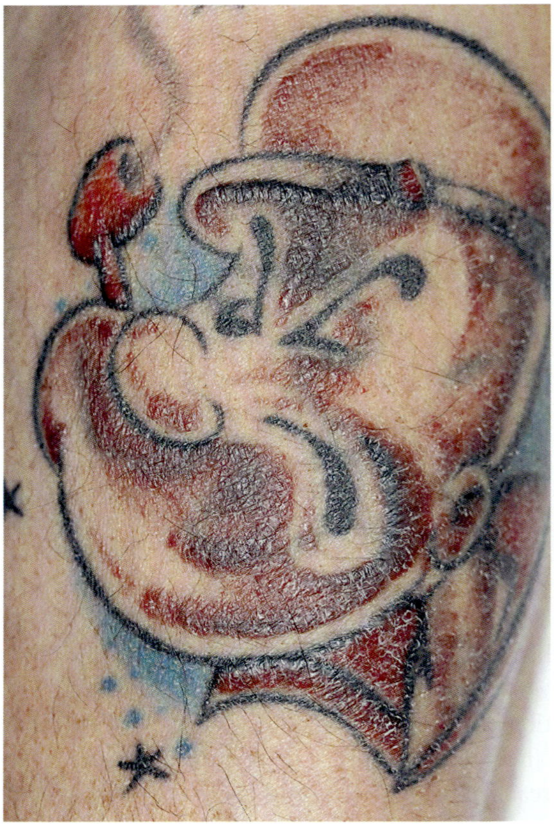

History
A red tattoo started to swell and itch after a period of 3 years, with the pathology limited to the red parts of the tattoo. Local corticoid was without convincing effect and could not be used for extended periods.

Comment
Parts of the red tattoo with denser pigment showed flat elevation, while milder allergic reaction was seen in other parts of the tattoo including reaction where only little pigment was installed. Some lichenoid scaly look was apparent on the surface. The normal skin surface microrelief was flattened or changed. The case illustrates that allergic reactions may sometimes vary in severity relative to the density of the culprit pigment tattooed into the skin.

Treatment
Treatment was dermatome shaving leaving very little scarring. This case was ideal for dermatome treatment because the red pigment was concentrated in the papillary dermis and thus sliced out of the skin with a few cuts. In this case the allergy was mild, and small remnants of pigment left in the skin might fall under a threshold and not cause further trouble.

Allergic Reaction in the Red Part of a Multicolored Tattoo: Type Plaque Elevation

History
The patient had a multicolored tattoo on the leg. Healing had been normal. After 7 months, the red part of the tattoo started to thicken and itch day and night, contrasting no reaction in any other color.

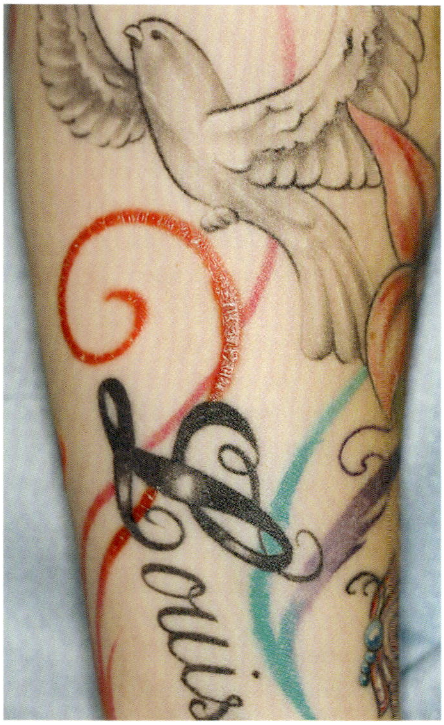

Comment
This case is typical. The raw punch biopsy showed red pigment deep in the dermis. This case illustrates the delayed onset of reaction during the period of pigment metabolism, hapten formation, and primary sensitization. It also illustrates the selectivity of reaction limited to one specific color, red, while various other colors, including red nuances, did not react and were without cross-allergic reactivity.

Treatment
Treatment was dermatome shaving, which relieved symptoms. However, a few small sites in the shaved field apparently had remnant pigment and required potent local corticoid for some months.

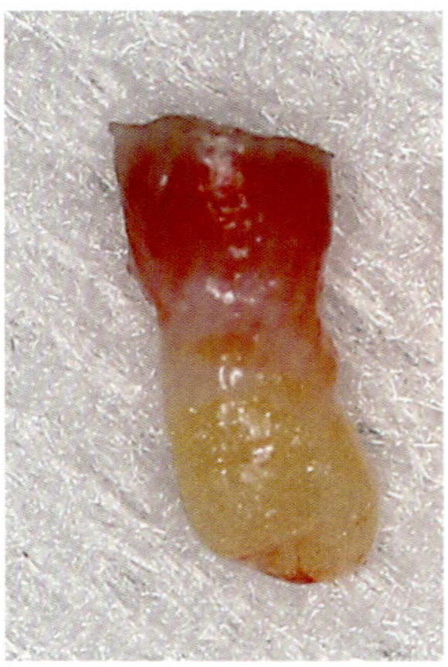

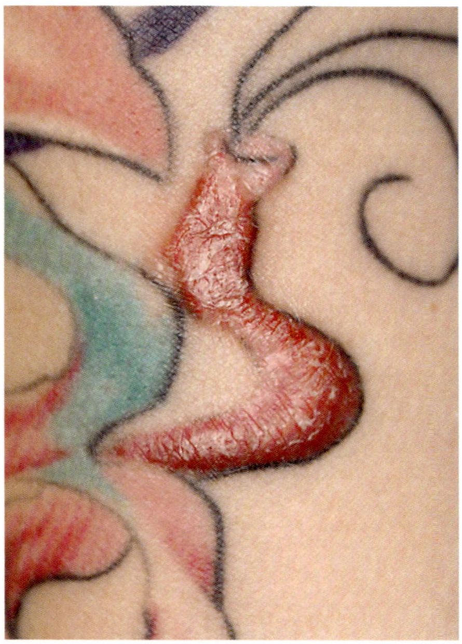

Allergic Reaction in the Bordeaux Part of a Multicolored Amateur Tattoo with Atypical Nodular Appearance

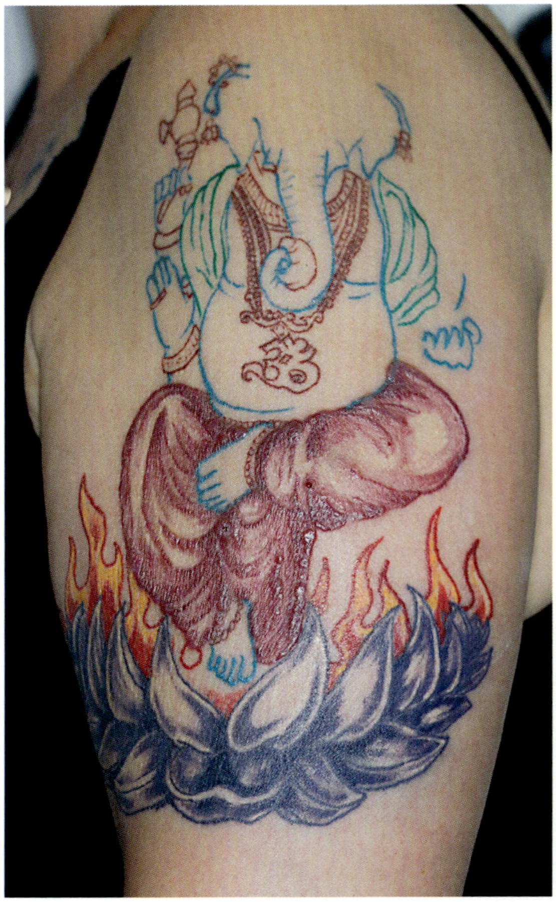

History
The patient had acquired a multicolored tattoo on the upper arm 2 years ago, performed by an amateur in a private home. Tattooing had taken 7 h and caused unusual bleeding. After a few months, variable skin thickening developed, which was limited to the bordeaux-colored fields; it was very itchy and disturbed the patient's sleep.

Comment
The reaction was allergic with dense lymphocytic infiltration. Biopsy also showed a few giant cells and fibrosis of the outer dermis. Allergic reactions are typically manifested as flat plaque type elevation. The nodular appearance in this case might be explained by amateur tattooing, which caused dermal fibrosis and had been performed with variable injection of tattoo ink in the tattooed field. Giant cells, but no granulomas, might indicate that the tattoo ink applied was a mix of pigments with red as the basis but including carbon black used as darkener. The carbon black pigment is typically the cause of papulonodular reactions, occasionally with granuloma formation.

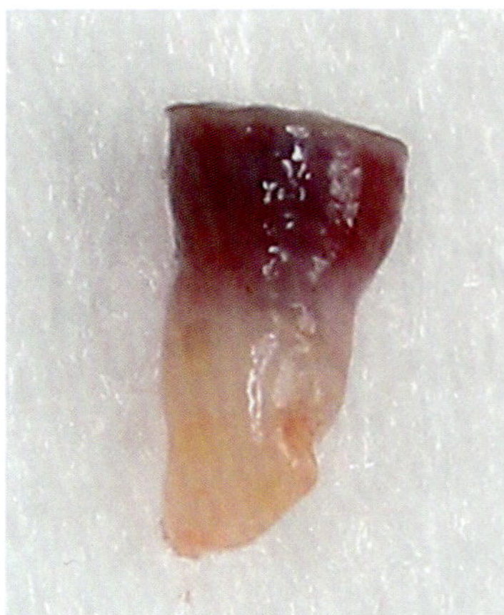

Treatment
Treatment was dermatome shaving down to the low mid-dermal level, which relieved symptoms and left acceptable scarring.

Allergic Reaction in a Red Tattoo: Type Excessive Hyperkeratosis

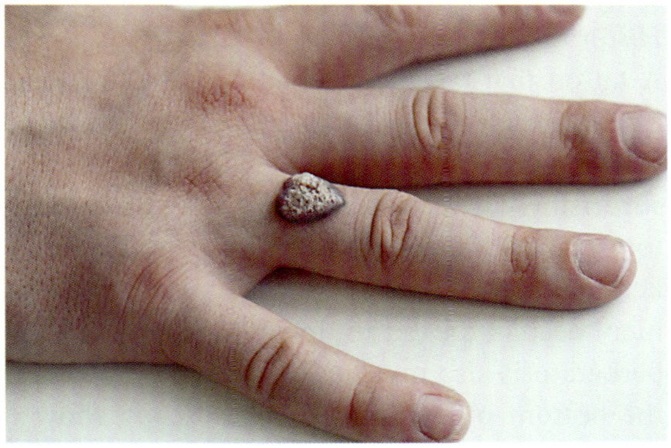

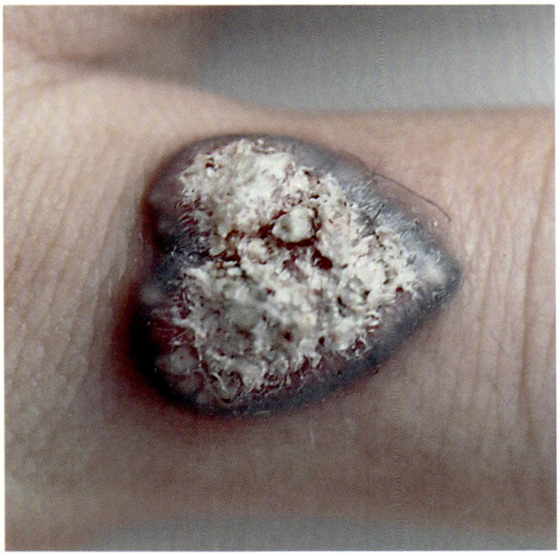

History
A red tattoo on a finger acquired 1 year ago started to thicken already 2 months after uncomplicated healing. The tattoo became covered by a thick layer of keratotic material. It itched and caused pain and discomfort whenever the finger was used.

Comment
The reaction was clearly an allergy to the red ink used, with severe inflammation in the dermis associated with a proliferative response of the epidermis. In excessive hyperkeratosis, the dermo-epidermal barrier to spontaneous pigment drift out of the skin is often leaking; minor pigment escape from the dermis to the basal layer and epidermis can happen as part of ongoing interphase dermatitis. A dyskeratotic secondary response of the epidermis on the top of a fiery allergic reaction in the outer dermis, where tattoo pigment is found in large amounts, is the clinical outcome.

Treatment
Treatment was dermatome shaving. Lasers are not efficient and rational in such thick lesions.

Allergic Reaction in a Red Tattoo: Type Excessive Hyperkeratosis

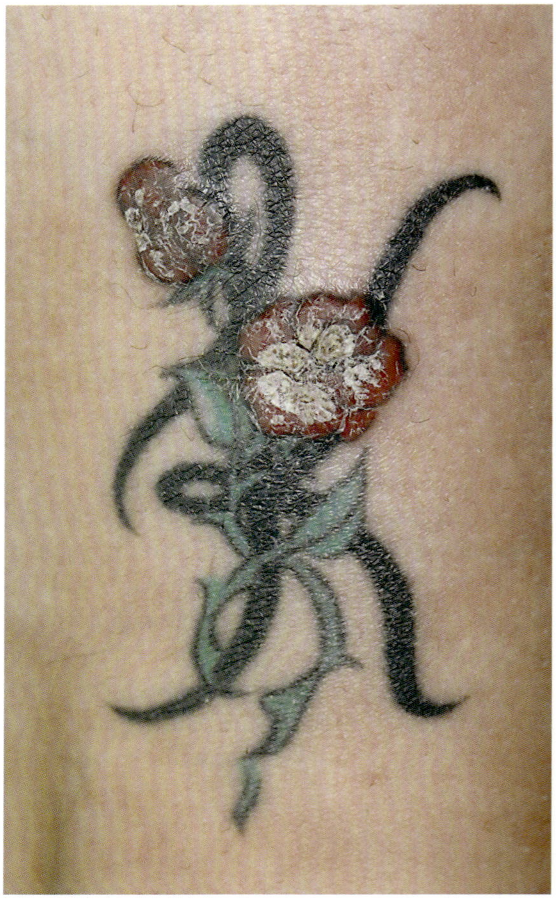

History
A tattoo that the patient had acquired 12 years ago and that had hitherto caused absolutely no problems abruptly became thickened and scaly, surprisingly without significant subjective symptoms. The raw punch biopsy showed thick hyperkeratotic material on the top and dense red pigment deep in the dermis towards the fat. The hyperkeratosis also involved a hair follicle down to the bottom of the dermis. Microscopy showed dense lymphocytic infiltration in the dermis going close to the interphase to fat.

Comment
Allergy to the red tattoo pigment can have years of latency and abrupt onset once the culprit hapten is formed in the dermis as a result of metabolic change of the pigment with formation of the specific epitope coding the allergy. Excessive hyperkeratosis is a secondary proliferative response of the keratinocytes of the basal cell layer. This response may involve hair follicles and sometimes extend deep into the dermis and seed epidermoid inclusions, which may proliferate and produce keratotic material that can complicate and prolong healing for months after dermatome shaving.

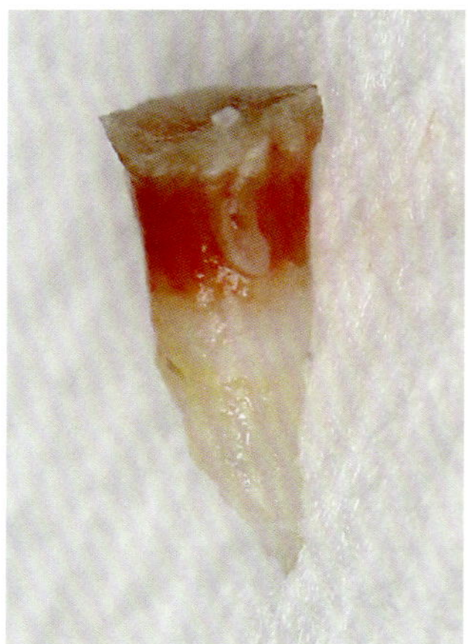

Treatment
Treatment was dermatome shaving performed to the level of the deep dermis. Lasers can burst the allergy and are not efficient and not applicable in such thickened lesions.

Allergic Reaction in a Red Tattoo: Type Excessive Hyperkeratosis

History
A red tattoo made 5 months ago, located on the lower leg. The tattoo did not heal normally and started to thicken, soon with marked swelling, major hyperkeratosis, and itching. Local corticoid showed no effect. The patient had many other tattoos including various red tattoos, which did not react. His normal skin, especially the palms and soles, showed signs of a predisposing hyperkeratotic state.

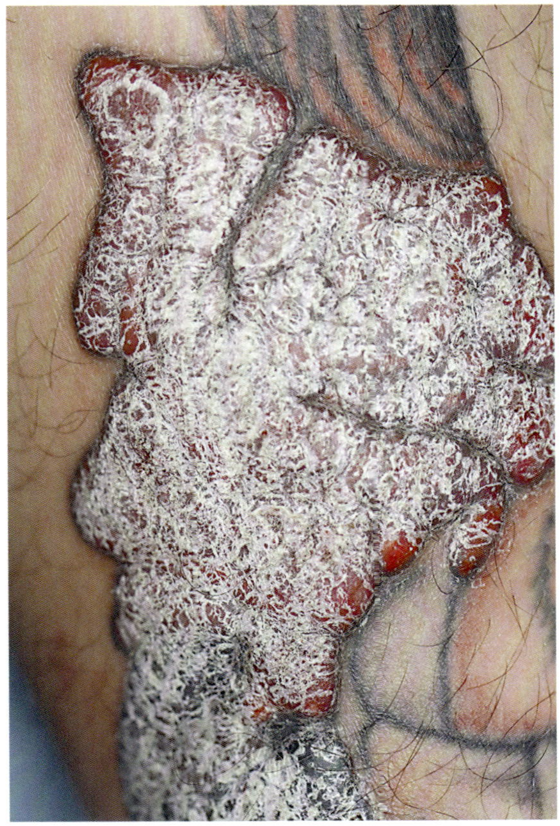

Comment
The skin was heavily thickened and infiltrated with lymphocytes as well as with interphase dermatitis and major hyperkeratosis. Pigment in the dermis was fiery and reached the deep part of the dermis. Deep furrows noted by clinical examination sometimes can reach the mid-dermis with formation of epidermal inclusions.

Treatment
Treatment was dermatome shaving performed to the deep dermis level. The patient healed with acceptable scarring requiring no further treatment. Symptoms were relieved.

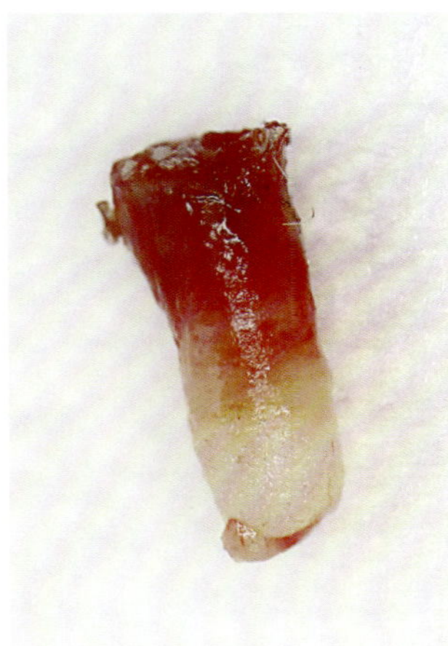

Allergic Reaction in a Red Tattoo: Type Excessive Hyperkeratosis

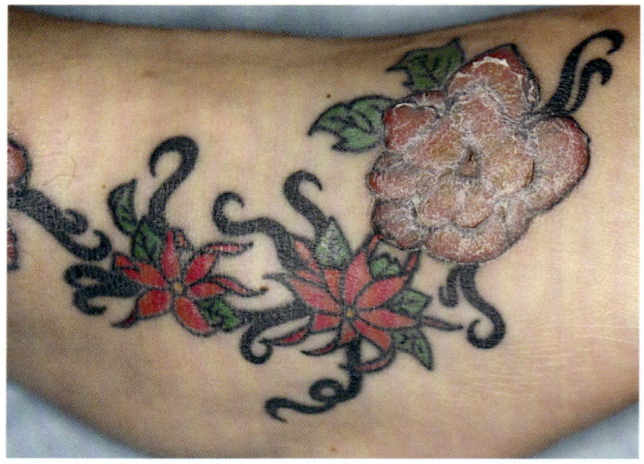

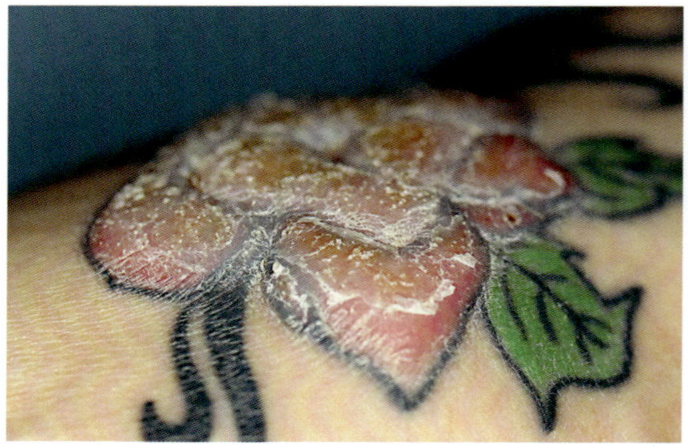

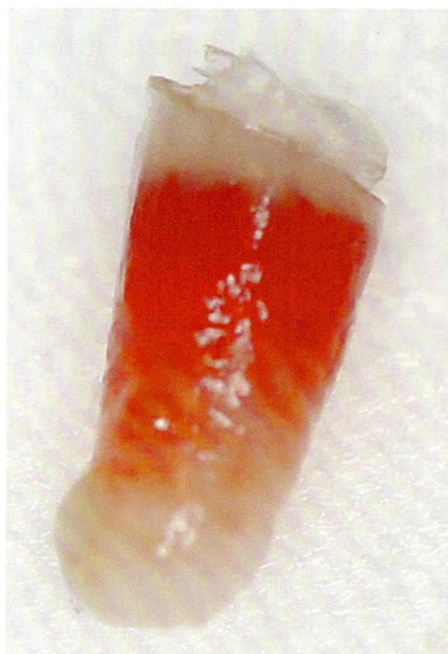

History

A few years after tattooing, tattoos on the leg and over the ankle joint of the patient had shown fading of color in one of the tattooed red flowers. The flower had then been refreshed with a red cover-up tattoo. After 4 weeks, the tattoo thickened markedly and started to itch day and night.

Comment

Hyperkeratosis was excessive and seen directly in the raw biopsy as a whitish layer under the surface of the skin with a major scale. Microscopy showed dense lymphocytic infiltration throughout the entire dermis.

Treatment

Treatment was dermatome shaving to the level of the lower dermis, with relief of symptoms but some scarring, which was treated with local corticoid.

Allergic Reaction in a Red Tattoo: Type Excessive Hyperkeratosis in a Case Predisposed to Hyperkeratotic Response to Physical Stimuli

History
The patient had a tattoo on his leg which had caused no problems for 4 years. Suddenly and almost overnight the red part of the tattoo started to thicken. The tattoo was covered with a horny material. It itched day and night. The patient scratched a lot and had to cover the tattoo reaction with a bandage to limit scratching. Local corticoids were of no effect. The patient was burdened by callosities for years and thus predisposed to hyperkeratosis.

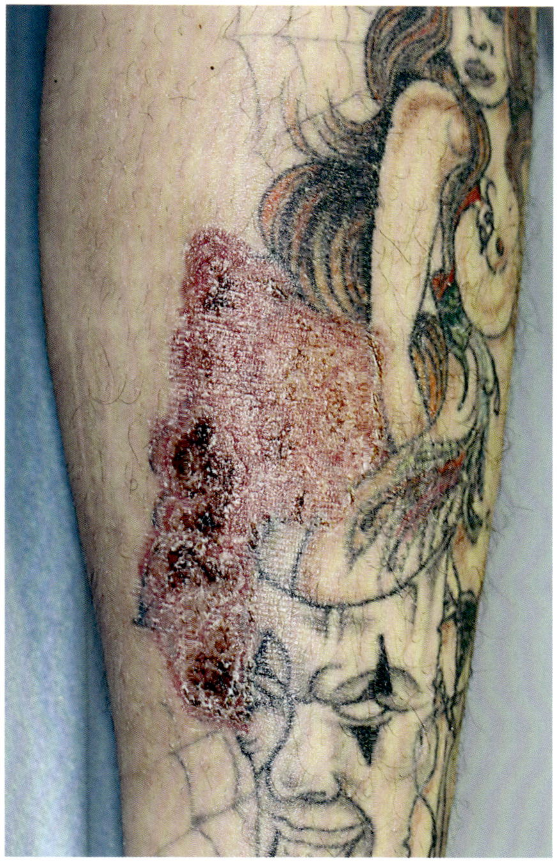

Comment
The reaction was concluded to be allergic with red pigment causing the allergy. The allergic reaction primarily took place in the dermis, where the tattoo pigment is situated, in the dermis manifested as lymphocytic inflammation and interphase dermatitis according to biopsy. The hyperkeratotic and hyperproliferative response of the epidermis was considered secondary and apparently dependent on the patient's individual predisposition to such a response.

Treatment
Treatment was dermatome shaving, which led to remission without complications and perfectly relieved the patient's itch.

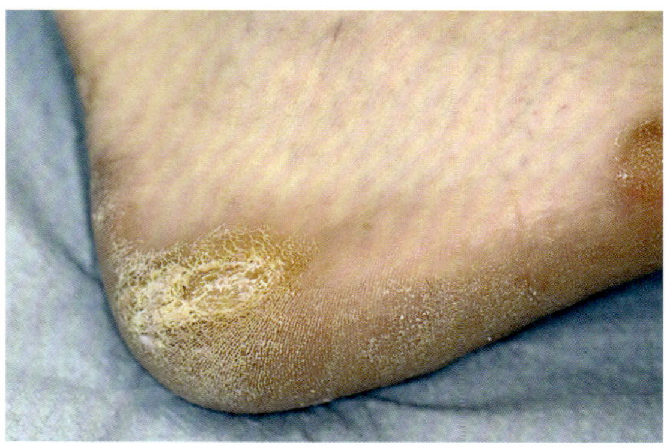

Allergic Reaction in a Red Tattoo: Type Excessive Hyperkeratosis, Acneiform Variant with Epidermoid Cysts

History

A tattoo on the leg was acquired 8 years ago and hitherto had caused no problem. After sun bathing a year ago, the tattoo started to react and thicken almost like a tumor, associated with itch and tenderness. It did not respond to local corticoid. Keratoacanthoma was considered.

Treatment

Therapy was dermatome shaving performed to a level under visible epidermal inclusions, approaching the whitish dermis devoid of pigment. Remnant epidermis with proliferative potential in the shave wound bed can result in recurrences and complicate and prolong healing.

Comment

The tattoo reaction was exclusively in the red color and concluded to be allergic, possibly with light-induced activation of the allergen and active sensitization. It presented with excessive hyperkeratosis and looked like inflamed acne lumps, with comedo-like openings. Microscopy of the shaved material (the photo on the bottom right shows a flipped-over dermatome slice with the interior surface presented) found a number of small cyst-like structures with epithelium and keratotic material. The epidermis was very hyperkeratotic.

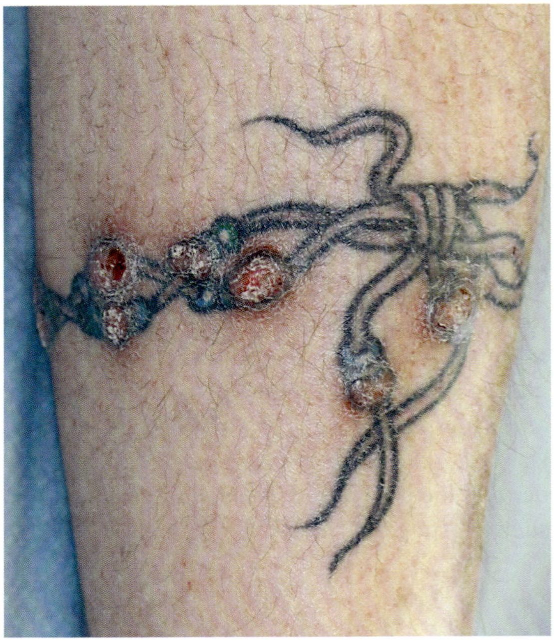

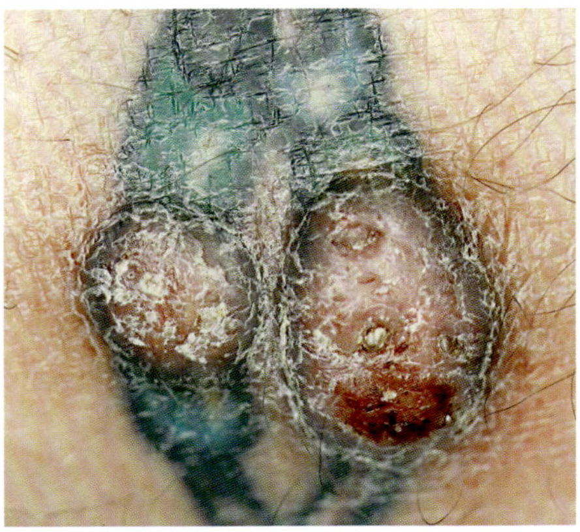

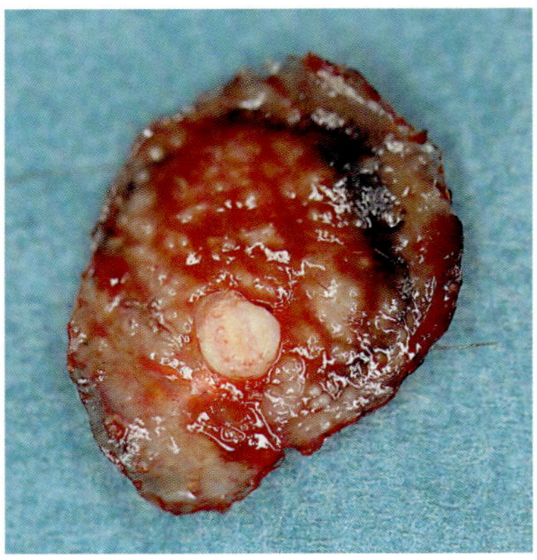

Allergic Reaction in a Red Tattoo: Type Excessive Hyperkeratosis, Acneiform Variant with Epidermoid Inclusions

History

Already 4–6 weeks after uncomplicated tattooing, the patient developed major thickening in the red-colored part of a tattoo, with keratosis and scales. Along with keratosis, whitish circular elements in the very outer dermis developed. The tattoo itched. He had many older tattoos but none reacted; thus, there was no evidence of a crossallergic reaction in other red tattoos. The reacting tattoo was the emblem of the Royal Danish Brigade, with the Danish banner and the crown.

Comment

Hyperproliferation of the epidermis was barely visible on the surface; nevertheless, it was massive with acneiform epithelial inclusions in the dermis as seen on close inspection of the skin lesions and already in the raw punch biopsy. This was confirmed by microscopy, which also showed interphase dermatitis and lymphocytic infiltration. Dermoscopy of the skin surface showed comedo-like circular openings, which were discrete and only visible on close-up view.

Treatment

Treatment was dermatome shaving, which in this case healed without complications and with no disturbance from the many epidermal inclusions in the wound bed having potential to hyperproliferate.

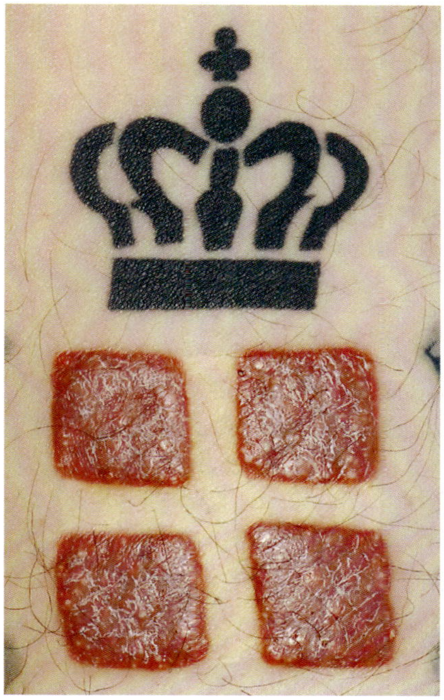

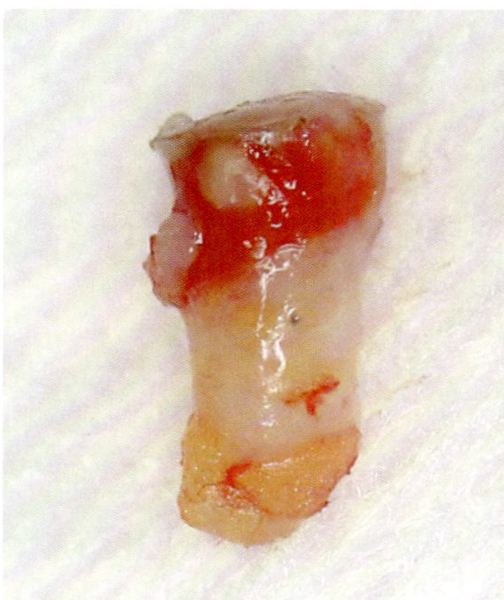

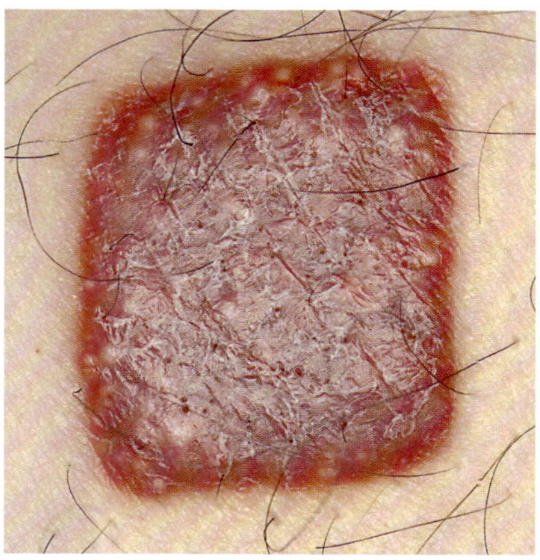

Allergic Reaction Provoked by Sun in Two Red Tattoos Made with Different Red Inks

History
The patient, who was himself a professional tattooist, had acquired a new tattoo on the arm made with 2 different inks, i.e. one for the main figure and another for red shades. After about a week, the figure started to react with thickening, whereas there was no reaction in the red shades. The pattern was plaque elevation in irregular lines like a magnified skin surface relief, thus not directly the papulonodular pattern. Years ago, the patient had acquired a small red tattoo on the leg, which had reacted for about 10 years until it faded spontaneously. Sun exposure while on holidays in Thailand had initiated the recent reaction.

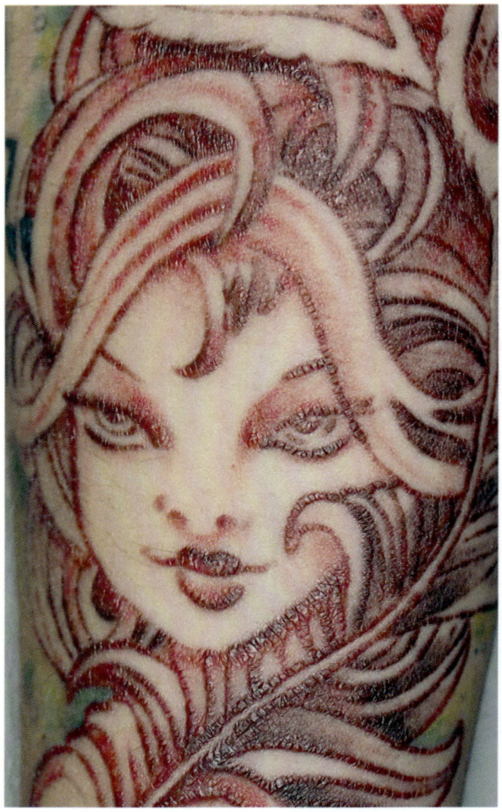

Comment
The allergic reaction occurred shortly after tattooing and affected one red color exclusively. The reaction might be seen as a cross-sensitivity reaction with his old tattoo being responsible for primary sensitization.

Treatment
Treatment was dermatome shaving. Local corticoid was ineffective.

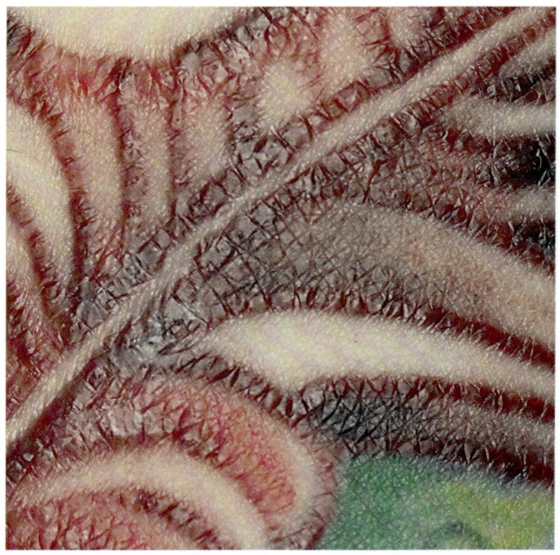

Allergic Reaction in a Red Tattoo: Type Plaque Elevation with Cross-Sensitivity Reactions in Other Red Tattoos Hitherto Tolerated

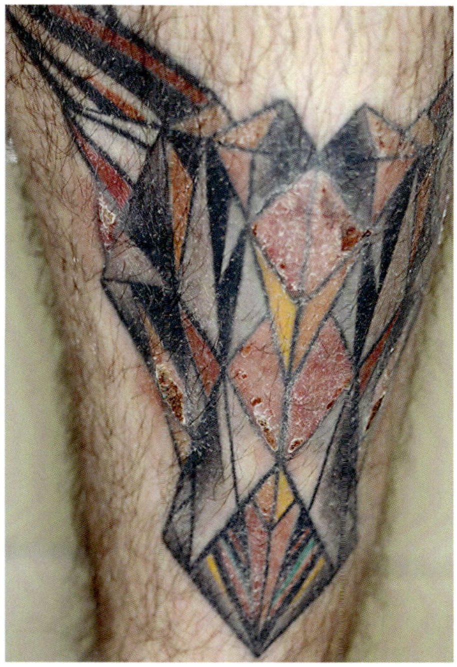

History

Three months after tattooing, which was reported to have been quite traumatic, the newly acquired red tattoo on the leg started to react with severe itching, which could not be controlled by local corticoid. Four weeks later, old tattoos on the trunk and on the arm also started to react, with itching. These old red tattoos had been made by the same tattooist a few years ago and had not caused any trouble in the past. The patient was severely burdened by the problem and suffered major itching.

Comment

This was a strong allergic reaction of the type plaque elevation in a recent red tattoo on the leg, which triggered cross-sensitization in other red tattoos that had been hitherto tolerated, with milder reactions in the responder tattoos.

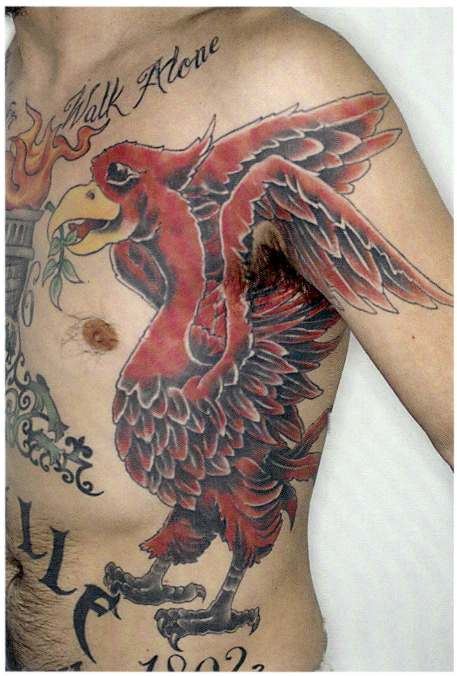

Treatment

Treatment was dermatome shaving of the trigger tattoo on the leg, with need of a second shave due to remnant pigment deep in the dermis. The trigger tattoo healed with no symptoms except for scarring. Responder tattoos on the trunk and the arm spontaneously and over about 8 months recovered and finally became normal. Active treatment of the trigger with ambiguous eradication of the culprit pigment in the skin is necessary. Laser removal is contraindicated due to the risk of acute allergic reaction or blowup of the reactions. Lasers cannot efficiently eradicate pigment deep in the dermis. Lasers work by dosing random spots and cannot systematically clean the skin for pigment in the horizontal plane. Laser light intensity declines in the dermis along with absorption and scattering.

Allergic Reaction in a Red Tattoo Triggering a Cross-Sensitivity Reaction in a Number of Red Tattoos Acquired in the Past

History
The patient had acquired a new red tattoo of a bird on her right shoulder. After 3 months, the tattoo started to thicken and itch. Two to three months later, all her red tattoos on the left leg thickened and became itchy, with increasing thickening towards the foot. These 'memory' tattoos made years before had not caused any problems before. The tattoos had been made by different tattooists. Local corticoid had no effect.

Comment
An allergic reaction in a new tattoo can trigger allergic reactions in tattoos of similar color despite being tolerated for years. The allergic reaction in secondarily reacting tattoos can be strong and even stronger than the reaction in the trigger tattoo. There must be some shared epitope fundamental for the class of pigment used in the different tattoos. Red azo pigments are especially prone to develop cross-sensitization.

Treatment
Dermatome shaving of the trigger tattoo only was performed with removal of the triggering pigment. Over a period of several months, the reacting tattoos on the leg gradually faded in activity and ultimately became nonreacting.

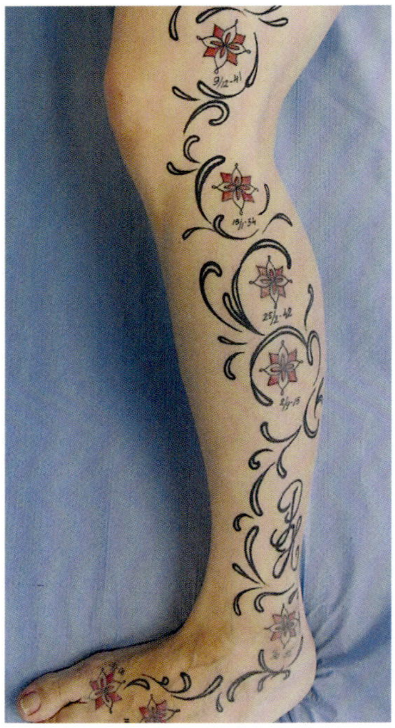

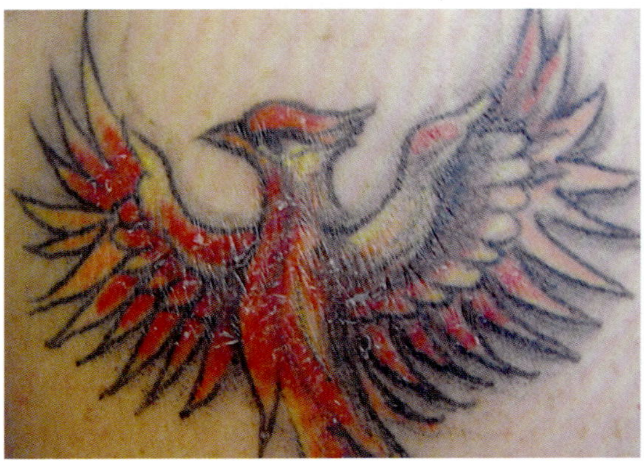

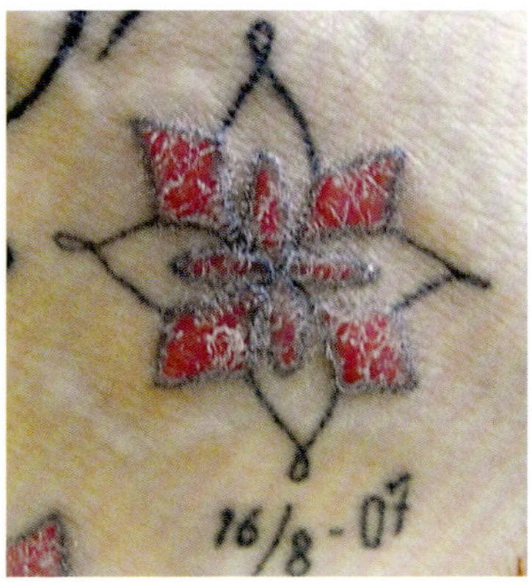

Allergic Reaction in a Red Tattoo Triggering an Allergic Cross-Reaction in Other Red Tattoos as well as in a Green Tattoo

History

The patient had acquired a multicolored tattoo on the arm 2 years ago. After 1 year, the part of the tattoo picturing a red ladybird started to swell and itch, which was after a few months followed by similar but milder reactions in another red-colored part of the same tattoo (picturing a group of two small birds) as well as in green parts of the tattoo. An old tattoo on the foot that the patient had acquired 5 years before also started to swell in the red and green parts. Other colors, such as blue, were completely nonreactive.

Comment

Azo chemical pigments can be red, yellow, green, and other tones. In this case one core chemical structure shared by different pigments seemingly contributed to the formation of the hapten in the skin that caused the allergy, triggered by the ladybird tattoo, with cross-allergic reactions in other tattoos.

Raw punch biopsies showed whitish epidermal hyperplasia and epidermoid cysts (red ladybird trigger tattoo, left), red pigment in the outer dermis only (tattoo of small birds on the arm, middle left; reaction on the foot, middle right), and more dispersed green pigment in the outer dermis with slight hyperkeratosis (reaction on the arm, right). Microscopy showed lymphocytic infiltration, interphase dermatitis, and variable hyperkeratosis in all biopsies including the one from the green tattoo.

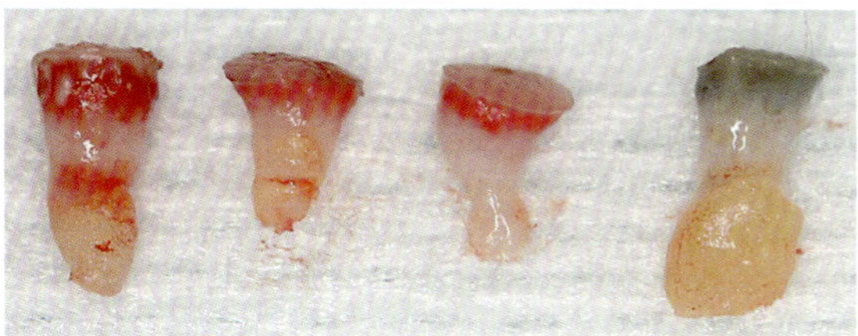

Treatment

Treatment was dermatome shaving of the ladybird trigger tattoo, which after a few months was followed by spontaneous remission of the reactions in the cross-reacting sites, which were not offered active treatment. Eradication of pigment from the trigger typically allows the responder reactions to heal spontaneously over time.

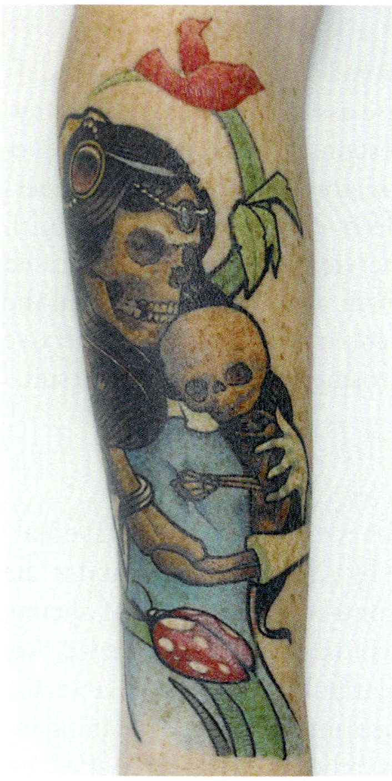

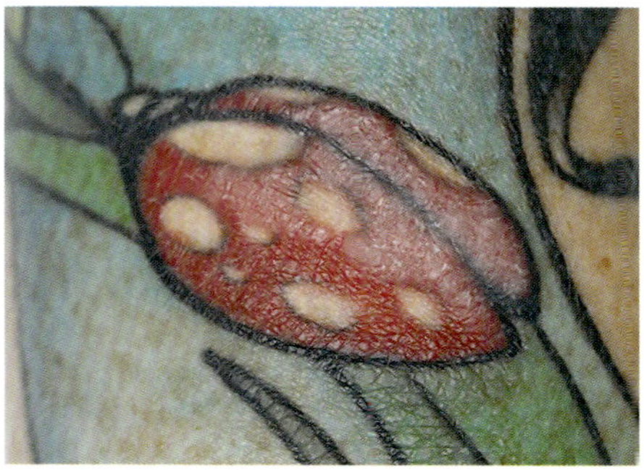

Allergic Reaction in a Red Tattoo: Type Excessive Hyperkeratosis – Uncomplicated Dermatome Shaving

History
The patient had 4 red roses tattooed on the leg. Shortly after initial healing, the tattoo thickened with roughness and furrows of the surface as well as pain and severe itching day and night. Biopsy showed lymphocytic infiltration, giant cells but no granuloma, and major epidermal thickening.

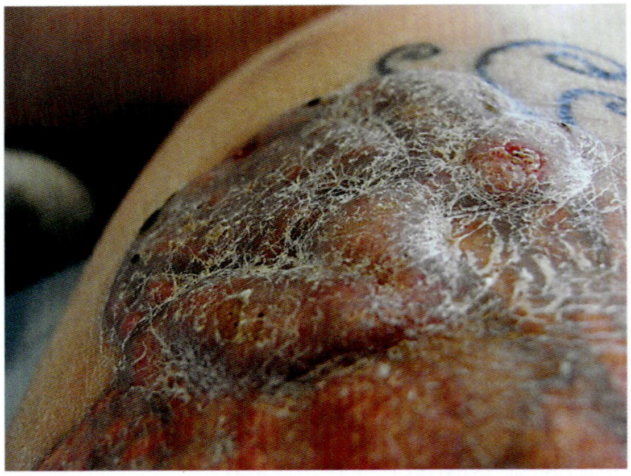

Comment
Allergic reaction to red tattoo pigment in the dermis was in this case associated with a severe hyperproliferative response of the epidermis. Despite furrows, dermatome shaving could be performed with a clean cut down to the whitish collagen of the inner dermis, with uncomplicated healing and regrowth of the epidermis from the adnexa. The patient ended with no subjective complaints and a cosmetically acceptable result.

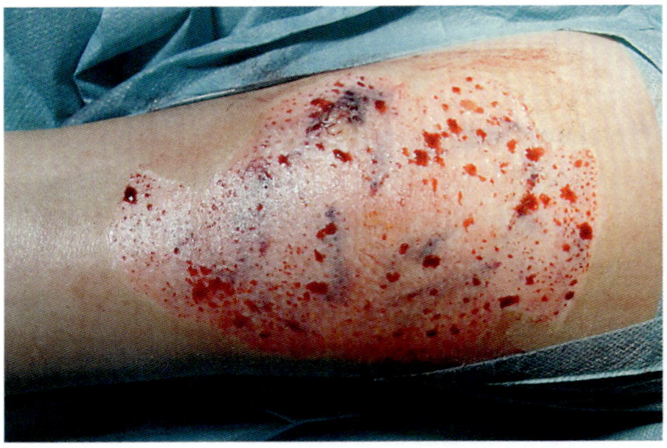

Treatment
With dermatome shaving, a clean removal of tattoo pigment slice by slice is possible under the surgeon's visual control of the depth of slicing, performed until whitish dermis is achieved. Lasers shoot in circular burn points or variable distribution in the horizontal plane, are of fading intensity, and have a rather unpredictable effect on pigment bleaching in the vertical plane.

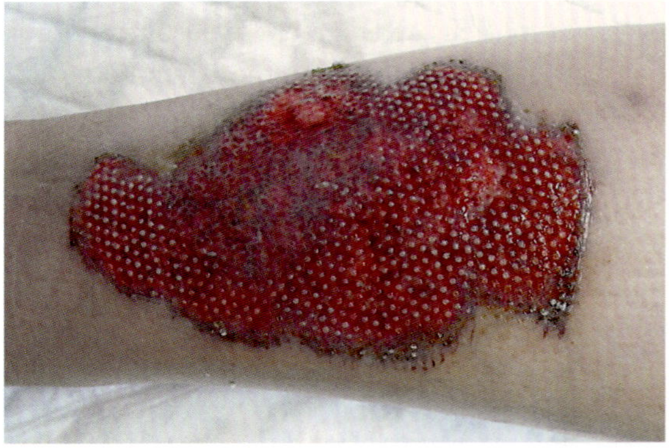

Allergic Reaction in a Red Tattoo: Type Excessive Hyperkeratosis, Acneiform Variant – Dermatome Shaving Followed by Epidermoid Growth and Prolonged Healing

History

Immediately after the healing phase, a red tattoo on the leg rapidly started to thicken with deep furrowing and comedo-like skin surface markings. The tattoo was painful and very itchy (fig. a). Biopsy showed excessive hyperkeratosis, fiery lymphocytic infiltration in the entire dermis down to the fat, and granulomas, which were not sarcoid. Dermatome shaving could not produce a perfectly pigment clean horizontal cut, and the surgical wound bed showed yellowish figures of little bleeding with seemingly epidermal inclusions very deep in the dermis. The wound took several months to heal, and masses of hyperkeratotic material grew in the granulation tissue interfering with healing (fig. b). After 6 months, the wound flattened (fig. c), and after 12 months it healed, however with a cosmetically unsatisfactory result (fig. d). Plastic surgeons denied corrective surgery.

Comment

Furrows of excessive hyperkeratosis and epidermal inclusions can go deep in the dermis and constantly proliferate and disturb healing. The allergic reaction to red pigment in the dermis triggers epidermal proliferation, which may be strong and entirely dominate the clinical reaction.

Treatment

Surgical excision and covering with a free transplant may seem preferable, but excisional surgery may result in aggressive necrosis of the surrounding tissues. Dermatome shaving is not ideal but practically without such a risk and preferable even if healing may take months. Local corticoid can be used to control hypergranulation. Laser treatment is not applicable and directly contraindicated.

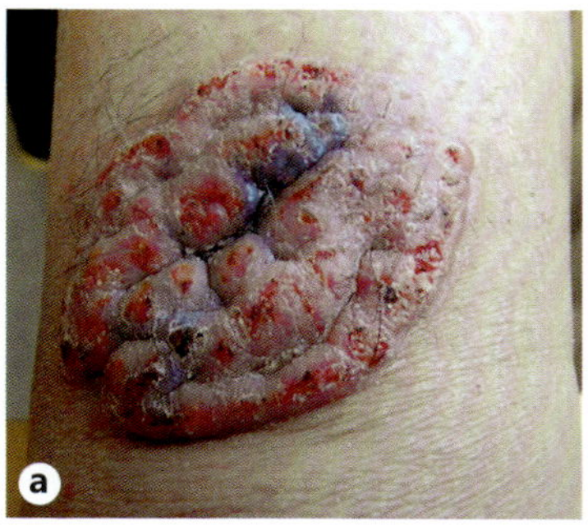
a

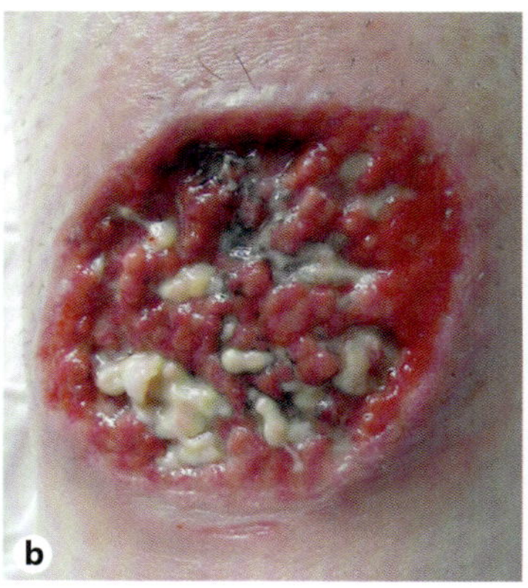
b

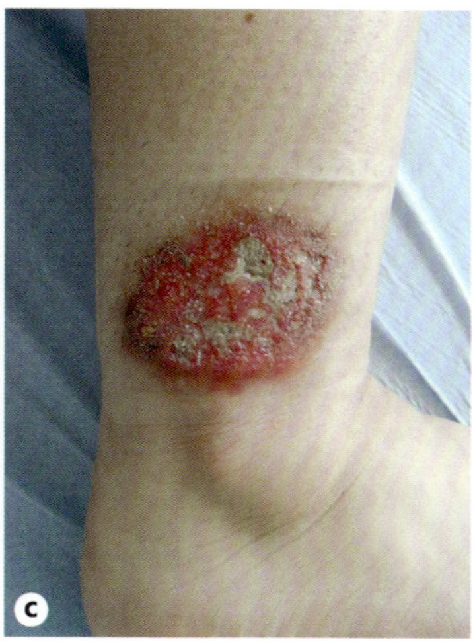
c

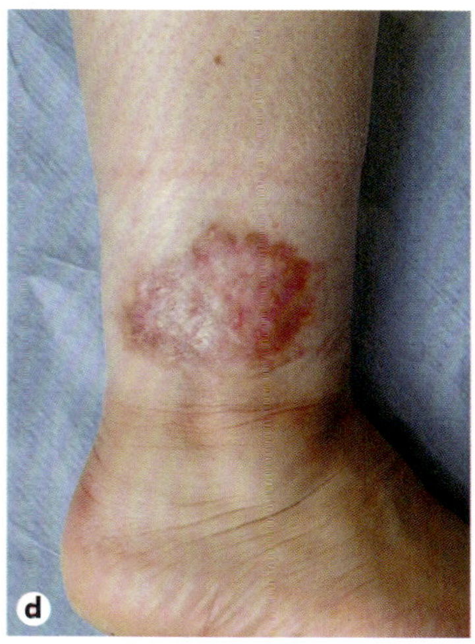
d

Aggressive Necrosis in a Multicolored Tattoo with Successive Amputations of the Leg, Chronically Impaired Wound Healing, and Generalized Dermopathy

History

At a tattoo convention in 1998, a 38-year-old previously perfectly healthy man acquired a large multicolored tattoo on one leg. The whole leg was swollen and healing prolonged. After 5 years, his tattooed foot suddenly started to become inflamed, followed by chronic deep ulceration, which gradually progressed over 2–3 years and involved most of his tattooed leg. Several excisions of necrotic tissue covered with transplants had failed. Amputation was done stepwise at the level of the forefoot, the ankle joint, over the joint, under the knee, and finally at the level of the thigh; however, ulceration was still present. The pathologist recorded visible red tattoo pigment on the muscle fascia of the amputated leg. Sampling of bacteria showed no special finding, and no mycobacteria. Several antibiotic treatments had failed. The amputated femur would not heal, and ulcerations constantly produced a hemorrhagic discharge. In 2006 he had an operation for a herniated disk. This wound remained open for years with hemorrhagic discharge. On the normal skin, circular wounds with a vasculitis-like look could appear, and occasional scratching of the skin caused excoriations that healed only after a long time. Histology on several occasions showed dermal inflammation, erythrocyte extravasation, no vasculitis, and no other specific findings. He was extensively evaluated for a specific underlying autoimmune disease and conditions causing delayed wound healing, with no result. No coagulopathy was found. In recent years, the disease appeared stationary with pain in the amputated leg.

Comment

The patient may represent a new and rare disease entity or mechanism not known from the literature. The tattoo of the leg involved a large local and systemic dose of tattoo inks, pigments, and other ink ingredients. The delay between tattooing and onset of complications might indicate an allergic mechanism as known from red tattoos made with azo pigments, and involvement of the entire skin might be interpreted as spread of the pigment-related allergen or hapten to the entire skin and other organs via the circulation, with chronic ulceration in other skin sites parallel to chronic ulceration and necrosis in the tattoo on the leg, which had started the disease. The aggressive course, attacking normal tissues, may indicate autoimmunity.

Treatment

The patient did not respond to oral prednisone, cyclosporine, and methotrexate given as monotherapy or in combinations. He also did not respond to biologic treatment with a TNFα inhibitor. He could not be offered efficient treatment other than medical relief of the chronic pain in his leg. His life was ruined because of the tattoo.

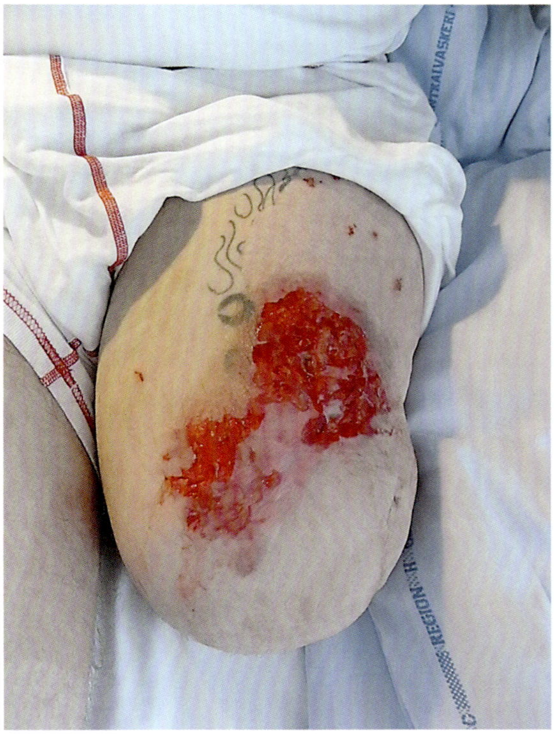

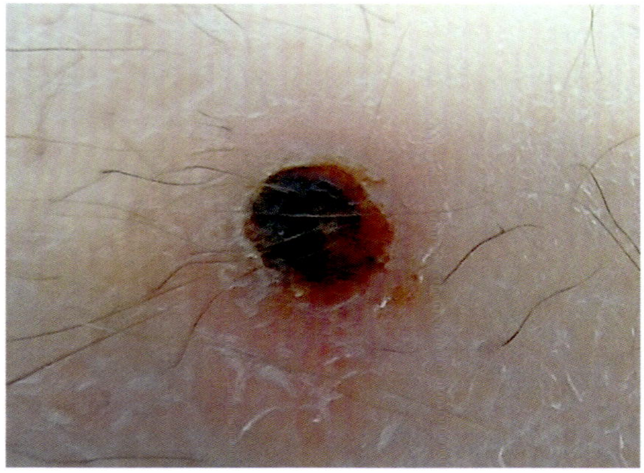

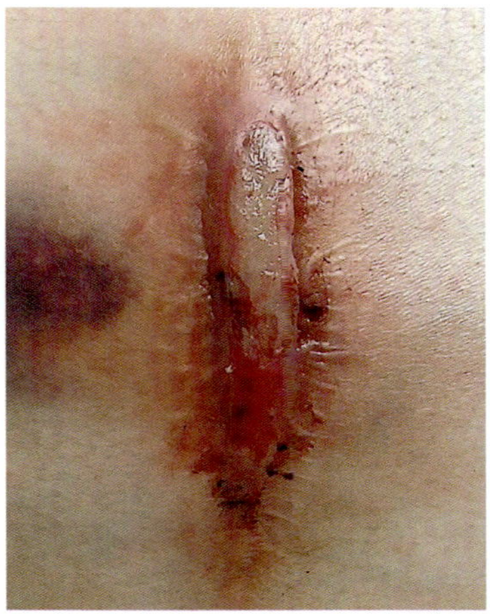

Allergic Reaction in a Red Tattoo: Type Ulceronecrotic Reaction, Severe

History
The patient's husband had bought a tattoo startup kit with a machine, needle, and inks over the Internet. He had tattooed a red heart over the ankle joint of the patient. After 10 days, the tattoo started to react, which soon turned into ulceration with necrosis of the entire dermis. The reaction and the ulcer were painful and constant for several months. There was no spreading or generalized involvement of the skin or other organs. Local corticoid was tried. The patient had no disease or condition predisposing to poor wound healing. Patch testing on the back with the culprit red ink and a brown ink from the same supply gave 2+ and 1+ reactions, with no ulceration under test chambers. Standard patch testing was negative.

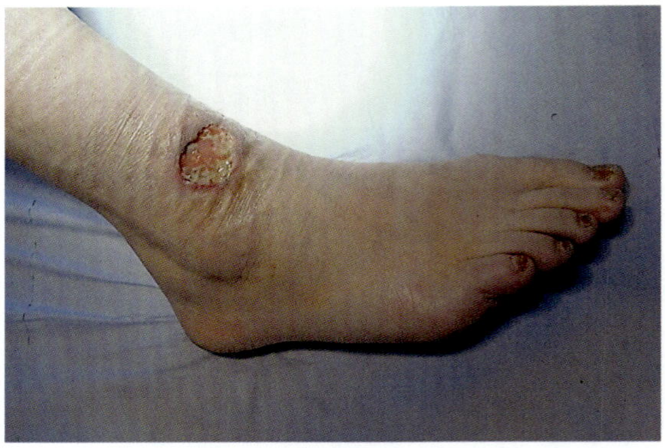

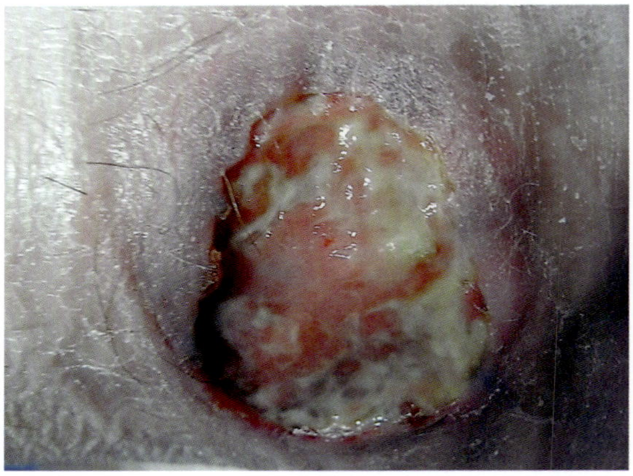

Comment
Aggressive allergy to tattoo ink ingredients may exceptionally cause deep ulceration and necrosis, which were in this case limited to the tattoo. The allergen was probably of rather poor solubility and thus remained in loco, apparently somehow related to the red pigment or a contaminant coming from primitive production. Allergy to red pigment is normally patch test negative when the ink is tested under standard test chamber occlusion.

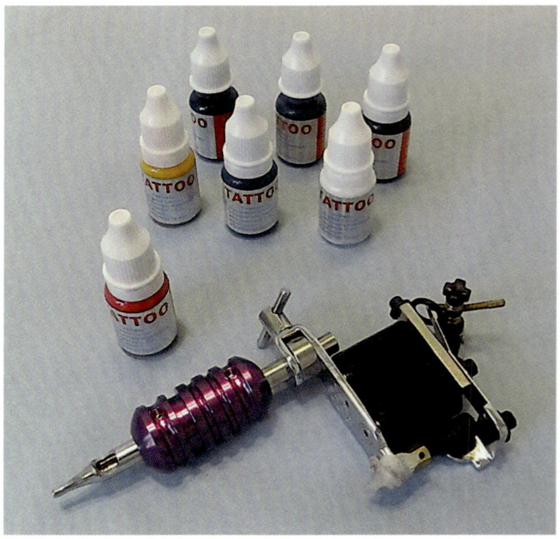

Treatment
Oral corticoid and immunosuppressant are the treatments of choice. This patient refrained from such treatment. Surgical excision is contraindicated since the allergen or, more precisely, the hapten may be embedded deeply in the tissue and also regionally beyond what is expected, with the risk of aggressive necrosis and even amputation helped by surgery.

Allergic Reaction in a Blue Tattoo Parallel to Spontaneous Color Shift in the Direction of Green

History
A multicolored tattoo recently acquired on the sun-exposed side of the upper arm developed itching and slight thickening in parts of the tattoo after about a year. The tattoo had undergone a spontaneous color shift from blue in the direction of green. The tattoo was made by a professional artist. Healing of the tattoo had been normal without any sign of infection.

Comment
The reaction was concluded to be allergic and suggested to be caused by a chemical breakdown product of the originally blue pigment while being metabolically altered and turning into a more green color variant. Only tattoos on normally sun-exposed sites reacted. The raw punch biopsy showed that the transition of color was limited to the outermost layer of pigment in the outer dermis, while the pigment deeper in the dermis, which is exposed to a reduced dose of light due to light absorption in the skin, remained blue. The color shift was likely to be due to ultraviolet light, which may induce both chemical and physical alteration of the original pigment.

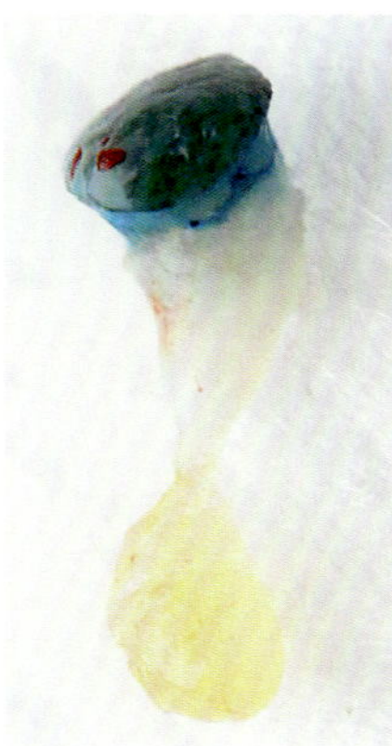

Treatment
Treatment was mid-potent local corticoid and use of sun blocker in the summertime.

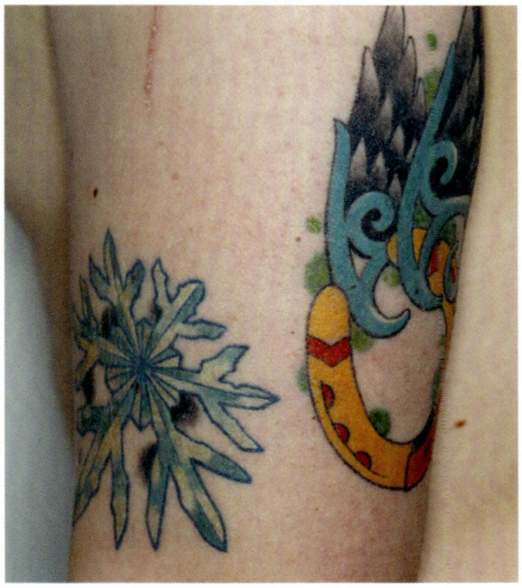

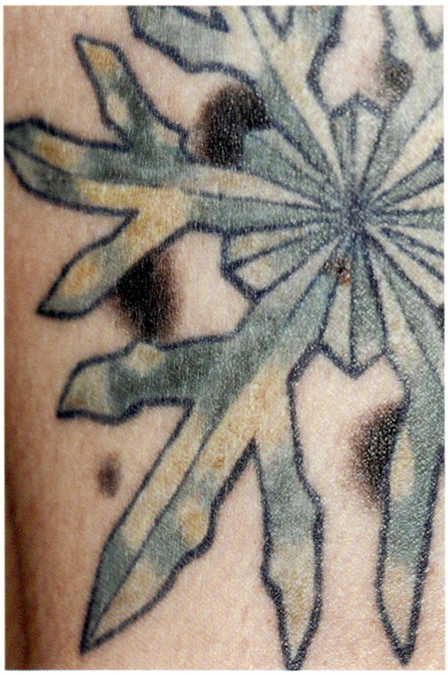

Allergic Reaction in a Blue Tattoo with Pigment Blowout

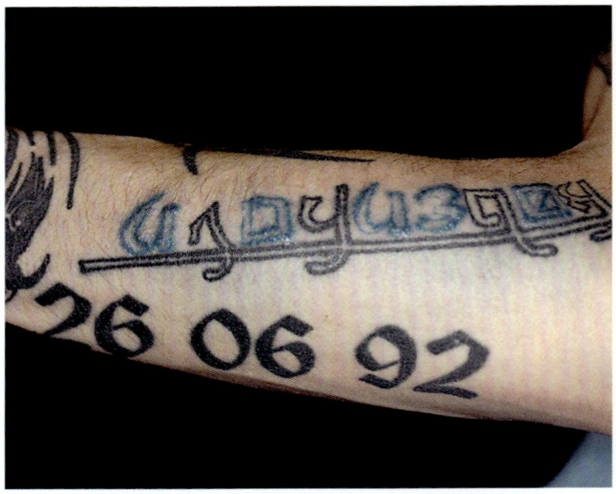

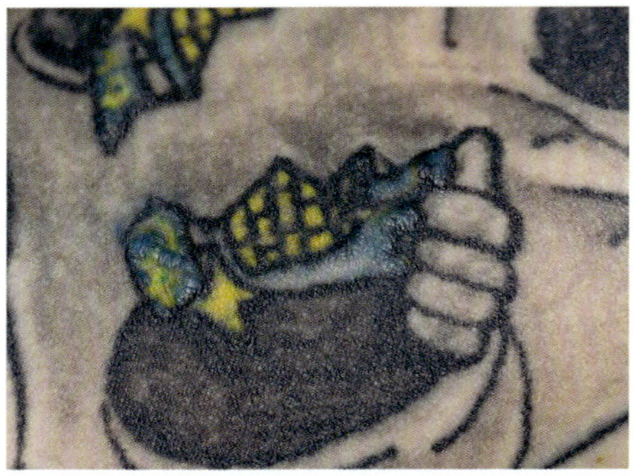

History
About 1 year after tattooing, a text made with a blue ink started to swell and itch, which was severe and disturbed sleep. The blue text presented a mix of papules, nodules, and plaque elevation. Parallel to the abnormal reaction or a few months before, the blue tattoo pigment started to diffuse to the surrounding skin, without noticeable reaction in the surroundings.

Comment
The reaction was allergic and classified as atypical plaque elevation. The reaction was manifested wherever the blue pigment was present in the tattoo and selectively in blue. No reaction in the surrounding skin with blue pigment blowout may indicate that there is a lower threshold for an allergic reaction to occur; or a metabolite or more disperse fraction of the blue pigment might not contribute to the specific hapten in the dermis causing the allergic reaction.

Treatment
Therapy was dermatome shaving. Local corticoid had been of no effect. The allergy was aggressive, and a second shave was needed for sites with remaining activity. The final outcome was satisfactory.

Allergic Reaction in the Lilac Part of a Multicolored Tattoo: Type Plaque Elevation

History

A tattoo started to thicken and itch 2 years after it was made. There had been no special exposure to sun, and the tattoo was not sensitive to light.

Comment

This case illustrates a selective allergy manifested in one color only. Histology showed lymphocytic infiltration to the mid-dermal level, with a few small epithelioid granulomas in the black lining. The epidermis showed mild acanthosis and hyperkeratosis, clinically with barely visible scaling.

Treatment

Treatment was dermatome shaving. Local corticoid had no effect.

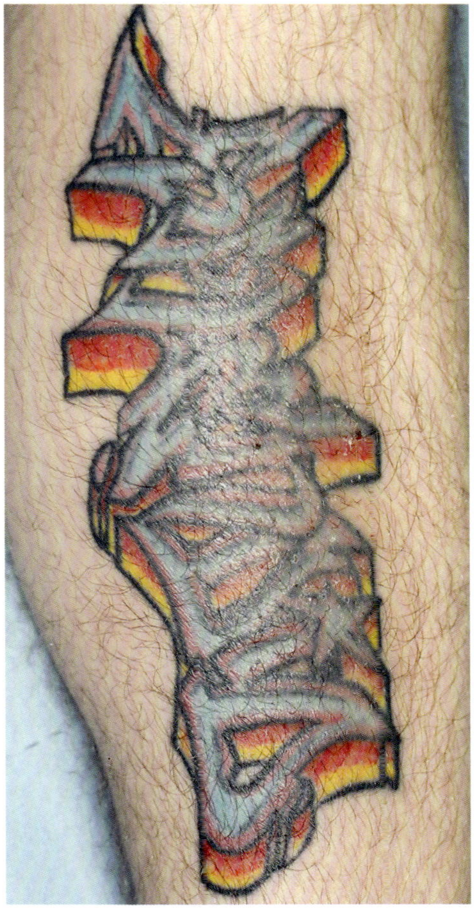

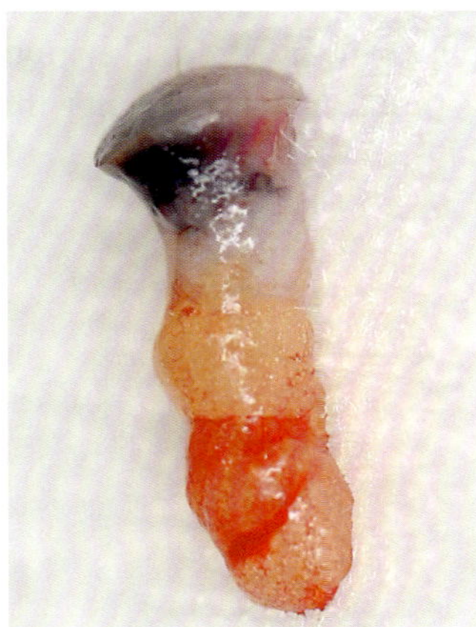

Allergic Reaction in a Lilac Tattoo: Type Excessive Hyperkeratosis with Parallel Reaction in Lymph Nodes

History
Two weeks after tattooing of the leg with lilac ink, the new tattoo started to thicken and itch, which became prominent. After a couple of months, the patient noted tender lymph nodes sized 2 × 3 cm in the inguinal fossa. Symptoms were constant over months with pain and itch in the tattoo and tenderness of the lymph nodes. There were no symptoms or signs of infection. PET scanning confirmed two enlarged lymph nodes and otherwise normal findings. Punch biopsy showed fiery lymphatic infiltration of the entire dermis, and epidermal thickening with parakeratosis and hyperkeratosis were also seen on the raw punch biopsy.

Comment
The allergic reaction was strong and, despite little surface scaling, clinically of the type excessive hyperkeratosis (mild grade, acneiform type). The surface showed follicular openings and comedo-like structures, and the punch biopsy excessive hyperkeratosis.

Enlargement of the regional lymph nodes, tenderness of nodes, and chronicity of symptoms exceeded the typical course of simple reactive lymphopathy. Tattoo pigment is primarily drained via the lymph to deposits in the regional lymph nodes. An allergic reaction to tattoo pigment with necrosis can occur in the lymph nodes parallel to the skin reaction, particularly in case of pigment overload of the tattoo as the raw punch biopsy showed in this case.

Treatment
Treatment was dermatome shaving of the tattoo followed by local corticoid. The lymph nodes were observed. In strong allergy with necrosis of the lymph nodes, surgical excision of nodes can be required.

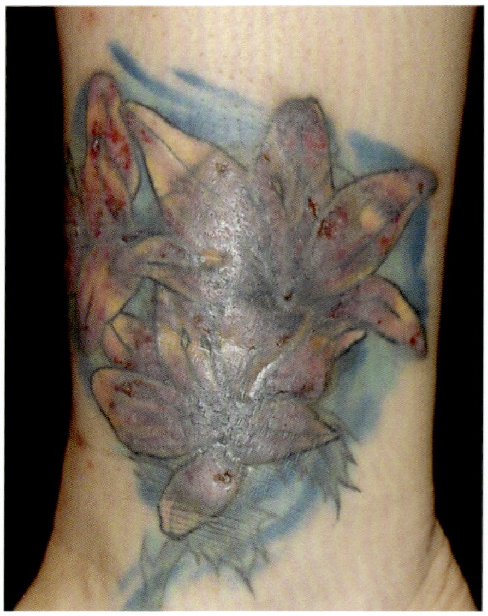

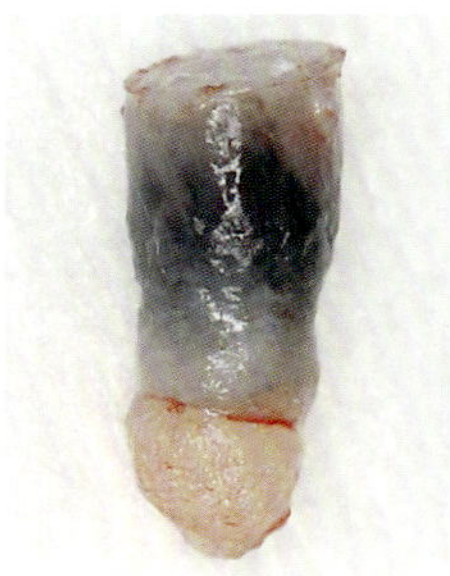

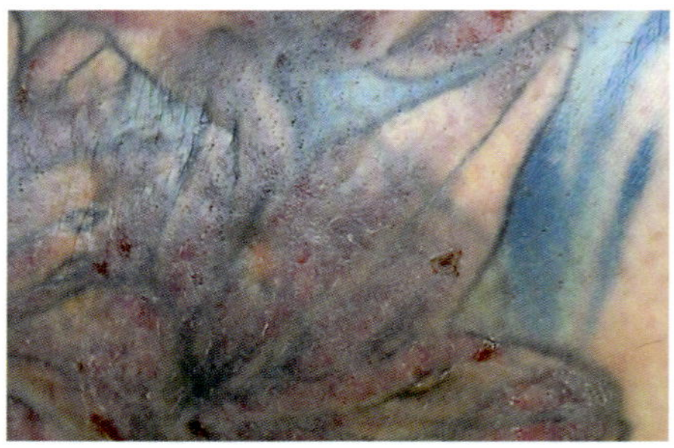

Allergic Eczema in a Cover-Up Tattoo with Progression into the Surrounding Skin

History

Within 1–2 days after cover-up tattooing of 2 old flower tattoos – with refreshment of black lining and pollen grains added to the motif and the surrounding skin – the patient developed inflammation in every tattooed spot including a rim of normal skin outside the tattooed area. Clinically, the inflammation had the appearance of a papulovesicular eczema. It had the look of a positive patch test reaction with 3+ reading. The reaction was completely independent of the existing colors of the tattoo. The patient had no history of allergy or eczema and tolerated metal contacts.

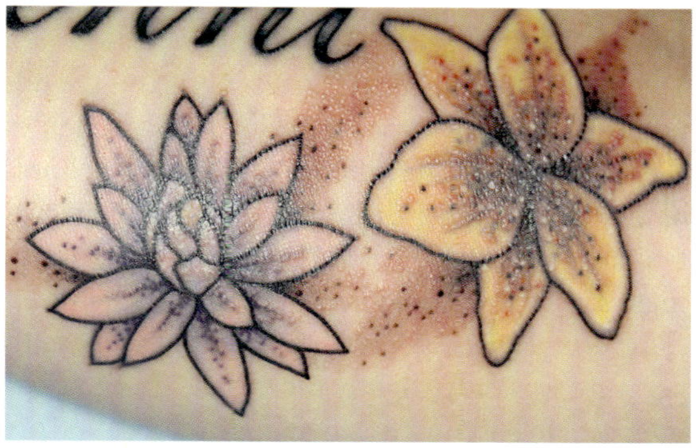

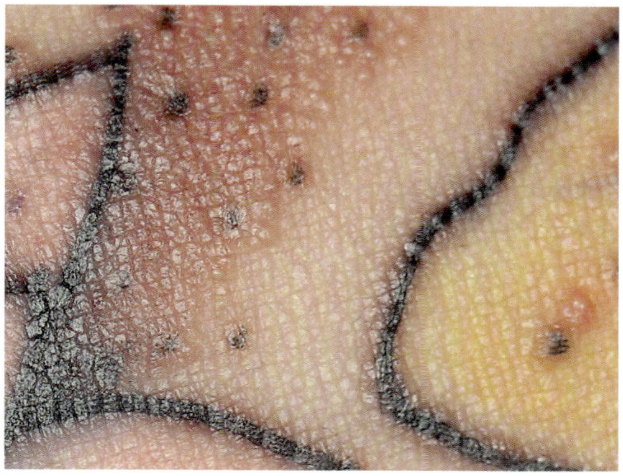

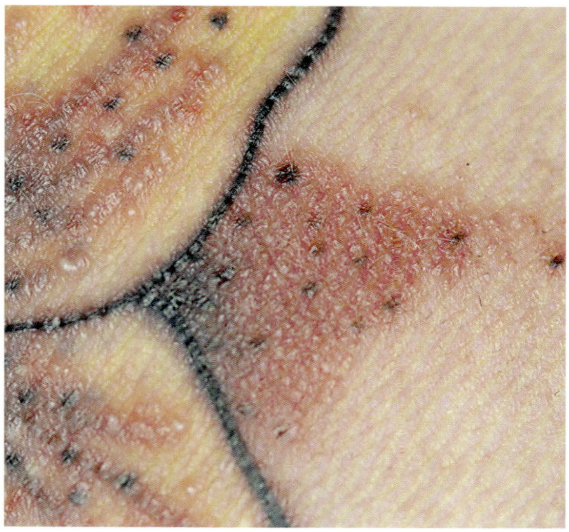

Comment

The clinical findings and the course of events indicated local allergic eczema by challenge through tattooing with an unidentified soluble allergen in the black tattoo ink, an allergen to which the patient was likely already sensitized without knowing it. The dermatitis persisted for several months and was quite resistant to treatment with local corticoid. Standard patch test was negative and the cause of the reaction was not found.

Treatment

For treatment, see above.

Generalized Allergic Eczema after a New Tattoo Caused by Primary Sensitization to Nickel

History
Two weeks after acquiring a new tattoo on the upper arm, the patient developed severe reaction of the tattoo within a few hours followed by redness of the surrounding skin and the entire skin, in particular the face with swelling of the eye surroundings. The rash was manifested as an exanthema on the trunk. He felt generally ill but the body temperature was only slightly increased. The itch was intense. He had no known allergic disease.

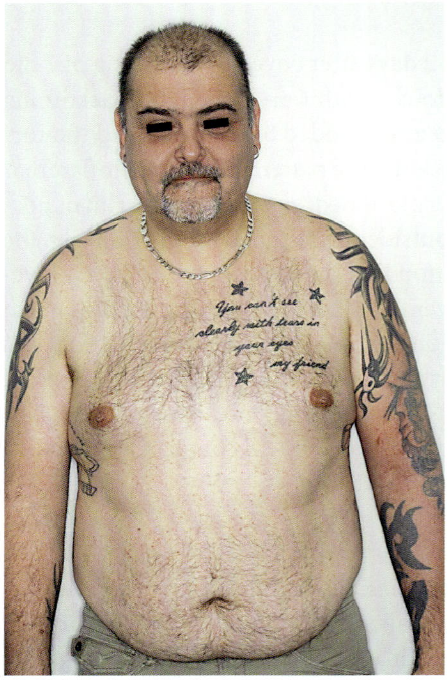

Comment
With the tattoo, the patient apparently became sensitized to a soluble allergen spread via the circulation; thus, the acute allergy was not directly due to the tattoo pigment. At patch testing after recovery he reacted strongly to nickel (3+++) and also to fragrances. Cobalt gave a doubtful reaction only. Preservatives came out negative. He was concluded to be sensitized to nickel by tattooing. The ink was the likely cause.

Treatment
Treatment was oral prednisone in high dose, taped out over weeks guided by stabilization and improvement of the clinical condition. After 5 months, he finally recovered completely with no local reaction in the tattoo.

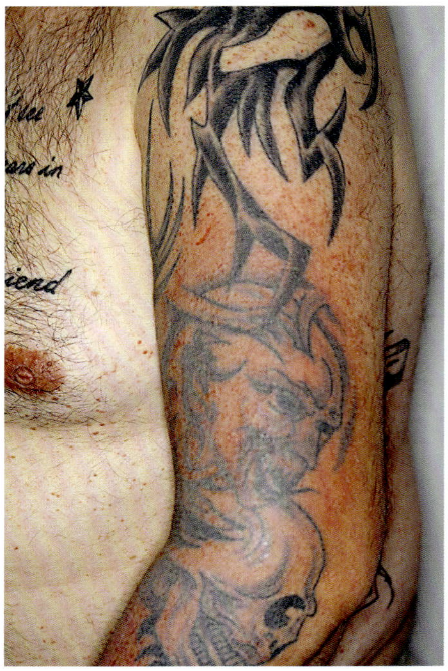

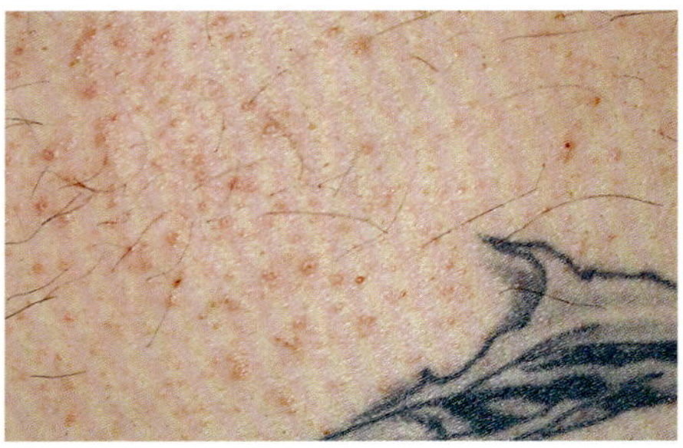

Generalized Allergic Eczema due to Primary Sensitization by Tattooing: Allergen Not Identified

History

Nine days after a new red tattoo was made and after normal initial healing, the red tattoo started to itch and swell within a few hours. The next day, spotty redness occurred in the surrounding skin and as an exanthematous rash in the thighs and other sites including the face. Some elements looked follicular. The patient felt malaise but had no fever.

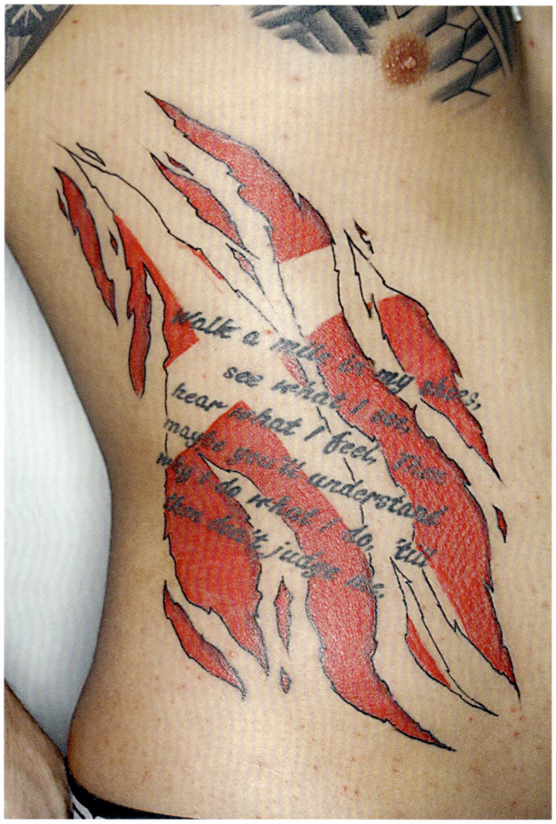

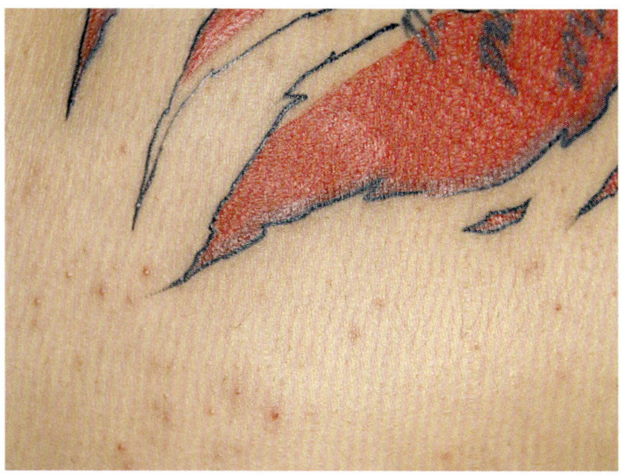

Comments

Because of the delay from tattooing to onset, the case was concluded to be allergic with primary sensitization acquired by tattooing. The allergen was probably some soluble tattoo ink ingredient spread in the body via the circulation and thus unlikely to be the red pigment, which follows the lymph. The tattoo was swollen and tender with inflammation and acute dermatitis. Patch testing after recovery showed no positive finding at all (standard tray including preservatives, textile series, and a panel of risk inks). The allergen could not be identified. Tattoo ink stock products are industrial products with many unknown chemicals and contaminants from production.

Treatment

Treatment was oral prednisone in high dose, taped out over 3 months, with complete recovery without sequels at the end.

Generalized Allergic Eczema the Day after Tattooing due to Preexisting Strong Allergy to Nickel

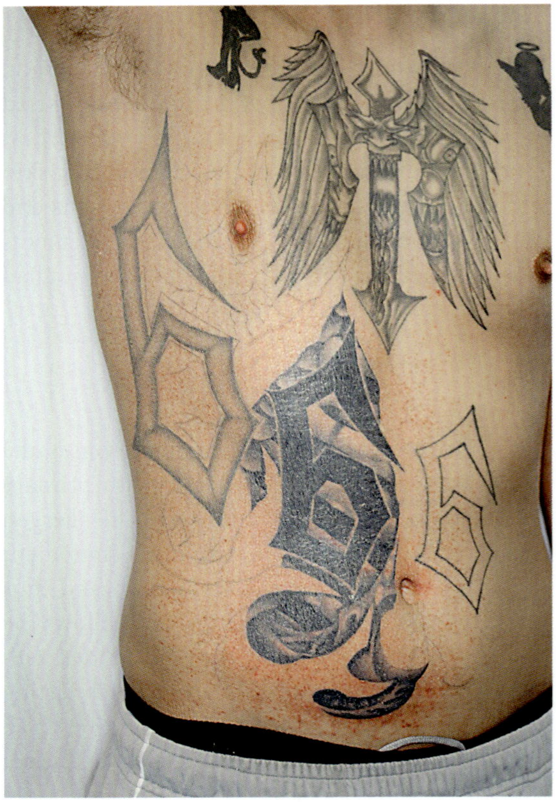

History
Within a day after a black tattoo was performed on the abdomen, the patient developed a universal rash, prominent in the skin surrounding the new tattoo, but also at distant locations such as the face and periorbital skin. The rash was strongly itchy, and the general condition was influenced. There were no signs of local or systemic infection. The patient had a history of skin reactions to metal contacts but no history of any other allergy.

Comment
A patch test with a standard panel performed after healing showed a 3+ positive reaction to nickel sulfate. The case was concluded a severe boost of preexisting strong nickel allergy, with soluble nickel contaminants likely to be present in the black tattoo ink stock product used. The local reaction in the fresh tattoo was prominent and strong, but the rash dominated. It is likely that nickel from the ink reached the circulation.

Treatment
Treatment was oral prednisone for a period of 3 months until the rash gradually healed.

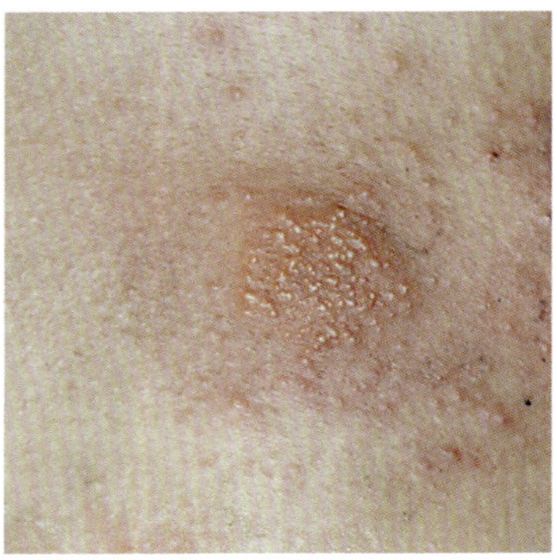

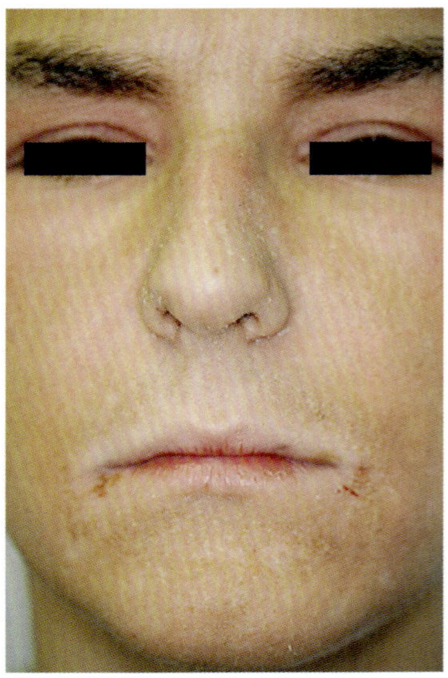

Generalized Dermatitis after Sensitization to Parabens from the Tattoo Ink

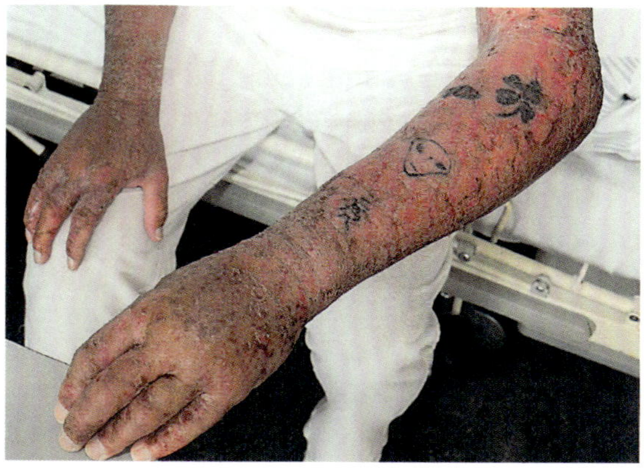

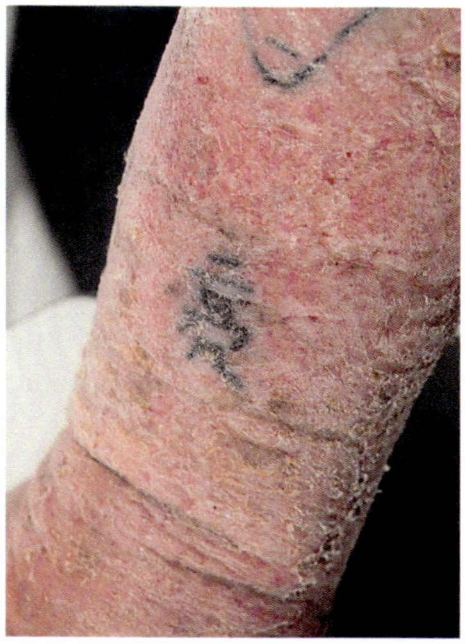

History

Two weeks after acquiring a homemade tattoo and within a day, the patient developed severe dermatitis of the tattooed arm, which soon spread to the entire skin. He had used a cheap tattoo ink from China that he had bought over the Internet. He was hospitalized and treated with oral prednisone. The dermatitis was active for several weeks, and treatment with cyclosporine was instituted. The dermatitis gradually improved over months with some remaining activity in selected sites. Patch testing showed strongly positive reactions against 3 parabens but no other relevant findings, including negative nickel and paraphenylene diamine (PPD) patch. He had not suffered from dermatitis in the past.

Comment

The dermatitis was concluded allergic with primary sensitization against parabens directly from the tattoo ink. The clinical course was protracted and maybe chronic and different from nickel sensitization from tattoo ink, which often fades in a few months. Cheap tattoo inks can be filled with preservatives such as parabens to camouflage dirty production. Clinical photos and case: courtesy of Dr. Carsten Saur Mikkelsen, Brønderslev, Denmark

Treatment

Treatment was oral high-dose corticoid and immunosuppressant, in this case cyclosporine.

Allergic Eczema in a Patient with a Tattoo Reaction and Known Hair Dye Allergy with the Rash Possibly Elicited by a PPD Analogue

History

Only 3 days after getting a new red tattoo, toned with a lilac dye, the patient presented with a widespread eczematous reaction in the skin with severe itching, which was intolerable. One day after tattooing, the tattoo reacted with major swelling associated with widespread active dermatitis in the normal skin. The reaction in the tattoo was more likely a chronic eczema and not a typical allergic plaque elevation of the 'lichenoid' type. The patient had been using hair dyes for years. She had stopped using a dark dye that had caused dermatitis a few years ago. There was no known metal allergy. She was given high-dose prednisone with limited effect, and the tattoo was dermatome shaved to eradicate the culprit pigment in the skin. Prednisone was needed for more than 6 months, but there was frequent flare-up of eczema in the neck and other anatomical sites including the hands, however, after shaving, only little in the tattoo. After 1 year, she still had sporadic activity in her eczema.

Comment

The clinical course of the allergic reaction with abrupt outbreak and chronicity was similar to paraphenylenediamine (PPD) allergy with generalized eczema. The patient reacted shortly after getting the tattoo and therefore must have been sensitized in the past. Her history indicated hair dye allergy. A patch test was positive to PPD (2+), textile mix (3+), and specified dyes, but negative to metals and preservatives. PPD is forbidden in hair dyes, but analogues are allowed and commonly used. She was presumably sensitized by a hair dye containing PPD analogue(s) and reacted within 1 day on challenge by the recent tattoo made with a tattoo ink that contained identical analogue(s) or cross-reacting chemical(s) somehow associated with the colorant of the ink.

Treatment

Treatment was oral prednisone and local corticoid for months as well as early dermatome shaving of the triggering tattoo.

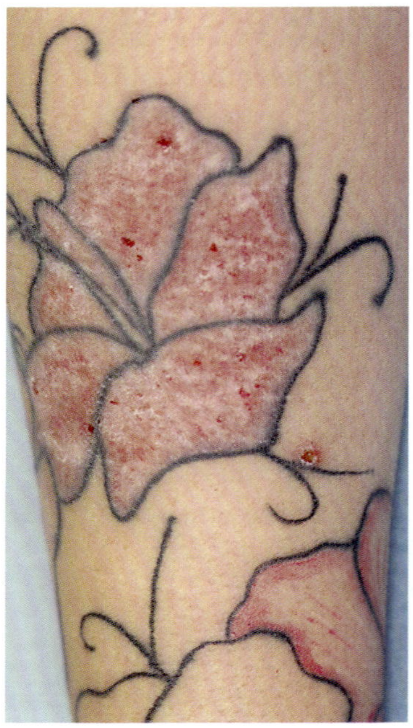

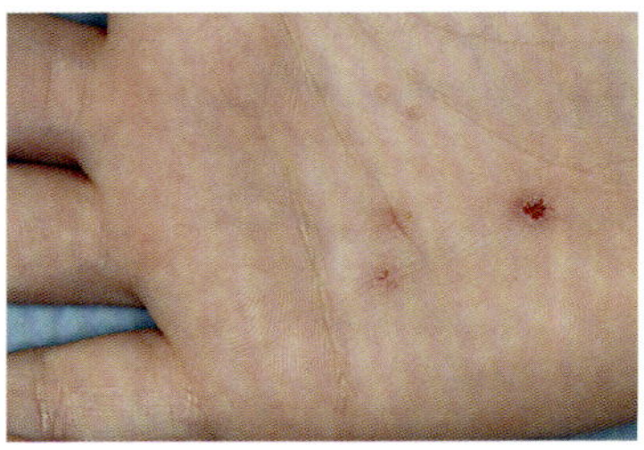

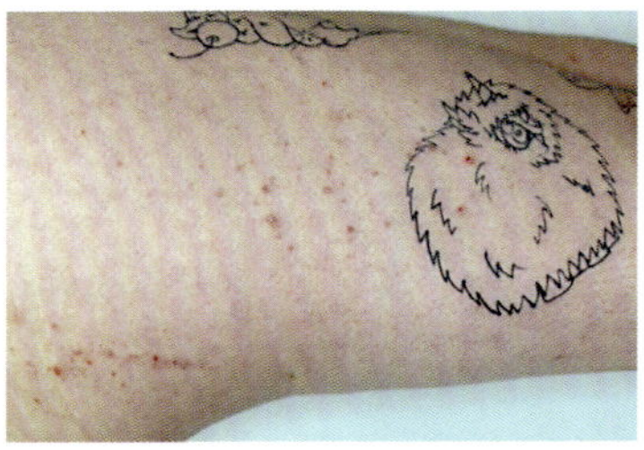

Henna Tattoo Reaction with Generalized Dermatitis: Is PPD Allergy Also a Potential Risk with Permanent Tattooing?

History

A young girl got a henna tattoo on her hand during holidays in Turkey. After 1 day, the tattoo started to react, and soon she developed a rash involving the entire skin including the face. Two years before, also during holidays, she had gotten her first henna tattoo, which after about 10 days had reacted with eczema in the tattoo. Her sister also got a henna tattoo on her hand on the same recent holiday in Turkey. She had a strong local reaction after 8 days, which in her case did not spread to other parts of the skin.

Comment

These cases illustrate contact allergy to 'black henna' enriched with the strong allergen para-phenylenediamine (PPD) used to darken the paint. One case already sensitized and challenged had a local reaction and rash after 1 day, the other case not allergic before became sensitized with a strong local reaction but no rash after 8 days.

Tattoo ink stock products on the market analyzed for PPD have hitherto not been found to have PPD as an ingredient or contaminant. However, some low-priced inks are produced scrupulously and under primitive conditions, and there is a constant risk that dark inks for permanent and cosmetic tattooing holding PPD or PPD analogues may show up in the future. The expected clinical manifestations of PPD-contaminated permanent tattoo ink used by amateur or professional tattooists for decorative tattoos are expected to match what is known from henna tattoos; however, generalized and severe dermatitis is expected to be much more common. Dermatologists should be aware and spot such a situation and patch test with PPD if tattoos cause a rash.

Treatment

Treatment was oral prednisone for about 6 months followed by local corticoids. However, after 2 years, minor flares of activity still occurred.

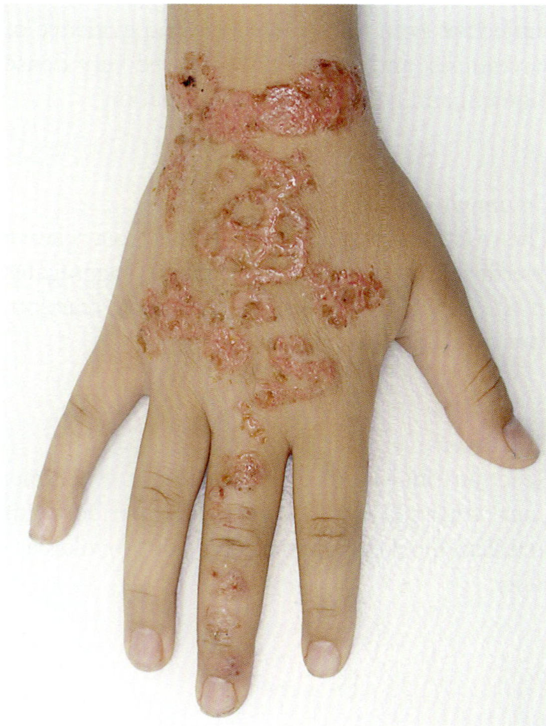

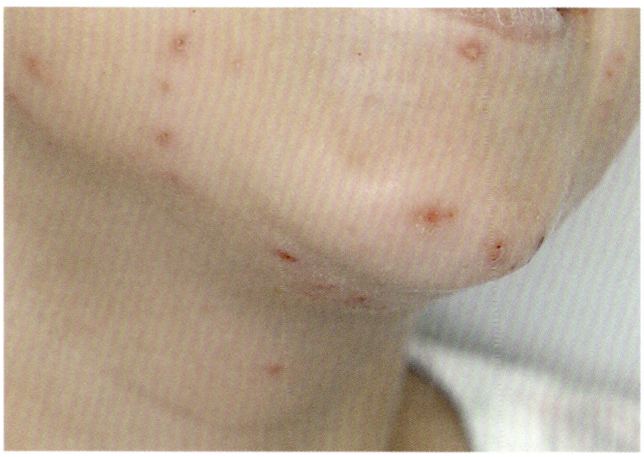

Reaction in a Black Tattoo: Type Papulonodular Reaction

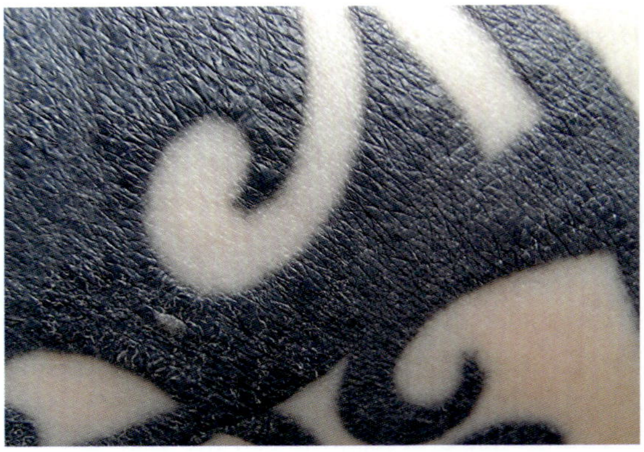

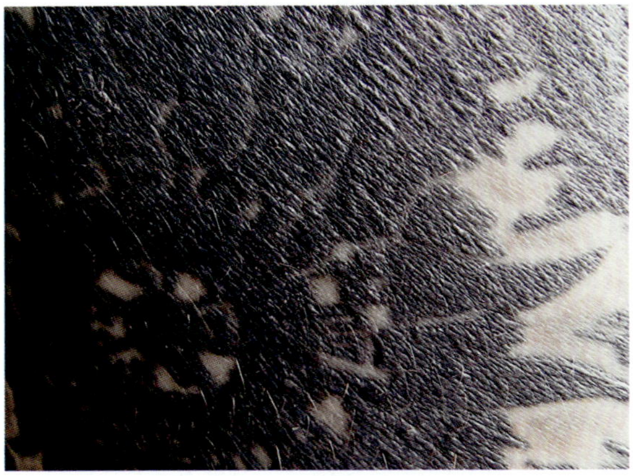

History
Over a period of 3–5 years, black tattoos gradually developed slight thickening as well as papules and small nodules. There were also parts of the tattoos with no change. Reactions intermittently were more active and generally caused only mild subjective symptoms. There was no evidence of sarcoidosis, and biopsy only showed very dense pigment and lymphocytic inflammation.

Comment
The reactions were probably related to a relative overdose with black pigment forming aggregates in the dermis with mild foreign body reaction, thus nonallergic in nature.

Treatment
Reactions may resolve spontaneously over time. Local corticoid can be used during periods with itch. Sun blocker can be used if sun provokes activity.

Pigment Overload Reaction in a Black Tattoo: Type Papulonodular Reaction Treated with Surgical Excision

History
A black bracelet tattoo on the distal forearm of a young woman developed prominent thickening with tenderness of the tattoo over 3–6 months. Healing of the tattoo had been without complications albeit maybe delayed. The tattoo looked bad.

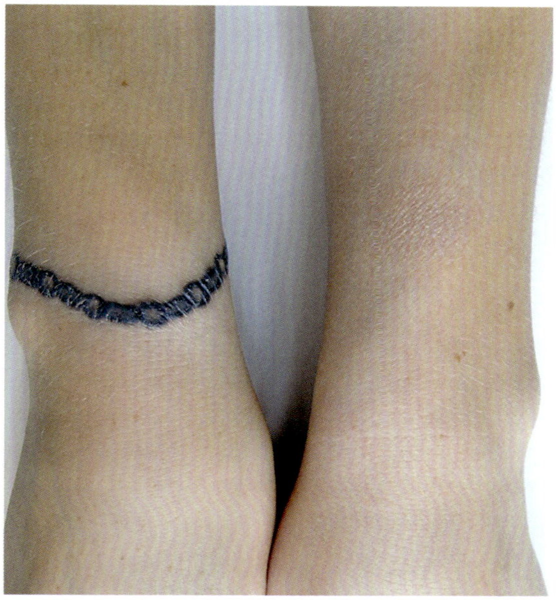

Comment
Punch biopsy showed dense pigment throughout the full thickness of the dermis and granulomatous inflammation interpreted as simple foreign body reaction to large aggregates of black pigment particles. Aggregates in the dermis biopsy were directly visible by the naked eye. Dermatome shaving sparing the deep dermis was not possible due to deep pigment deposits. Surgical excision with primary suture was performed. The excised skin (the lower part of the photo of excised skin with the skin strip flipped over shows the inner side of the dermis towards the fat) showed black pigment directly at the interface to the subcutaneous fat.

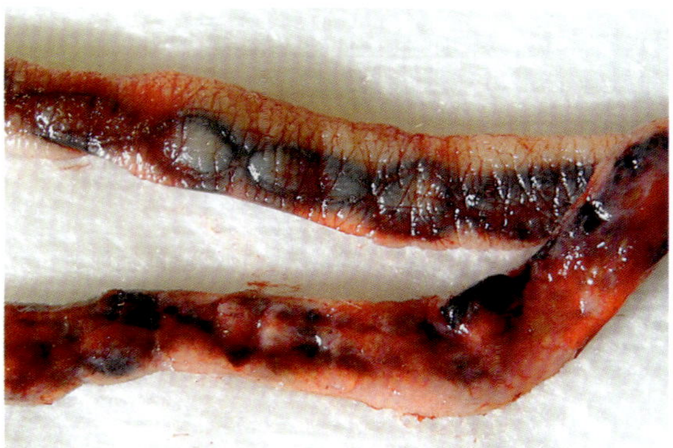

Treatment
For treatment, see above.

Pigment Overload with Mild Papulonodular Reaction and Sensitivity to Sun

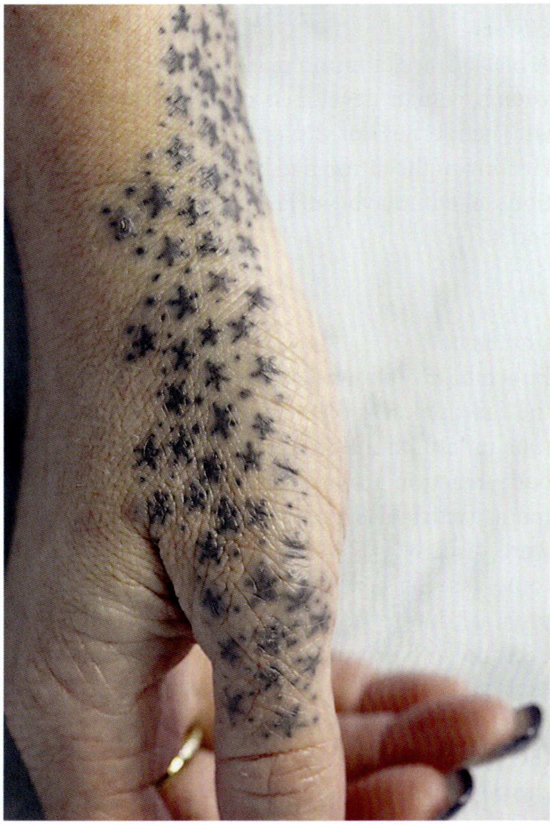

History
A black tattoo made by a professional tattooist 8 years ago. For 3 years, there were constant papular and nodular swellings of some tattoo elements but not of others, with intermittent activity and itching especially at summertime.

Comment
The dermis is heavily packed with black pigment, apparently more than the skin can accept. Pigment is aggregated with visible minor aggregates by visual inspection of the raw biopsy. Histology showed mild lymphocytic infiltration and no granuloma formation.

Treatment
Treatment was local corticoid in periods of complaints and sun blocker on sunny days. The problem may recover spontaneously over time. Ultimately, laser removal can be applied.

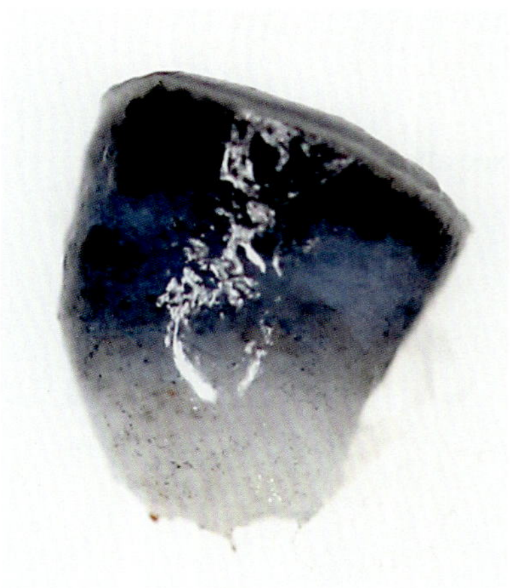

Pimples after Tattooing with Black Ink

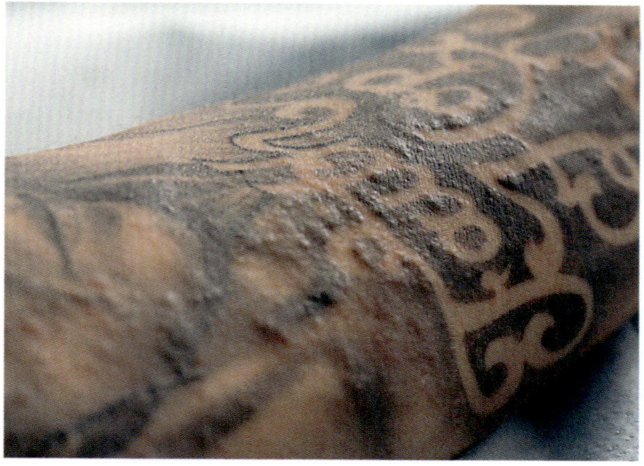

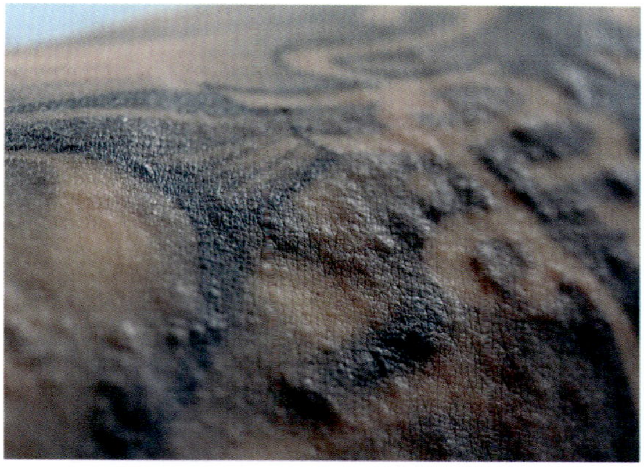

History
Three weeks after acquiring a new black tattoo and at the end of an uncomplicated healing process, pimples appeared scattered in the tattooed skin. Pimples were not associated with subjective symptoms.

Comment
Biopsy of a pimple on the tattoo showed an eczematous reaction with acanthosis and parakeratosis as well as a lymphocytic reaction in the outer dermis. Lesions were not vesicular. There was no evidence of a granulomatous reaction. In this case, pimples healed after only 1 month without treatment.

Pimples now and then may occur a few months after tattooing. They may be intermittent and reoccur for several months but ultimately spontaneous healing will occur. Pimples may also show up after laser removal.

Treatment
Treatment is observation. Pimples are not associated with subjective symptoms.

Black Tattoo with Pigment Blowout

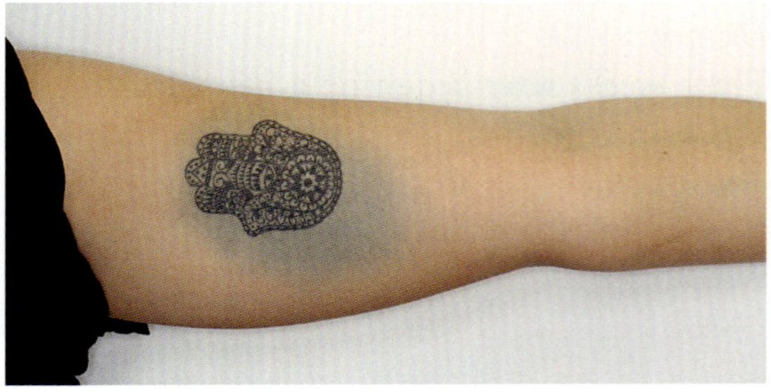

History
A few weeks after having acquired a new tattoo on the inner side of the upper arm, the patient observed staining of the surrounding nontattooed skin. The pigment blowout was not concentric and not in the direction of the central lymph flow but apparently followed gravitational forces. The tattoo had healed normally. The tattooist was an amateur. A normal ink bottle had been used, not printer ink. The patient's friend had acquired a black tattoo the same day made by the same tattooist using the same ink bottle, but she showed no blowout.

Comment
Pigment drift to the surrounding skin can happen and is somehow unpredictable. Predispositions seem to be black ink, thin and soft skin, including the eye lids, and amateur tattooing with a too deep injection of pigment.

Treatment
Treatment is by YAG laser, which is often successful after a few treatments only. The density of pigment particles is low. Pigment blowout is self-limiting over time and once cleared further drift is unlikely to occur. Remnant blown out pigment in the lower dermis is barely visible.

Black Tattoo with Pigment Blowout to the Surrounding Skin with a Halo Nearby the Tattoo

History
A black amateur tattoo made in a private home by a friend of the patient. Tattooing had been very painful and with bleeding, followed by delayed healing but seemingly with no infection. Over time, the tattoo acquired a slightly blueish tone indicating deep deposition of pigment, i.e. Tyndall effect. After a few months, the normal skin around the tattoo started to darken concentrically, with the dark zone propagating further in the adjacent skin followed by a pale-looking transition zone, i.e. a halo, in the skin nearby the tattoo.

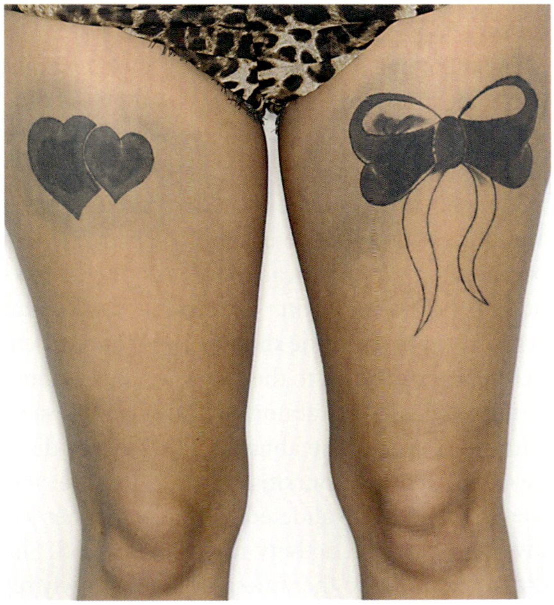

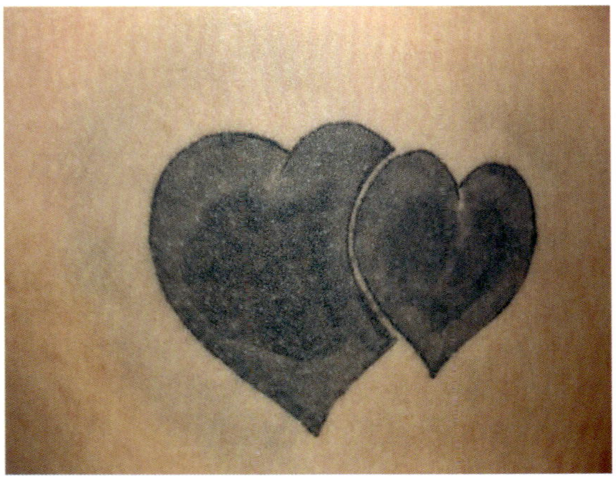

Comment
The blowout of pigment from the tattoo was apparently driven by diffusional particle movement in the subcutaneous fat, thus indicating that the black pigment had been placed too deep in the dermis and maybe directly in the fat. Movement of pigment emptied the original deposition of pigment available for passive displacement, and a halo appearance turned up. Pigment drift in this case was not determined by lymph flow or gravity but concentric.

Treatment
Treatment was observation. YAG laser treatment may be a treatment option and camouflage the color change; however, the bulk of pigment of the blowout is located very deep.

Black Tattoo with Pigment Blowout to Underlying Structures, Subcutaneous Inflammation, and Painful Shoulder

History

The patient had a tattoo made over the left shoulder, with pain and bleeding followed by swelling of the shoulder region as well as green and yellow coloring, indicating subcutaneous bleeding. After healing of the tattoo, the shoulder started to swell and hurt, and the tattoo became thickened with a papulonodular reaction and visible pigment blowout in the normal skin. Ultrasound showed an echo-free mass over the shoulder joint about 1 cm in thickness adjacent to the supraspinatus tendon. X-ray confirmed the abnormal finding of the subcutaneous space. The abnormality was not diagnosed as a simple bursitis. Pain and tenderness were heavy and invalidated the patient in her job involving physical activity for a long period. She did not respond to therapies but finally slowly recovered after 2 years.

Comment

Tattooing had been traumatic and complicated with subdermal bleeding and spreading of pigment both seen as blowout in the normal skin and as scattered pigment granules found in the deep dermis and in the subcutaneous fat by microscopy. Dermal fibrosis and some deep flow of pigment to the fat were seen already in the raw biopsy. The patient reacted to black pigment manifested as a papulonodular reaction in the skin, accompanied by abnormal appearance of the fat by ultrasound and X-ray. Movements in the shoulder were very painful and invalidating for a long period, with no effect of NSAID but some help of intralesional corticoid and oral prednisone. Morphine was needed for a period. The patient finally recovered slowly supported by physiotherapists, with parallel improvement of the local reaction in the tattoo and the pain in the shoulder. Tattoo pigment can blow out not only to the surrounding skin but also to the structures under the tattoo and cause problems. Pigment blowout normally causes no reaction; however, if pigment in the skin causes a reaction, a parallel reaction in other sites with the pigment can take place.

Treatment

Treatment is difficult as described above.

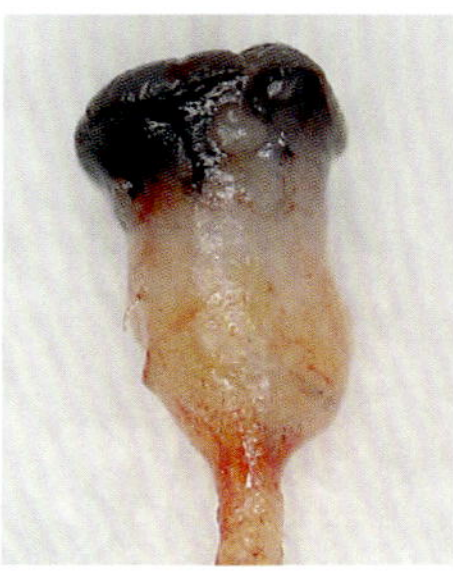

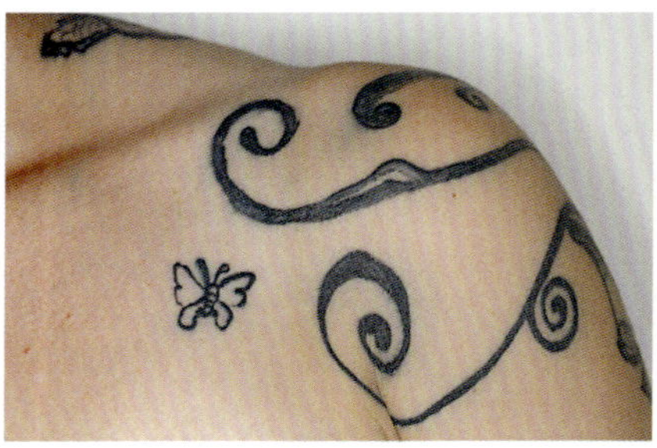

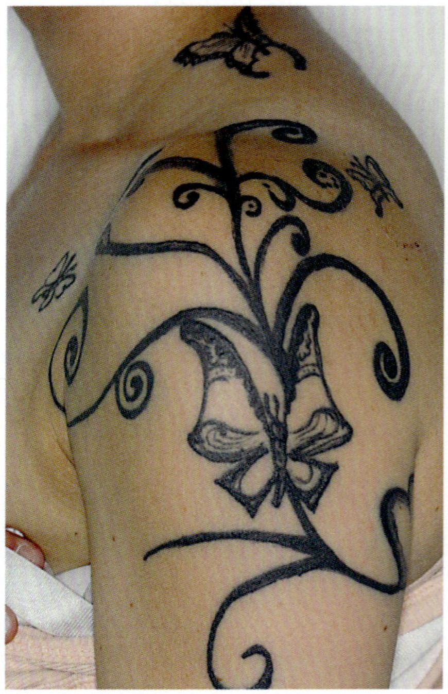

Sarcoidosis Locally in a Black Tattoo with a Papulonodular Reaction

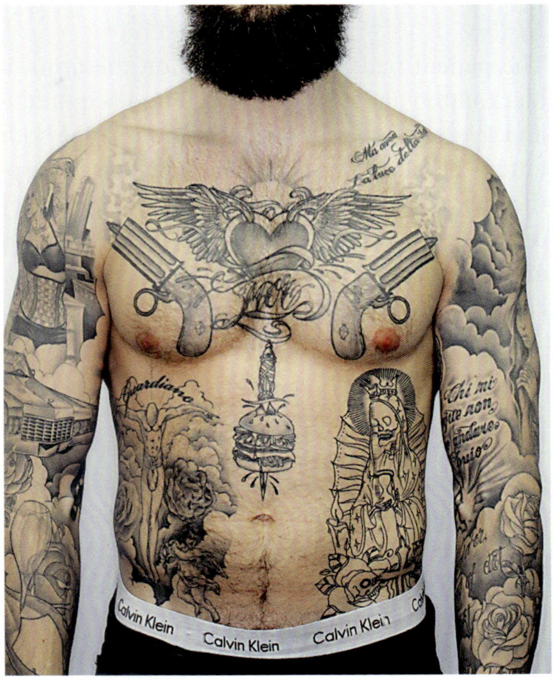

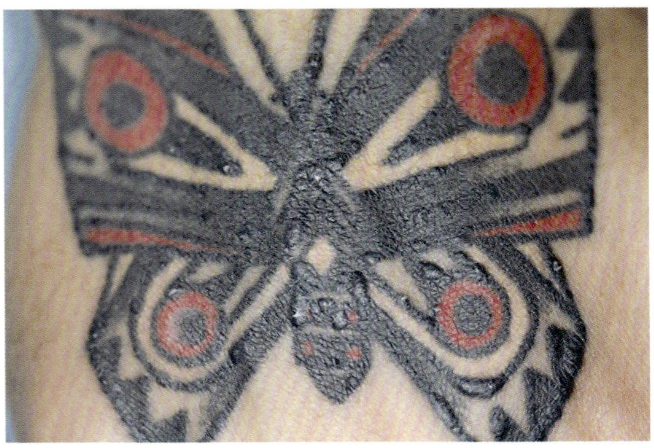

History
In 2 tattoos that had been performed 1 year ago on the back of the hand, papules and nodules developed in the black lines of the tattoos after 2–3 months, while red parts were unaffected. The patient had extensive tattoos for several years, which had never caused any complications. The recent reaction on the hands triggered no reaction in other tattoos, and there were no signs of pulmonary or ocular disease. Joints and other parts of the skin were normal without erythema nodosum or scar sarcoidosis.

Comment
Biopsy showed sarcoid granuloma. X-ray of the chest indicated enlarged hilar glands, but high-resolution CT did not confirm active sarcoidosis. The case was concluded to be sarcoidosis locally in 2 tattoos on the back of the hands. Apparently the used black tattoo ink stock product had triggered the same reaction on 2 independent sites made with the same ink, while various other black inks used in the past had been tolerated. The tendency of black pigment to agglomerate and form foreign bodies in the skin is supposed to vary from one ink stock product to another depending on raw materials, ingredients, and production. In this case the reaction did not trigger autoimmunity and second organ affection.

Treatment
Treatment was potent local corticoid over a few months, which relieved symptoms but not papules. The patient has an increased risk of suffering an outbreak of systemic sarcoidosis later in life.

Sarcoidosis in Black and Brown Tattoos with Erythema Nodosum

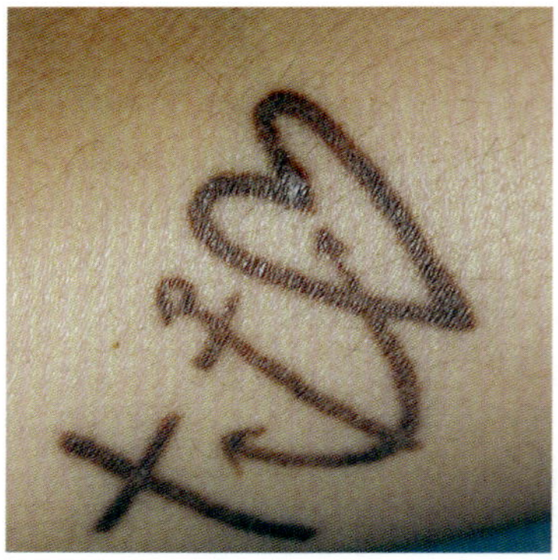

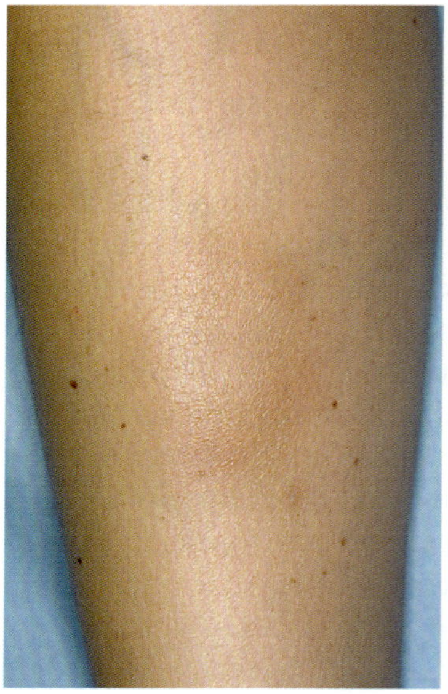

History
The patient had 2 small tattoos on the arms, a black tattoo and a dark brown tattoo acquired 8 and 4 years ago, respectively. Six months ago both tattoos developed nodules, and 1 month ago erythema nodosum was developed on the leg. On debut of the symptoms, the patient had felt tiredness and shortness of breath. There had been no joint complaints or ocular symptoms.

Comment
Biopsy from nodular change of the tattoo showed sarcoid granuloma, and biopsy from the leg confirmed the diagnosis of erythema nodosum. X-ray of the chest was normal. The case was concluded to be tattoo sarcoidosis. It was suggested that the autoimmune predisposition of the patient triggered the reaction locally in the tattoos, with local reaction to pigment particle agglomerates. The brown tattoo ink may have been a mixture of black pigment toned brown with red pigment.

Treatment
Treatment was potent local corticoid for a period of time. The condition healed spontaneously over about 6 months with no signs of internal organ involvement.

Sarcoidosis in a Black Tattoo Associated with Scar Sarcoidosis and Erythema Nodosum

History
Within a few months, the patient developed papules and nodules in a 10-year-old tattoo in the sacral region. At the same time, she had nodules in old scars over the knee joints, some minor discomfort of the joints, and felt a discrete, flat, and tender abnormality in the leg located directly under the skin. For about 3 years, she had noticed some minor shortness of breath.

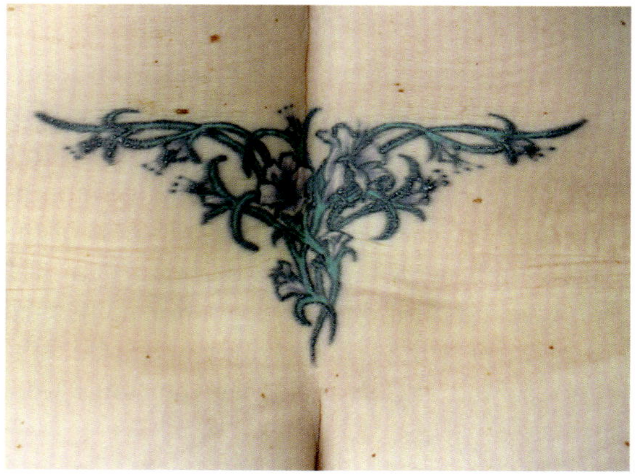

Comment
Biopsy from the black tattoo in the sacral region and from the scar over the knee showed sarcoid granuloma with inflammation. Biopsy of the discrete change on the leg confirmed the diagnosis of erythema nodosum. X-ray of the chest showed hilar gland enlargement but unaffected lung parenchyma. Examination of the eye and the joints was normal.

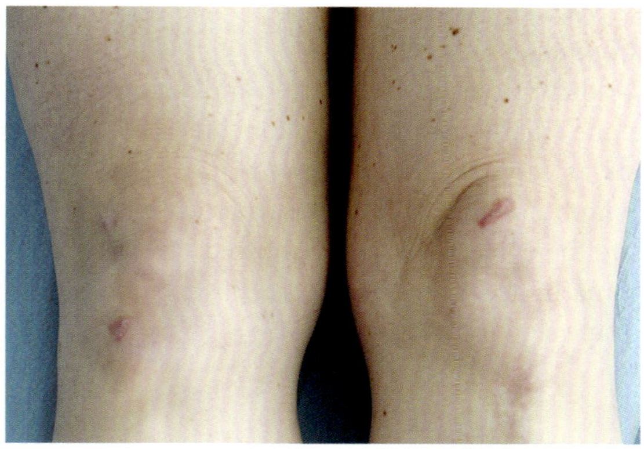

Treatment
Therapy was observation with no medication, according to the patient's wish. Symptoms spontaneously declined over a period of 2–3 years, however, without being completely cleared.

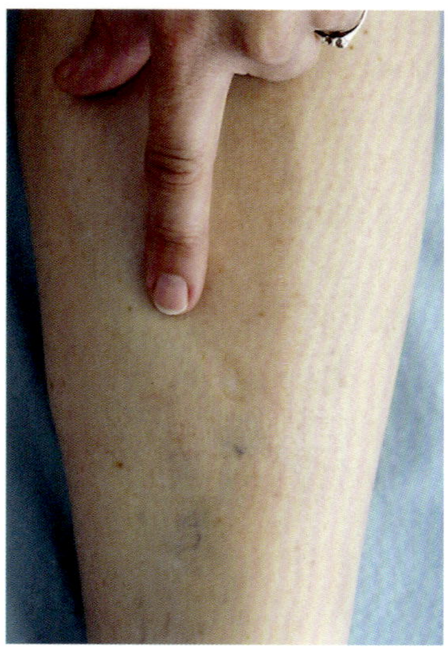

Sarcoidosis in Black Tattoos with Enlarged Regional Lymph Nodes and Associated Iridocyclitis

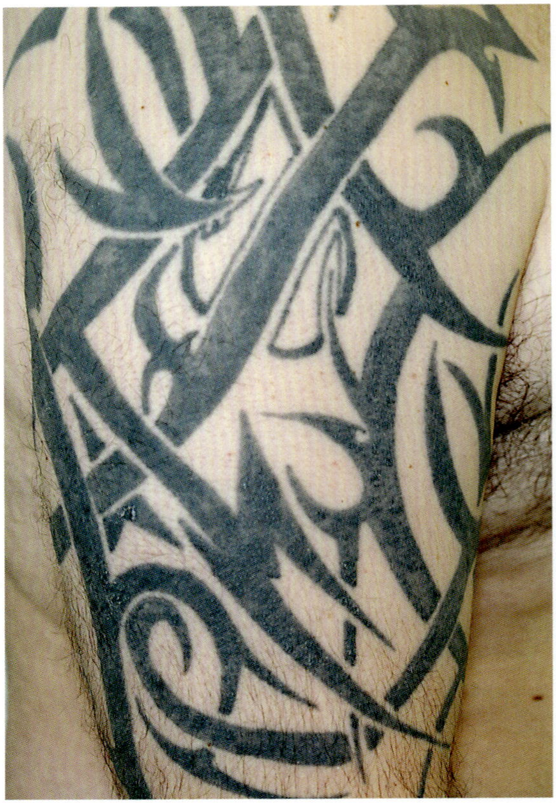

History

For 13 years, the patient had suffered from recurrent iridocyclitis treated by ophthalmologists. For 10 years, he had observed recurrent nodules in a black tattoo on the right shoulder. Three months ago, he observed swelling and tenderness of the right armpit, with lumps sized about 3 cm. CT scanning and ultrasound examination confirmed enlargement of the axillary lymph nodes, but other nodes and organs including the lungs were normal.

Comment

Nodular reaction of the tattoo and regional lymph node enlargement, finally, concluded his diagnosis as sarcoidosis manifested in a black tattoo, lymph nodes, and for years intermittently affecting the eyes. Microscopy showed sarcoid granuloma in accordance with the observed bunch of grape sign in the raw biopsy.

Treatment

Treatment was oral prednisone adjusted to a proper dose relative to effect and side effects. Other systemic immunosuppressants were second choice.

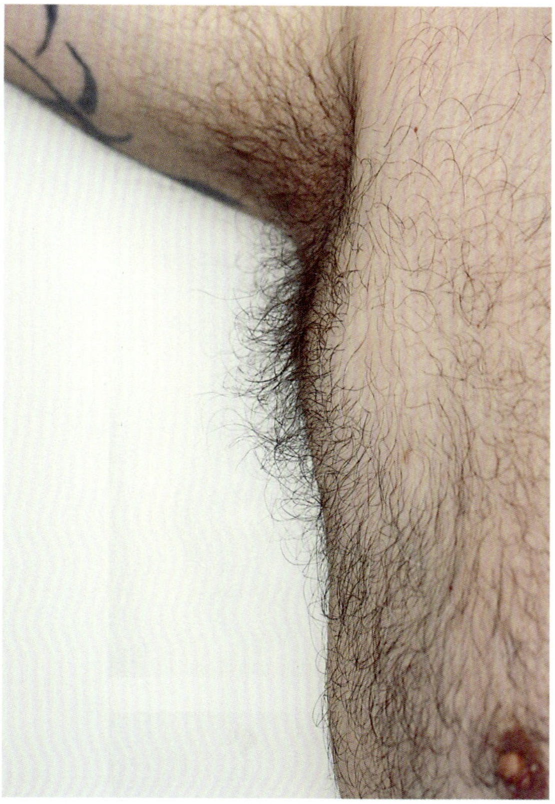
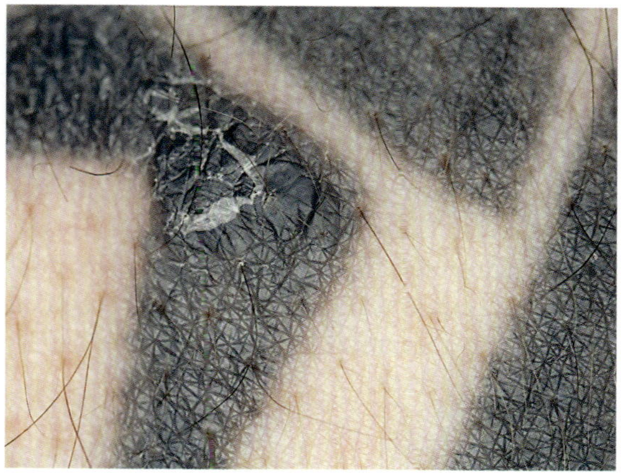
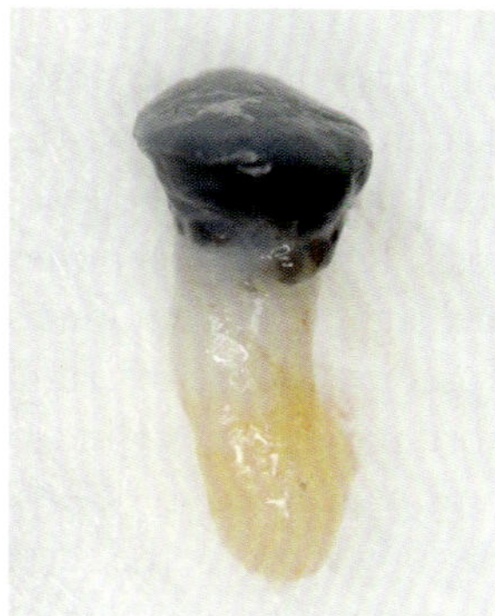

Sarcoidosis in Black Tattoos Accompanied by Erythema Nodosum, Joint Affection, and Involvement of the Lungs with the Tattoo Reaction as the Clue to Diagnosis

History
The patient had for 6 months observed nodular thickening of 2 black tattoos acquired 37 years ago. He had also noticed redness and tenderness on the legs associated with pain and swelling of the major joints for 3 months. He had no diagnosis and consulted the dermatology clinic simply because of tattoo problems. Until 2 years ago, he had been a marathon runner, now limited by shortness of breath.

Comment
The patient suffered from systemic sarcoidosis, which had been overlooked in the past but was finally diagnosed with a papulonodular tattoo reaction as the clue to diagnosis. Raw punch biopsies showed a 'bunch of grape' sign, and granulomas were confirmed by microscopy. Biopsy of crural redness showed an extraordinarily large cylindrical punch of fat, which was confirmed to be erythema nodosum by microscopy. X-ray of the chest showed large hilar glands and minor affection of the lung parenchyma. There had been no eye symptoms. His flare of disease with shortness of breath as the initial symptom seconded by other manifestations, including the pathology of the tattoos, was seen as autoimmune activity occurring first, triggering manifestations of sarcoidosis including a granulomatous tattoo reaction.

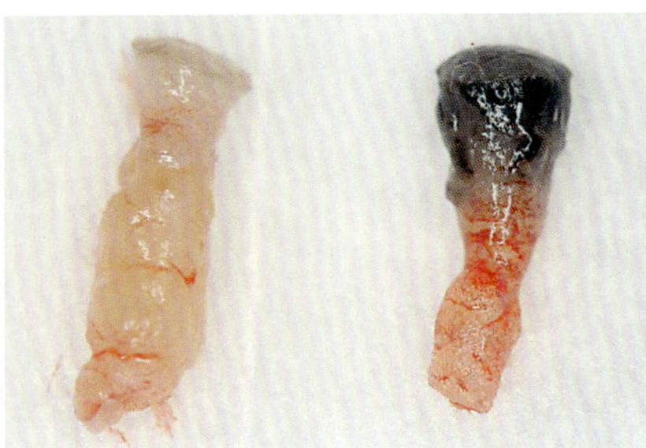

Treatment
Treatment was oral prednisone, which after a few months almost normalized his condition, with flattening of his tattoos.

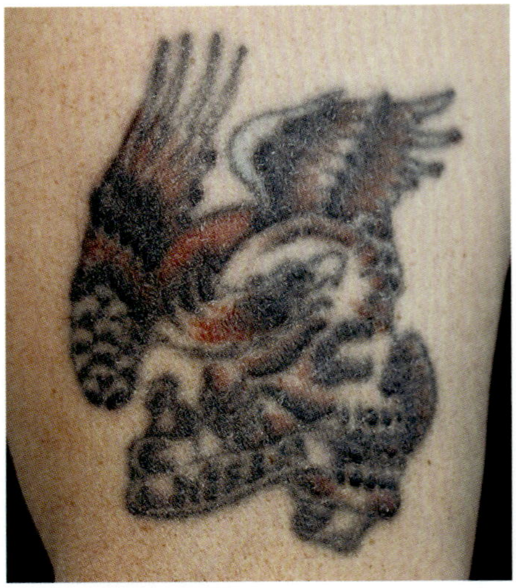

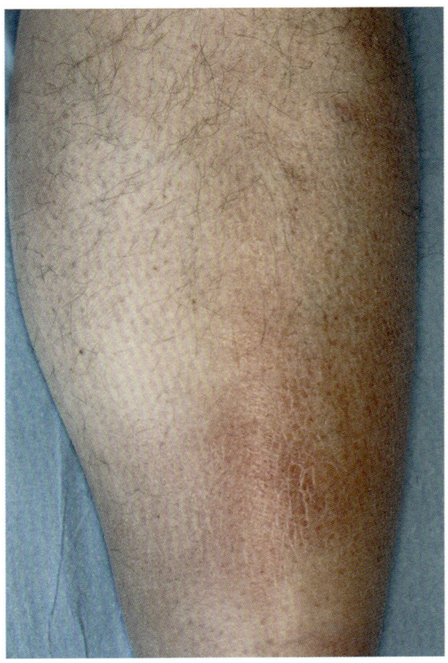

Sarcoidosis in Black Tattoos Manifested as a Rush Phenomenon

History

The patient had several black tattoos, which he had acquired over many years and which had been performed by at least 5 tattooists. A 6-year-old tattoo on the wrist suddenly started to swell with formation of a nodule. After 2 weeks, nearly all of his black tattoos started to develop similar nodules, amounting to at least 50 nodules. He had no symptoms in the lungs, joints, eyes, and other organs and no erythema nodosum. X-ray of the lungs was normal.

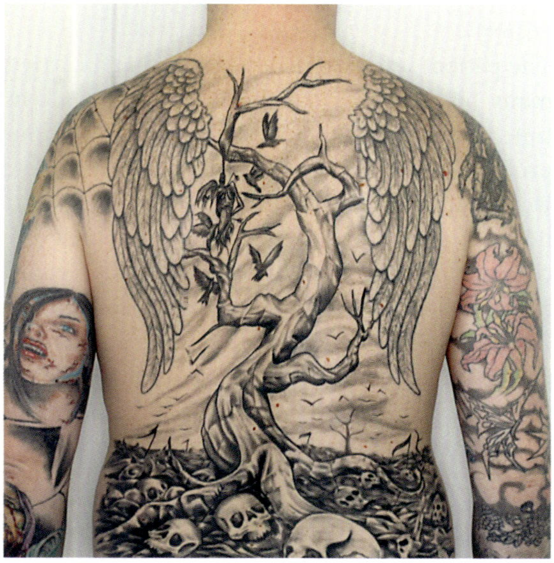

Comment

Raw punch biopsy showed a bunch of grape sign, and microscopy confirmed the finding of sarcoid granuloma. His sarcoidosis was manifested in tattoos only and occurred as a rush phenomenon in nearly all black tattoos irrespective of the age of the tattoos, the tattooist, and the ink used. All sorts of black tattoo pigments have the tendency to aggregate, agglomerate, and form large physical foreign bodies, which can induce a tissue response with granuloma formation. The tattoo on the wrist was the trigger or the forerunner. An autoimmune mechanism is supposed to lie behind the rush phenomenon, which is manifested as unexpected and simultaneous affection of several tattoos at the same time.

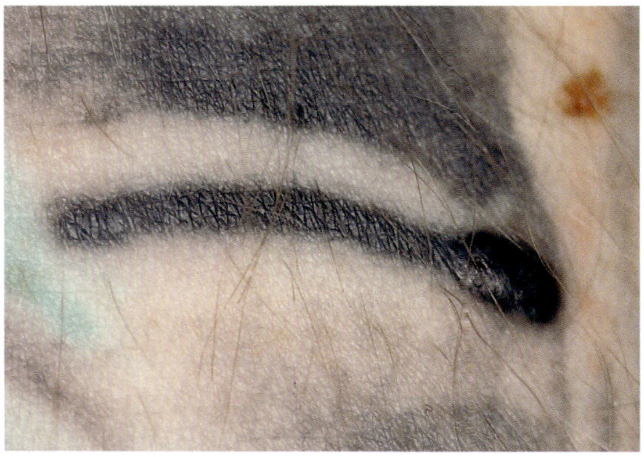

Treatment

Therapy was ultrapotent local corticoid according to the patient's preference. Oral prednisone is the preferred first-line treatment.

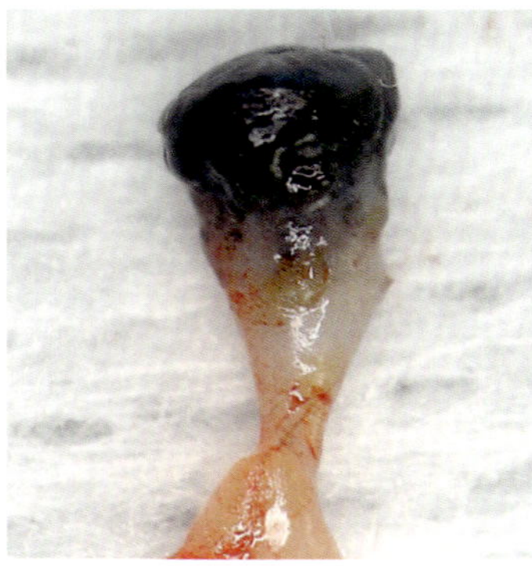

Sarcoidosis in Black Tattoos Starting Abruptly as a Rush Phenomenon in Every Black Tattoo

History
The patient was extensively tattooed and carried many black tattoos dating 20–30 years back in time, which had hitherto been tolerated with no problem. One year ago and abruptly within a few weeks, all tattoos started to react with papules and nodules, and at the same time the patient felt discomfort in his skin and more tired. Papules could itch. He had no shortness of breath and no eye complaints; however, for 10 years, he was having joint pain understood to be osteoarthrosis. Over the years, he had been tattooed by some 10 different tattooists and, therefore, with different brands of black ink.

Comment
The black tattoos all over the body started to react at the same time, with nodules, papules with swollen outer skin, and accentuation of the skin surface relief with symptoms depending on the density of the installed pigment, i.e. simultaneous reactions manifested as a 'rush phenomenon'. Raw punch biopsy showed a 'bunch of grape' sign, which was confirmed to be sarcoid granuloma by microscopy. X-ray of the chest was normal, and he had no other manifestations of sarcoidosis. The general activity in his skin was probably initiated through an autoimmune mechanism attributed to some common property of black ink particles despite their origin from a number of different industrial producers. As known from vaccines with aluminum, physical foreign bodies can have adjuvant function and trigger autoimmunity and sarcoidosis. The reaction in his skin occurred first in the Sigmund Freud tattoo (pictured) on his thigh.

Treatment
Treatment was oral prednisone for a period of time, which efficiently brought his skin back to normal.

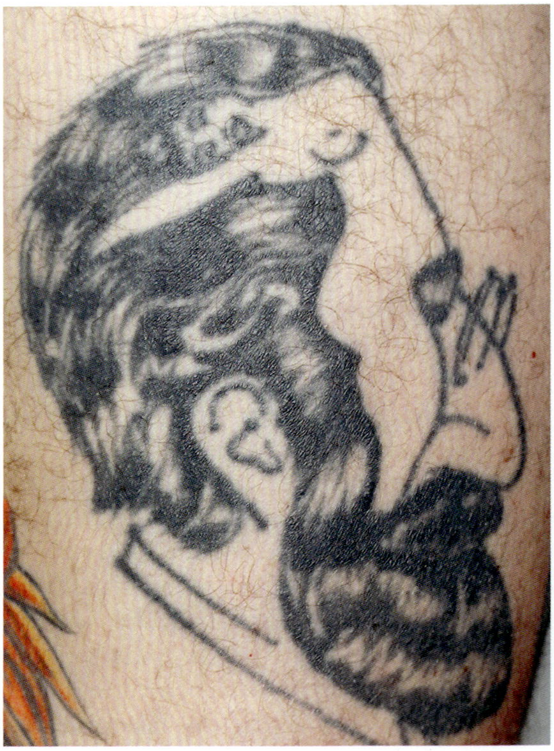

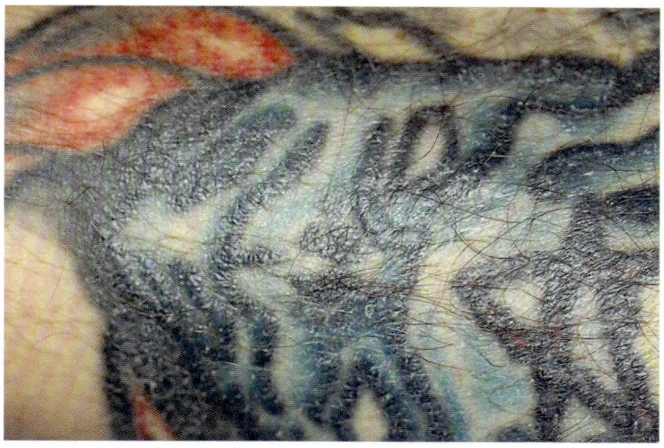

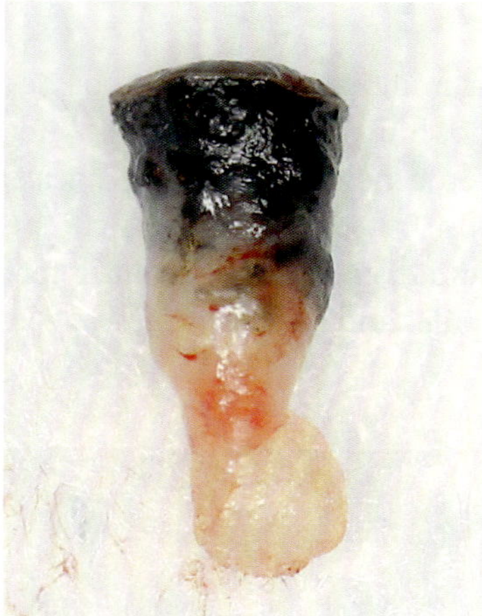

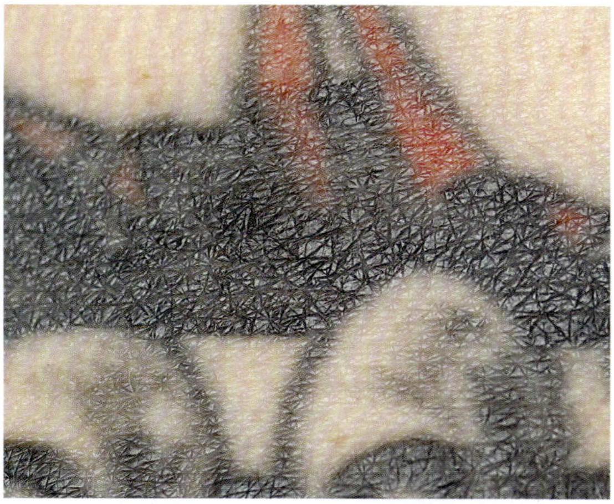

Sarcoidosis in Black Tattoos with Associated Rush Phenomenon in Other Black Tattoos and Affection of the Ankle Joints

History
The patient had a number of black tattoos acquired 20 years ago, hitherto nonreacting. After the patient acquired a new black tattoo 3 years ago, all black tattoos started to swell and itch, the itch being severe and disturbing sleep. Black tattoos developed papules and nodules selectively in black parts contrasting no reaction in other colors. Symptoms developed from intermittently to daily. Sun did not provoke a reaction. There were no pulmonary or ocular complaints, but the ankle joints became swollen and painful; alkaline phosphatase was increased. The patient suffered from insulin-dependent diabetes.

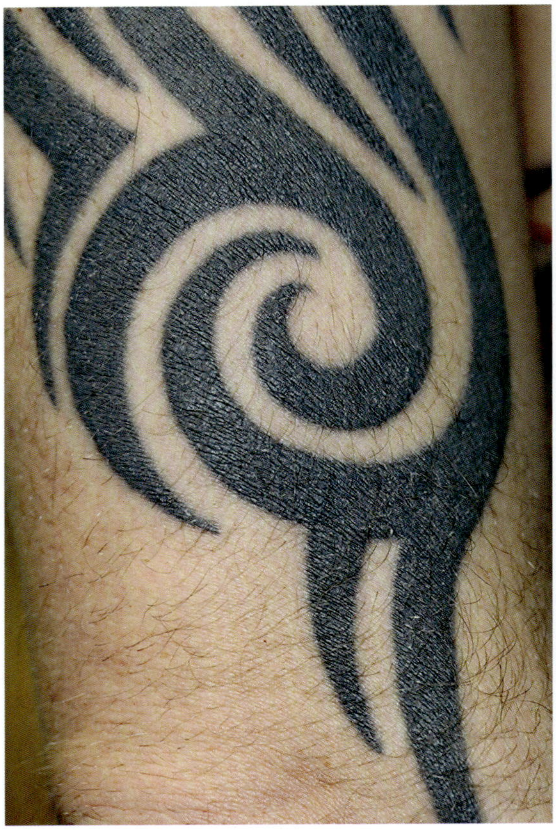

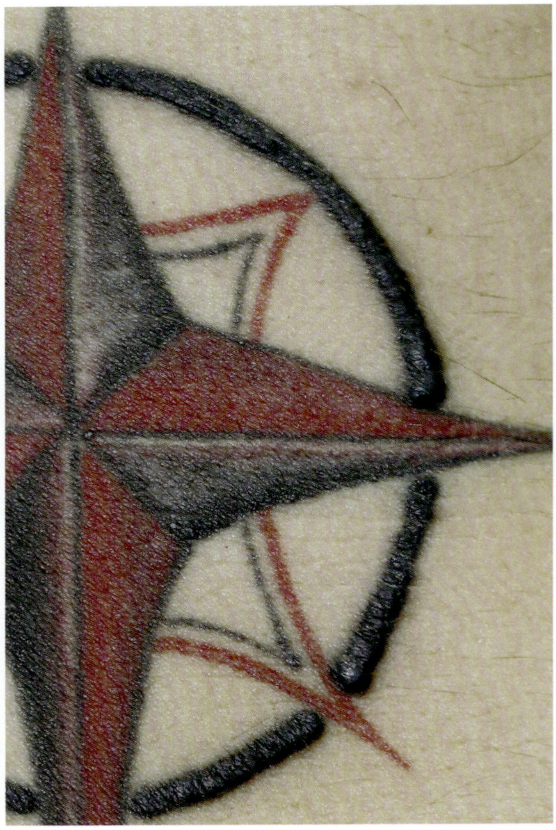

Comment

Raw punch biopsies showed a 'bunch of grape' sign with granulomas, which were confirmed to be sarcoid granulomas by light microscopy. X-ray of the lungs was normal. The case was concluded to be sarcoidosis primarily manifested in a recent tattoo (the trigger); however, over a period of time, similar reactions occurred in the patient's other black tattoos despite having been acquired years ago and hitherto having been silent. It was likely that the sarcoidosis flare also became manifested in joints. The case was seen as autoimmune activation of sarcoidosis triggered by a recent black tattoo, where agglomerated black tattoo pigment had developed into physical foreign bodies that exerted an adjuvant effect resulting in autoimmunity and generalized activation of sarcoidosis to which the patient might be predisposed. His brother already had a diagnosis of sarcoidosis.

Treatment

Treatment was ultrapotent corticoid locally, and the patient was referred to rheumatologists. His diabetes was a relative contraindication of oral prednisone, which would have been the preferred treatment.

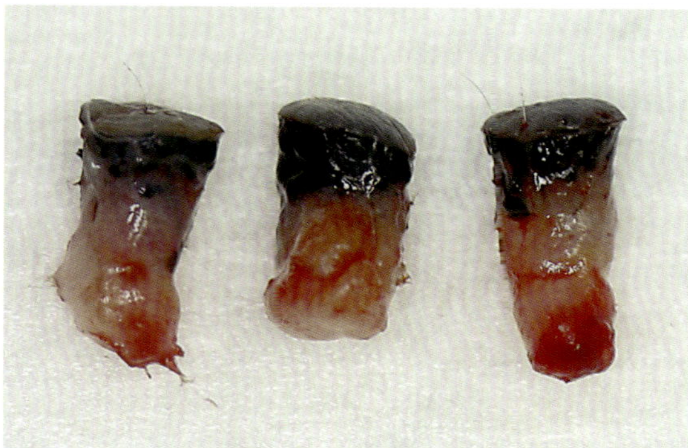

Sarcoidosis in Black Tattoos with Rush Phenomenon and Pulmonary Affection

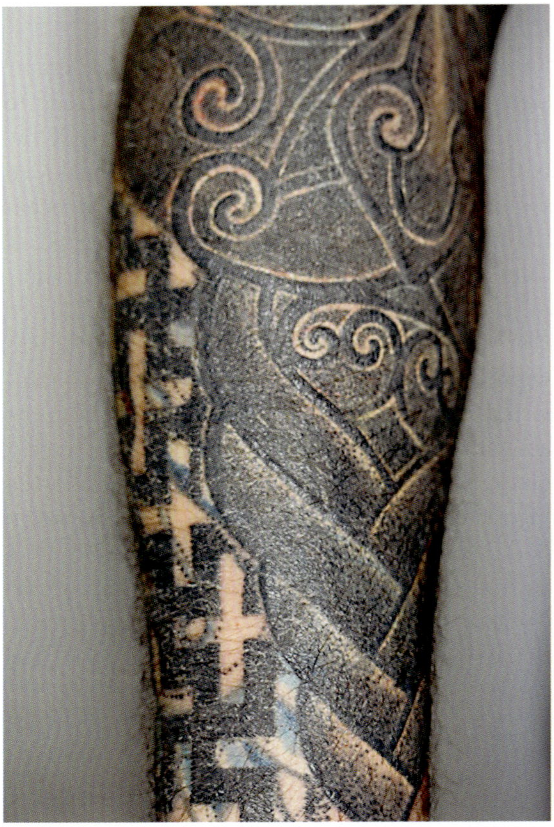

History

The patient, who had no special medical history, had acquired several black tattoos over about 10 years without any previous complications. About 6 weeks after a recent black tattoo on the forearm, the new tattoo and all old black tattoos in any anatomical site started to react with papules, nodules, itching, and discomfort. Other colors were unaffected. About 3 months after the recent tattoo, he noticed shortness of breath while walking, particularly while taking the stairs.

Comment

Raw punch biopsy showed a 'bunch of grape' sign with granulomas, which were confirmed to be sarcoid with fiery lymphatic inflammation by light microscopy. X-ray of the chest showed enlarged hilar glands, but high-resolution CT showed no significant affection of the lung tissue. Symptoms from the newly acquired tattoo (the trigger), general reaction in all black tattoos manifested as a 'rush phenomenon', and dyspnea and hilar gland enlargement came up during the same period indicating triggering by the new black tattoo causing autoimmune activation of a predisposition to sarcoid granulomatosis in any tissue, which the patient probably already carried at a subclinical level. Triggering is supposed to be due to agglomerated black tattoo pigment forming physical foreign bodies with an adjuvant effect.

Treatment

Treatment was oral prednisone combined with ultrapotent local corticoid. The patient gradually recovered over a period of 2 years.

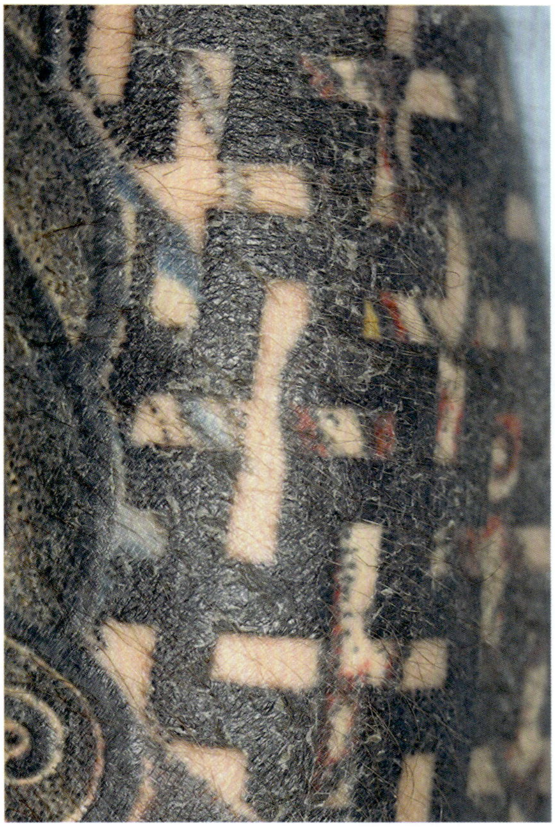

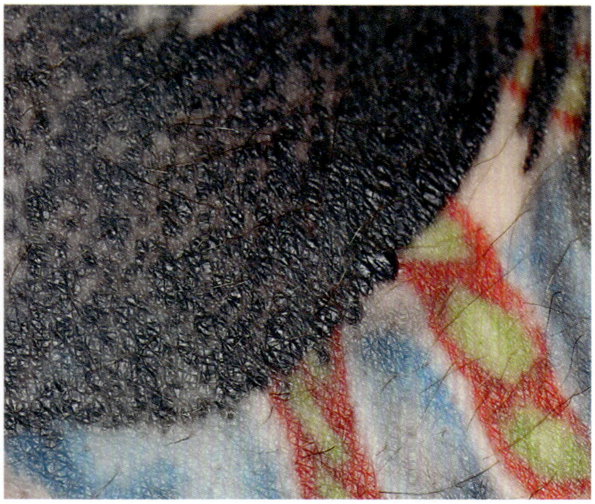

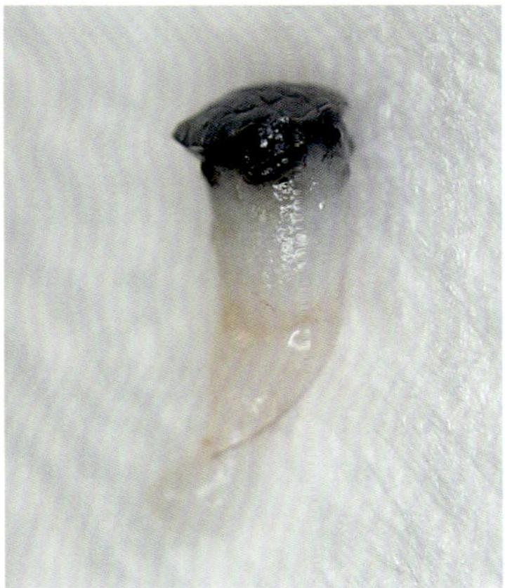

Neurosensitive Tattoo Reaction in a Red Tattoo with Constant Itch and Pain

History
The patient was happy with his previous tattoo in the pectoral region showing the national Danish banner. This tattoo showed no complications. Three years ago, he got a similar banner on his leg, which was made by another tattooist and using another red ink. The new tattoo had to be tattooed thrice since the skin would not accept the particular tattoo ink used. Healing was normal. After 1 year, the tattoo started to itch and became painful when touched, complaints which worsened and became constant. There was no thickening of the tattoo or any other abnormal finding. He decided against having a gray-shadowed frame added to the tattoo as done on the chest.

Comment
The injected red ink was scarce, and only a thin band was in the very outer dermis. There may have been a spontaneous mechanical barrier of the skin making tattooing difficult, with the skin taking up little of the ink. Microscopy showed no abnormal lymphocytic infiltration, and an allergic reaction was unlikely. Itch and pain were not secondary to inflammation. The particular tattoo ink product used on the leg may have been composed of industrial red pigment, which after some time and through metabolism of pigment released neurostimulatory substance(s). Parallel to the onset of itch and pain, the tattoo became sensitive to sun and photochemical pigment breakdown may have contributed.

Treatment
Treatment was dermatome shaving and removal of the pigment, which effectively relieved symptoms. In this case with no allergy and a superficial band of pigment, laser removal could also have been applied.

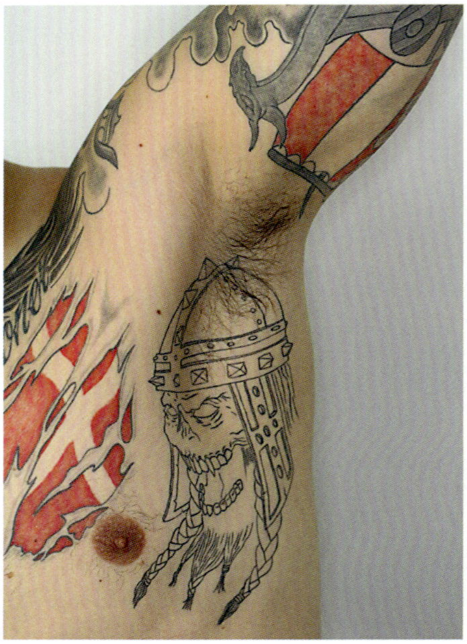

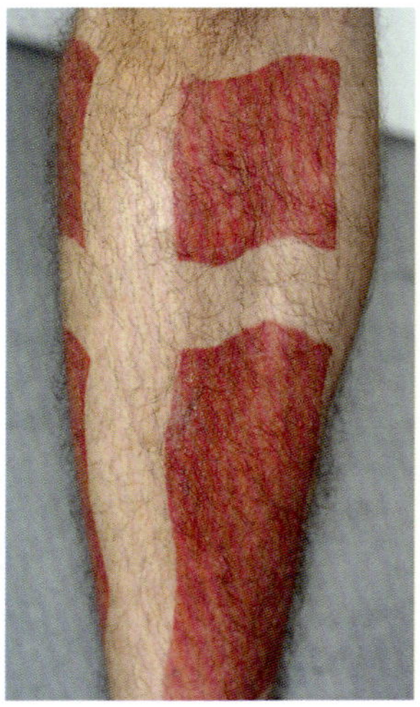

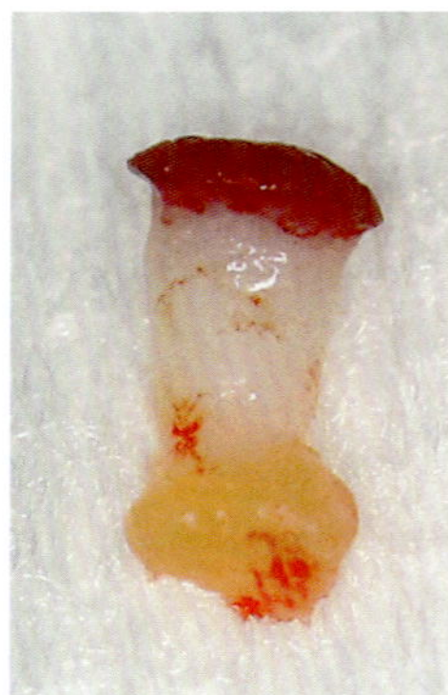

Neurosensitive Tattoo Reaction Associated with Exercise Addiction Threatening the General Health

History

Parallel to the development of an addiction to physical exercise with hours of training and sports every day, the patient developed intense itch and discomfort in large tattoos hitherto tolerated, with intermittent swelling. The patient had lost weight and menstruations had stopped. Blood biochemistry was disturbed with elevated muscle enzymes. The heart was enlarged with hypertrophy on the cardiogram.

Comment

Tattoos were independent of color and slightly swollen with loss of the normal triangular surface relief. Biopsy showed a minute lymphocytic infiltrate.

Treatment

Treatment was a change of lifestyle, with reduction and strict check of physical activity, helped by the patient's family. Over months her biochemistry became normal, and menstruation came back. Tattoo complaints faded in parallel, with no need for local treatment.

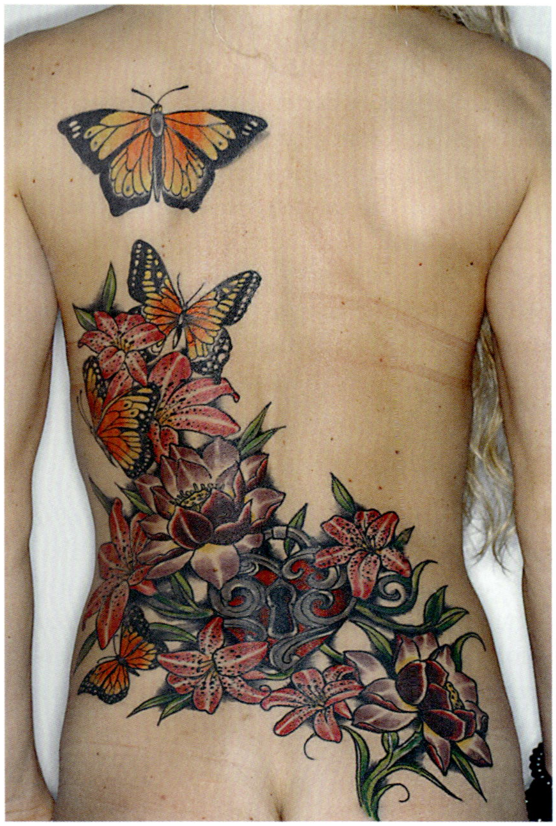

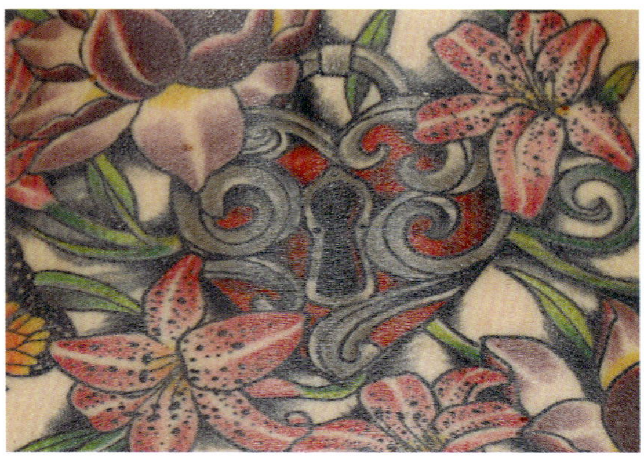

Neurosensory Complaints and Color Change after Bacterial Tattoo Infection

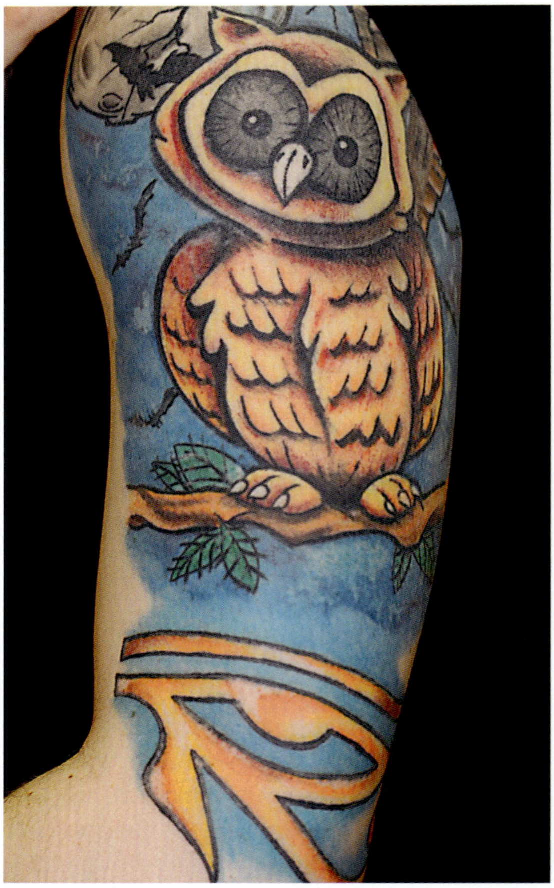

History
Already 1 day after tattooing, the arm started to swell with signs of bacterial infection all over the tattoo, independent of color. The patient had experienced the same problem of infection in a previous tattoo. The tattooist was professional and careful and used clean utensils, gloves, and disinfection. Treatment with fusidic acid cream had been given by the general practitioner, and signs of infection gradually disappeared. Culture had shown *Staphylococcus aureus.*

Comment
Infection was followed by chronic change of sensation in the tattoo with dysesthesia and abnormal sensation of touch. Pigment extrusion had occurred leaving whitish spots, disturbances of colors, and minimal scarring. Sometimes the blue pigment may switch in the direction of green following bacterial infection.

Treatment
Therapy could not be offered. Symptoms of altered sensibility were unchanged after 1 year but might decline over years.

Neurosensitive Reaction in a Blue Tattoo in a Case with Known Urticaria

History
For years, the patient had suffered from urticaria and often needed antihistamines. Two years ago, she got a cover-up tattoo on the abdomen tattooed in a blue color (the original color was lilac). Tattooing was technically difficult since needle trauma caused urticarial swelling more than usual. After the cover-up, she suffered constant pain in the tattoo, and it could now and then swell, which was, however, independent of urticaria activity in other parts of her skin. The tattoo reaction was resistant to antihistamine treatment.

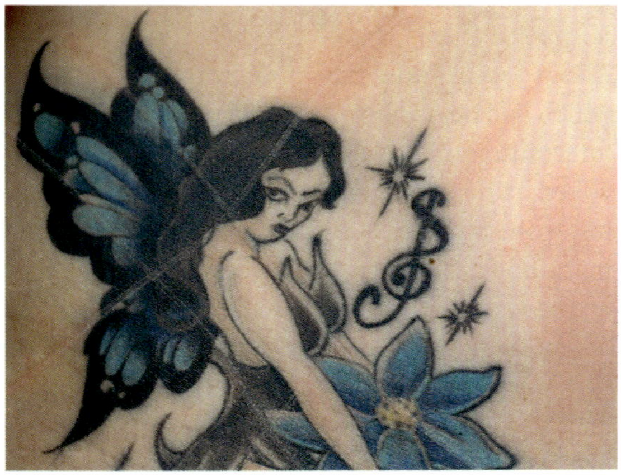

Comment
The tattoo reaction was not typical urticaria. A scratch test of the tattoo and the surrounding skin showed a wheal-and-flare reaction, with a full triple response in the normal skin but a linear wheal only and no flare in the tattoo. The flare response seemed to be absent or suppressed in the tattoo. The flare is neuron mediated and an axonal reflex. The test with suppressed axonal reflex in the tattooed skin, in contrast to pain in the tattoo, may indicate altered local neurophysiology in the tattoo. The tattoo showed no signs of scarring or other physical sequel of tattooing.

Treatment
Treatment was by observation. Antihistamines had no effect. Dermatome shaving is optional.

Disturbed Sensitivity and Urticarial Reaction in a Red Tattoo

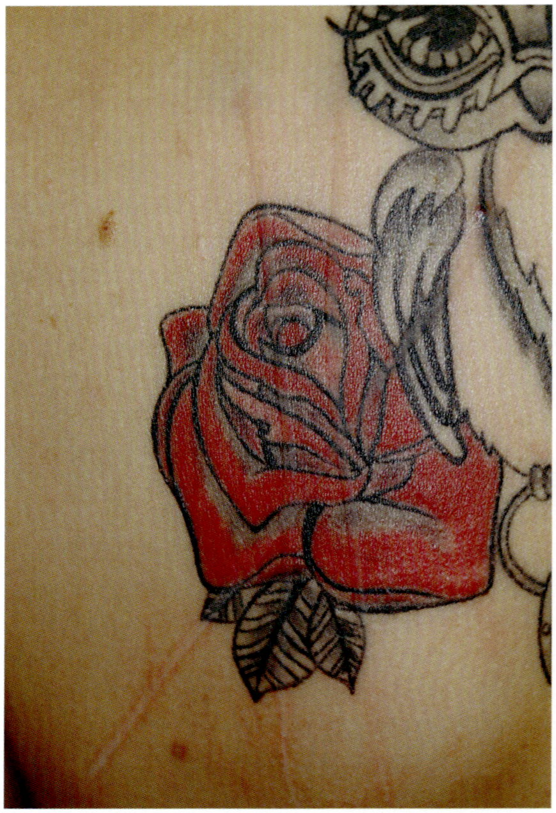

History
About 3 weeks after having acquired a new tattoo, which had healed normally, the patient developed intermittent urticarial swelling in the tattoo provoked by heat including sun exposure and sweating from physical activity. She gave up running marathons. Reaction to touch and friction from textile was abnormal. She had not suffered from urticaria or allergy in the past, and the general skin was normal.

Comment
The red part of the tattoo was minimally swollen. A factitia scratch test showed a normal wheal-and-flare response similar to the response in the surrounding skin, thus was negative. Sensation by touch was abnormal with dysesthesia. The disease mechanism was unclear. The patient felt limited in her life and needed active treatment.

Treatment
Treatment with YAG laser could not be offered due to the potential risk of inducing or boosting allergy. Local corticoid had no effect. Dermatome shaving was performed, which resulted in abnormal scarring but relieved symptoms. Observation with no active therapy might have been the best treatment.

Basal Cell Carcinoma in a Tattoo by Coincidence

History
The patient presented with a large basal cell carcinoma on the back (fig. a). The cancer had been treated with curettage about 10 times but relapsed in the margin toward normal skin. It partly covered a large tattoo made 27 years ago.

Comment
The patient claimed, and his wife witnessed, that the cancer had started in the normal skin above and thus outside the tattoo. It had expanded over a long time with overgrowth of the tattoo. Relapse at the tumor margin with keratosis and ulceration appeared similar over the tattoo and in the normal skin and was thus not worse in the tattoo. The relapsed lesions did not follow lines and shades of the tattoo and were appeared completely independent of the tattoo pigment, with the pigment apparently not acting as inductor or promotor of malignancy.

International consensus, a review of the literature [Kluger, Lancet Oncol 2012;13:161–168], and an EU/JRC report (EUR 27247 EN) conclude that skin cancers in tattoos are rare and not documented related to the pigment, thus coincidental. Pigment is located in the dermis and not in the basal cell layer, which may anyhow and independent of the tattoo pigment start to proliferate. Sun is the paramount trigger of skin carcinomas.

Treatment
The patient was treated with radiotherapy, which was efficient (fig. b). A pretest indicated no interaction between radiation and tattoo pigment. Radiation dermatitis was mild, independent of the tattoo, and within the normal range. In the healed lesion with chronic sequels of radiation, the original tattoo displayed through the atrophic skin showed up unbroken, thus with no disfiguring consistent with overgrowth of the tattoo with the basal cell carcinoma coming from outside the tattoo.

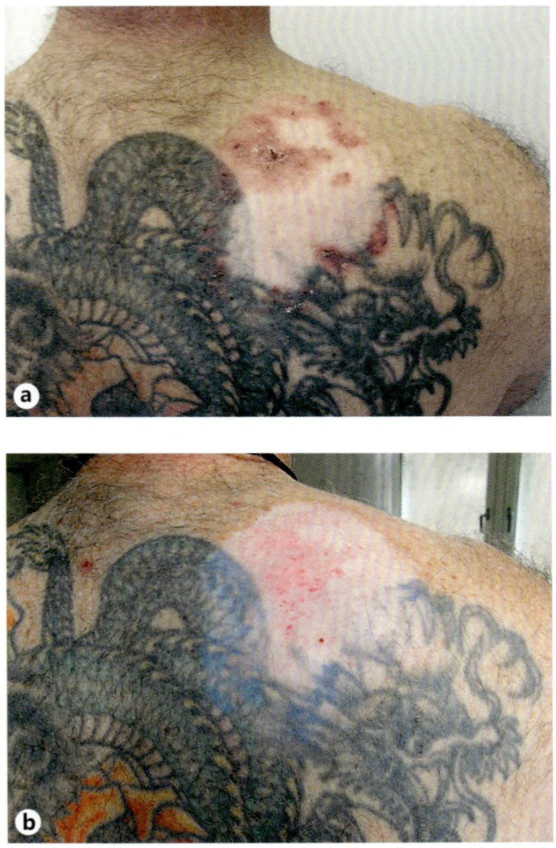

Keratoacanthoma in a Tattoo with Spontaneous Recovery

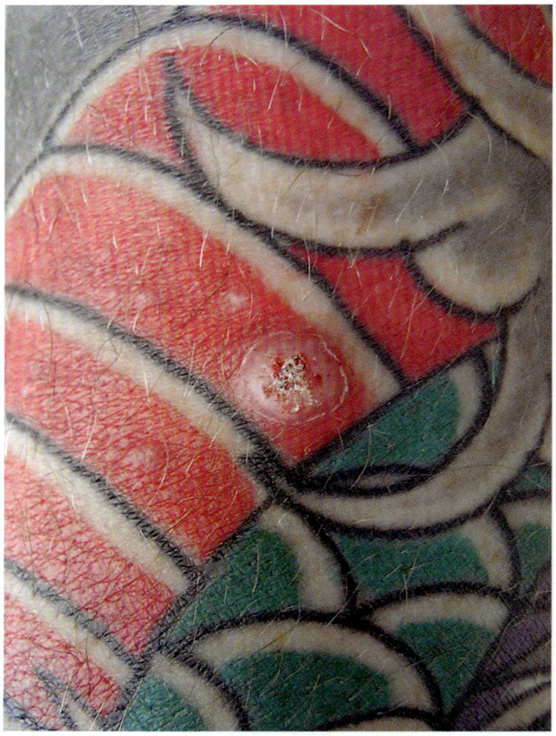

History

Already 1–3 weeks after the patient had acquired a new tattoo on the arm and shoulder, small round lesions sized 1–8 mm grew in the red parts of the tattoo. The lesions were keratotic and red, indicating an undisturbed outer dermis and unbroken distribution of the red pigment under the lesions, thus no invasive growth. Healing was otherwise normal. The patient had several other tattoos but had never experienced such lesions before.

Comment

Biopsies from a larger lesion and a small lesion both showed keratoacanthoma with the known reservation that squamous cell carcinoma could not be excluded. All lesions regressed spontaneously over a period of 2–4 months, helped by a potent corticoid, thus with no clinical indication of malignancy. Keratoacanthoma may be provoked by skin trauma including the tattoo operation.

Treatment

Keratoacanthoma is clinically benign and requires no active treatment other than observation and follow-up. Corticoid may be applied. Excision will damage the tattoo.

Keratoacanthomas in a Tattoo with Spontaneous Recovery

History

A new tattoo was made on the leg of the patient 6 months ago. Healing was normal. After about 7 weeks, 5 small circular lesions with keratosis rapidly grew in the red part of the tattoo. His dermatologist made a biopsy, which showed keratoacanthoma albeit squamous cell carcinoma could not be excluded. Meanwhile, the progression of the lesions had stopped. He had generally sun-damaged skin and another lesion in normal skin on the back of his hand. In the past he had had a basal cell carcinoma on the back.

Comment

In his recent tattoo, keratoacanthoma verified by biopsy and concentrated in the red part of the tattoo was diagnosed. As can be seen from the photos, the acanthomas carried no red pigment and thus appeared entirely epidermal in origin with an uninterrupted dermal-epidermal interface and undisturbed pigment residing below in the outer dermis. With pigment as tracer the lesions appeared not invasive. The patient was predisposed both to keratoacanthoma (photo of 2 lesions on the normal skin on the back of his hand) and skin malignancy.

Treatment

Therapy was observation only with no active treatment. The lesions in the tattoo spontaneously resolved over a few months leaving hardly any visible alteration of the tattoo. Surgical intervention would damage the tattoo.

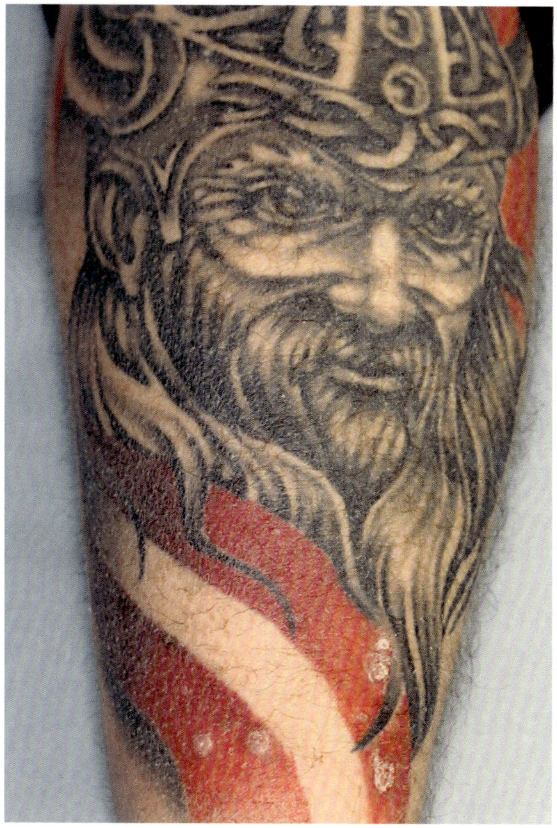

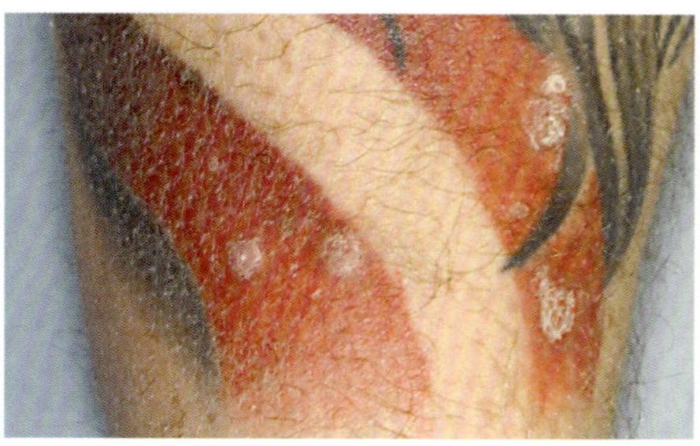

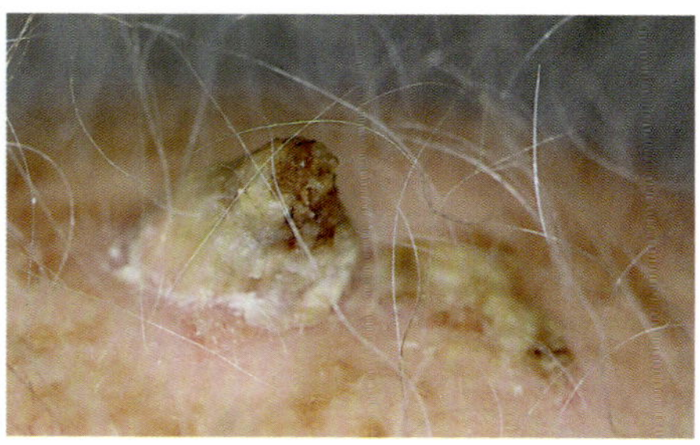

Paraneoplastic Reaction in a Multicolored Tattoo Provoked by Malignant Lymphoma

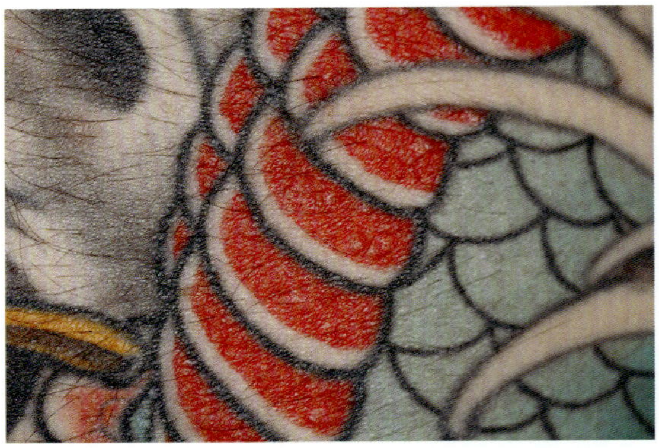

History

Shortly after getting a large tattoo on the trunk with the colors red, green, and black, the patient developed an unusual urticaria-like reaction in the tattoo and the surrounding skin with swelling and itch treated with oral antihistamine and prednisone by his practitioner. Infection was not suspected. Over a few weeks the reaction had faded leaving small papules in the tattooed skin distributed independent of tattoo color. Papules, which were not typical pimples, caused minor itch and discomfort and remained rather constant. As a very recent observation, the patient felt swelling of his abdomen and tiredness. He was referred to internists for medical diagnostics.

Comment

Malignant lymphoma with major affection on both sides of the diaphragm was diagnosed having a size and distribution that could not be secondary to the newly acquired tattoo. Thus, the reaction was concluded to be paraneoplastic. Skin biopsy was not conclusive, with mild inflammation. The reaction could be seen as multiple atypical pimples following a more general reaction in the tattoos. The reaction did not resemble Köbner psoriasis.

Treatment

The skin discomfort was treated with a potent local corticoid. Oncology treatment had priority.

Köbner Provocation of Psoriasis in a Recent Tattoo

History

The patient had suffered from psoriasis for years. She was under treatment with a biologic but still had some small plaques on sites exposed to pressure and friction. After normal healing, a new tattoo around the elbow manifested new psoriasis lesions in the tattooed black text. No general activation of psoriasis was observed outside the tattooed skin.

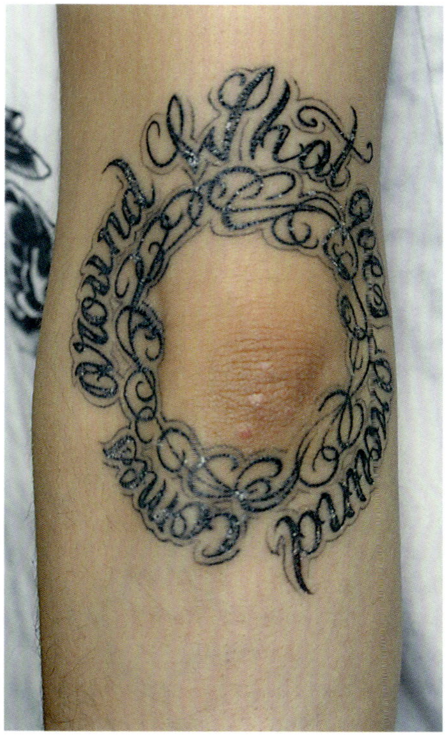

Comment

The needle trauma of tattooing can activate psoriasis in the tattooed site, but tattooing hardly ever causes general activation of psoriasis. Köbner psoriasis in tattoos often heals spontaneously over a few months, unless there is an abnormal reaction in the tattoo such as papulonodular reaction to black pigment maintaining psoriatic activity. The original publication on Köbner reaction from 1876 included a case of Köbner psoriasis by tattooing.

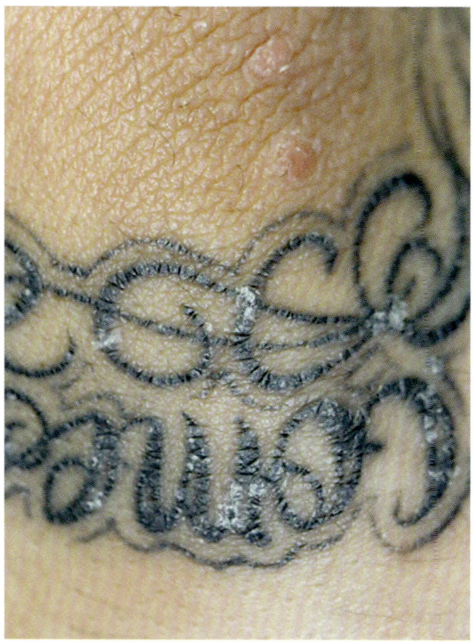

Treatment

Treatment is observation or local standard treatment of psoriasis with a corticoid or a D-vitamin analogue.

Köbner Provocation of Psoriasis in a Tattoo with a Papulonodular Reaction in Black Pigment Maintaining Local Psoriatic Activity around the Tattoo

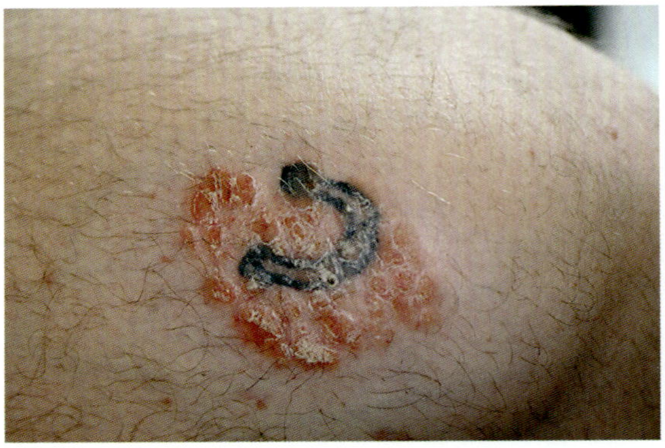

History

The patient had been suffering from stable plaque psoriasis for a number of years with constant plaques over the elbows and knees but in no other site. After normal healing, a black tattoo on the shoulder was after a few weeks followed by psoriasis primarily in the tattoo only but later with progression into the surrounding skin. The Köbner psoriasis in the tattoo remained constant for 2 years parallel to the known constant activity over the extensor side of joints, where skin is subject to constant mechanical frictions.

Comment

Physical trauma of tattoo needles can cause a psoriatic Köbner reaction in the tattoo. However, since tattoo needle trauma is limited and transient, the reaction will typically fade spontaneously over a few months or be easily cleared by local treatment without recurrence once it is healed. In this particular case, the patient had, partly hidden and under scales, a chronic papulonodular reaction to black pigment, which might act as a chronic trigger of psoriatic activity in the tattoo comparable to chronicity of his psoriasis over joints exposed to constant mechanical friction. Tattooing as a mechanical trauma is unlikely to trigger a generalized outbreak of psoriasis, but stress and pain of tattooing might. Worsening of psoriasis can at any time coincidentally affect a tattoo.

Treatment

The patient was treated with calcipotriol and later, indicated by his general needs, oral methotrexate.

Tattoo Needle Trauma of the Skin Followed by Abnormal Healing of the Tattoo

History

The patient and his wife had similar chameleons tattooed on their forearms. The tattooists worked hard to make an artistic soft shift of multiple colors over the body of the animal, and in the process overworked the skin with the needle (fig. a). The patient and his wife had similar complications during healing with a traumatic wound, a phase of heavy crust formation and inflammation (fig. b), and finally delayed healing with thickening, scar formation, and loss of pigment (fig. c). The artistically elegant work was gone albeit the chameleon ended up looking quite natural. There had been no infection and antibiotics had not been given.

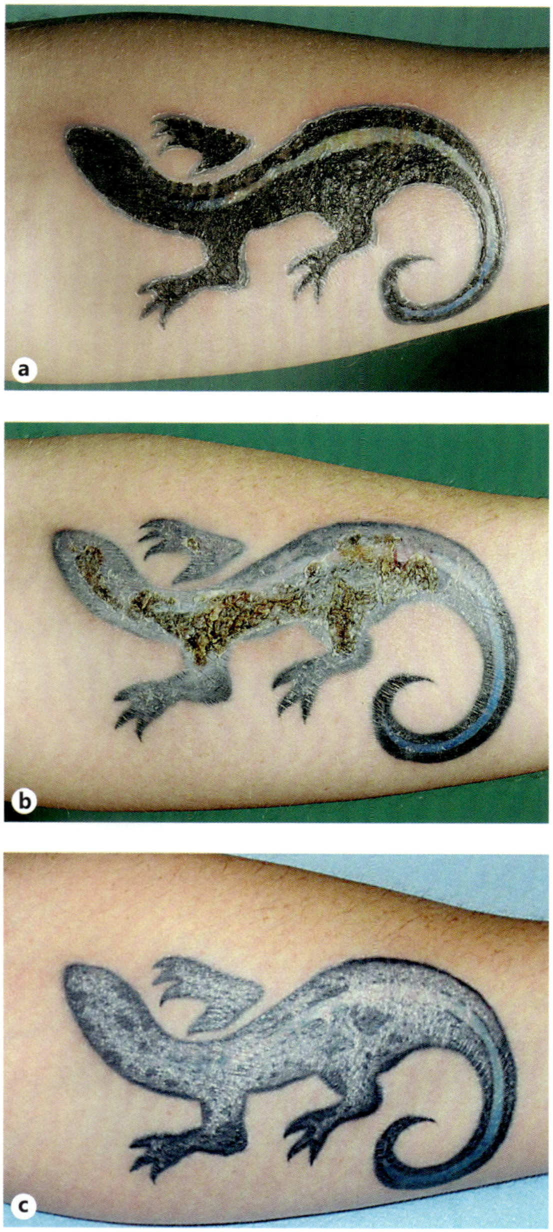

Comment

With thousands of needle pricks applied to a minute skin site, the risk of traumatic damage of the skin can be high. The enthusiastic tattoo artist may be unaware of this risk. Making overlapping color shades and thus mixing colors in the skin instead of in the ink cups carries a special risk of hazardous tattoo needle trauma.

Treatment

Proper wound care sometimes supplemented with oral antibiotics is the treatment of choice.

Traumatic Tattooing with Severe Local Damage and Chronic Sequels

History
The patient had acquired a multicolored tattoo on the arm, made in a professional parlor equipped up to good standard. Hygiene precautions had been taken. Tattooing had lasted 5 h and had been very painful with more bleeding than normal. The tattoo machine was low noise and apparently the tattooist recently had switched over from a traditional coil machine to a new rotary machine. The arm continued to be painful and swollen, and healing was abnormal with wounds in about 50% of the tattooed skin, independent of color (fig. a). The patient developed no fever. After 1 week, his general practitioner prescribed an oral antibiotic. The tattoo healed slowly over 6–8 weeks. During healing, much pigment had escaped from the tattoo, with visible green staining of the bandage (fig. b, c).

Comment
Tattooing was hazardous and a major physical skin trauma with wounds in the tattooed skin independent of color. It is likely that the tattooist was a rotary machine novice and trained with this recent device. It was malpractice. Luckily, pyogenic infection did not happen. The tattoo was destroyed. There were large fields with pigment loss and minor scarring seen as whitish skin and loss of the normal skin surface relief (fig. d, e).

Treatment
Treatment was wound care and oral antibiotic to prevent secondary infection.

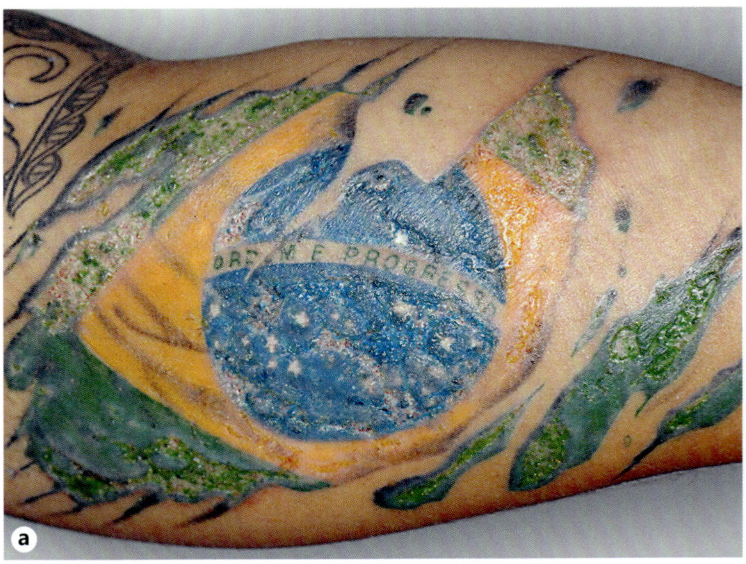

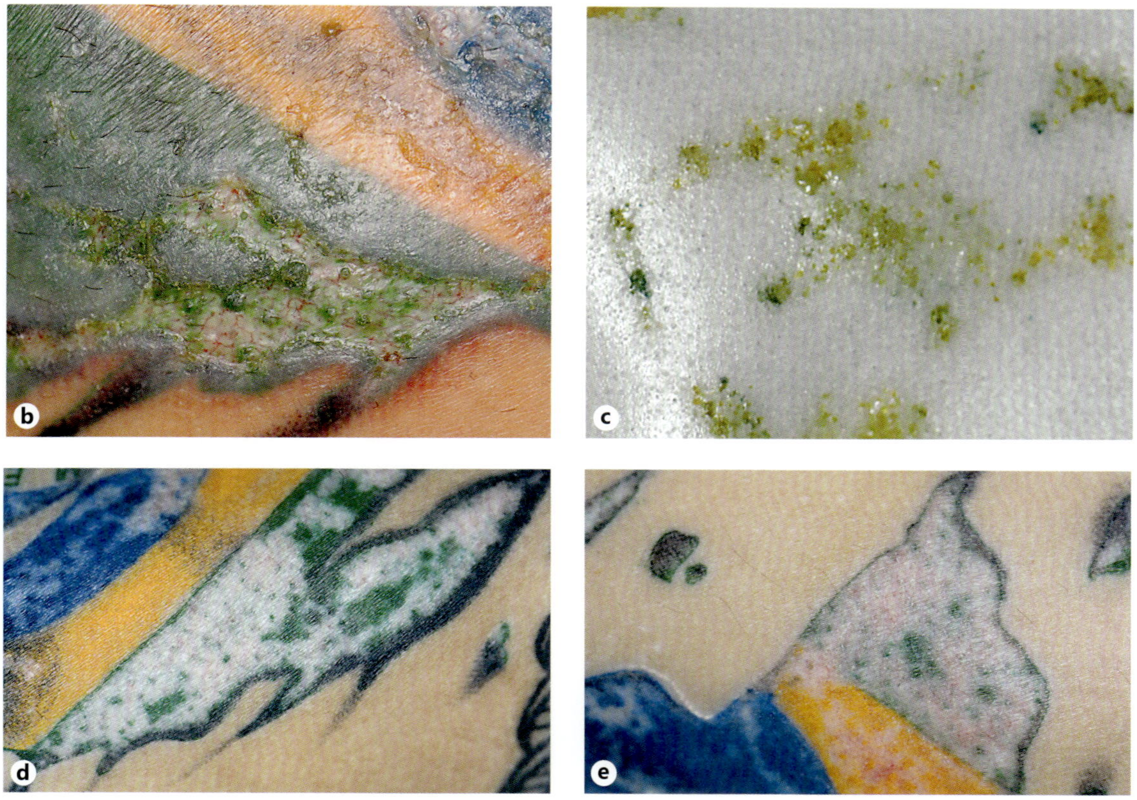

Tattoo Inflammation of a Newly Acquired Tattoo from Physicochemical Insult

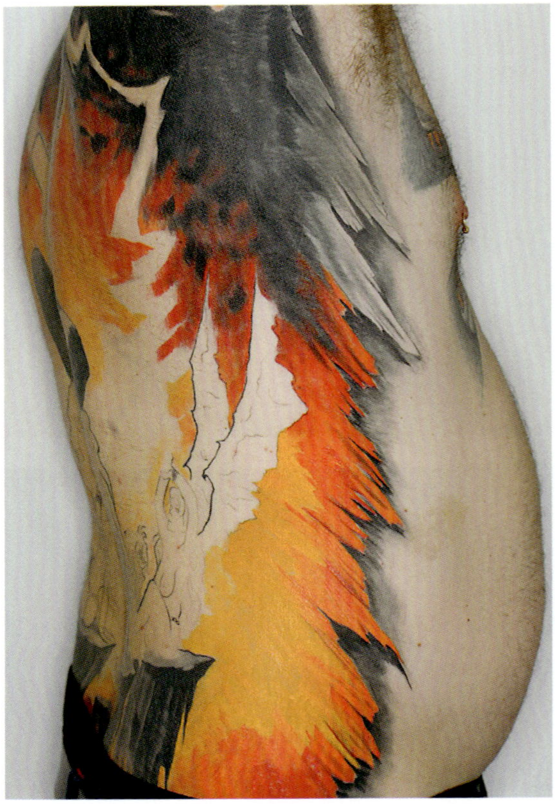

History
The patient had multicolored tattoos on both flanks, illustrating fire. Tattooing had been straightforward. After 3 days of seemingly normal healing, the red parts but also orange and yellow parts of the tattoo started to swell and itch, without signs of infection. Minor swelling continued for months and caused itch. Potent local corticoid only gave little relief. Allergy patch testing with a standard tray, textile colors, and a series of tattoo inks came out negative.

Comment
The cause of the reaction was unclear. The cause might be chronic chemical or physical irritation by tattoo pigments in the dermis in a person susceptible to such type of reaction. Allergy acquired with the tattoo was unlikely, since symptoms had an early onset within a few days after tattooing, and patch testing was negative including no reactions to nickel, preservatives, and a selection of disperse dyes and tattoo inks.

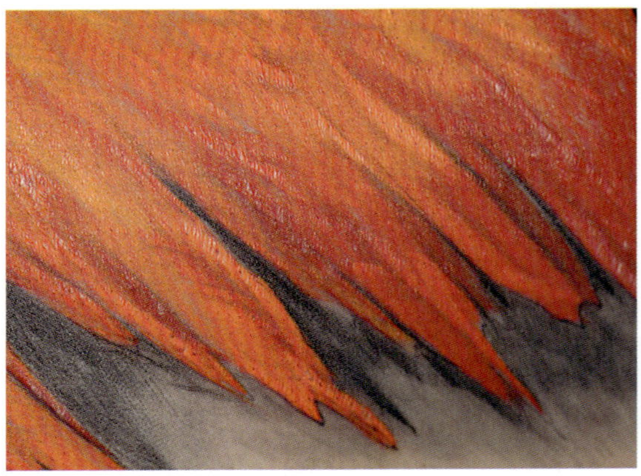

Treatment
Treatment was a potent local corticoid over months. The severity of symptoms and the patient's wish not to destroy the elegant tattoo by dermatome shaving or laser removal made these treatments not applicable following a pro-and-con conversation with the patient.

Amateur Tattoo of the Oral Mucosa with Unintended Tattooing of the Lip

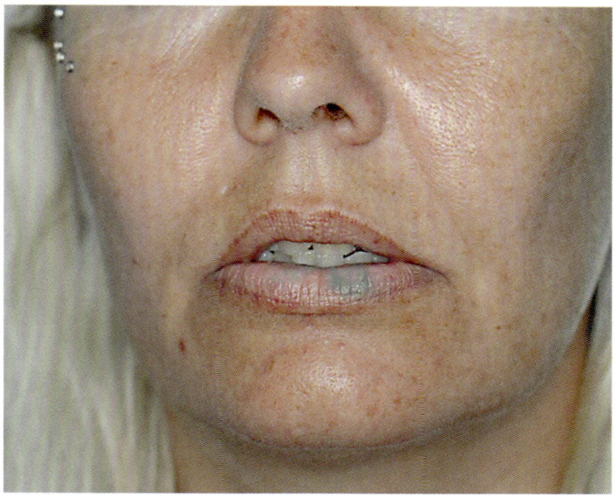

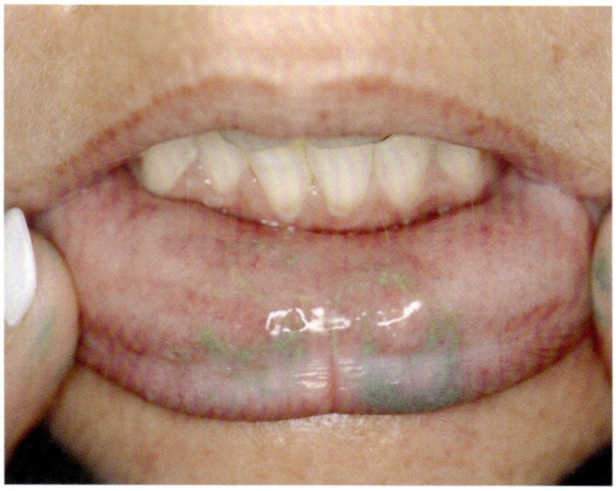

History

Under rather uncontrolled conditions, the patient had allowed a friend to tattoo a text on the oral mucosa of her lower lip. The lip was held between the fingers of the left hand of the operator, under stretching of the lip, while the right hand operated the tattoo machine. The outcome was not a readable text on the mucosa but a highly visible colorful tattoo on the lower lip!

Comment

Tattooing is craftsmanship that requires skills and long training. It has to be learned over a period of supervised training. Amateurs easily may malpractice and make trivial mistakes that professional tattooists would not make. In most countries, tattooed individuals have no legal protection and no insurance covering hazards and malpractices, which also include neglected hygiene precautions and use of unsafe tattoo inks.

Treatment

The treatment option in this case was laser removal; however, green is one of the most difficult colors to remove.

Tattoo and Risk of Keloid

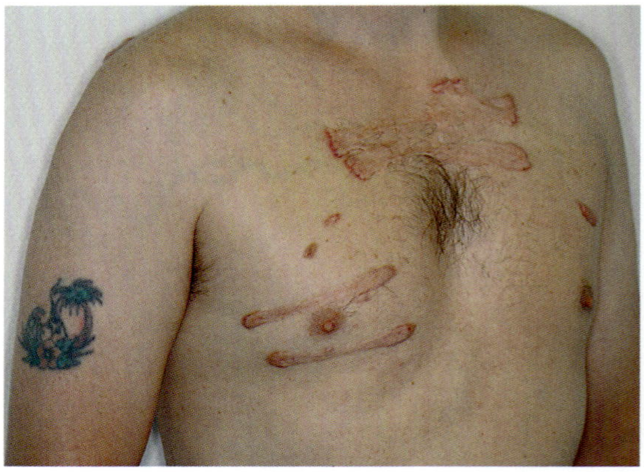

History
In 1984, the patient got a tattoo on his upper arm without complications, specifically without abnormal scar formation in the tattoo. Five years later, he started to develop spontaneous keloids on the chest, upper back, and shoulders. He could not indicate any physical trauma behind the keloids except, possibly, sunburn. Keloids were treated with intralesional corticoid over 12 months without any result. Contracture in the neck developed.

Comment
The case shows, remarkably, no keloid or abnormal scar formation in the tattoo contrasting severe abnormal scarring on the trunk. Despite severe needle trauma with thousands of needle pricks down to the mid-dermal level as well as minor dermal fibrosis in tattooed skin commonly found by histologic examination, tattooing is only rarely reported to result in keloid formation. The risk of keloid seems to be overestimated in the medical literature.

Treatment
Treatment was intralesional corticoid over 1 year, which did not help. Fractional CO_2 laser was considered inapplicable. Treatment with surgical excision of the larger keloids followed by radiotherapy was instituted already during the healing phase, so far with good results.

Keloid following Dermatome Shaving on the Chest, a Region Predisposed to Abnormal Scarring

History
A tattoo over the sternum with a text regretted by the patient, who insisted on complete removal of the tattooed text over the sternum, after having been explained the risk of abnormal scarring. The text showed no sign of abnormal scarring despite the needle trauma of tattooing. The patient had no indication of abnormal scarring in other parts of the skin except maybe in the tattoo on the shoulder. Laser surgeons were reluctant and preferred to refrain from treatment, which would involve a course of 8–10 treatments. Finally, dermatome shaving was performed after informed consent.

Comment
Surgery including laser removal on the chest carries a known general risk of abnormal scarring. In this particular case tiny spots of scarring on the shoulder and visible subepidermal scarring in the preoperative raw punch biopsy signaled some risk of scarring. The risk that tattooing itself causes keloid is surprisingly low even in anatomical sites predisposed to abnormal scar formation as illustrated with this case.

Treatment
Treatment was a series of intralesional corticoid injections, which had limited or no effect. The patient had his primary aim of treatment fulfilled and accepted and preferred the final outcome despite being medically unsatisfactory for the doctor.

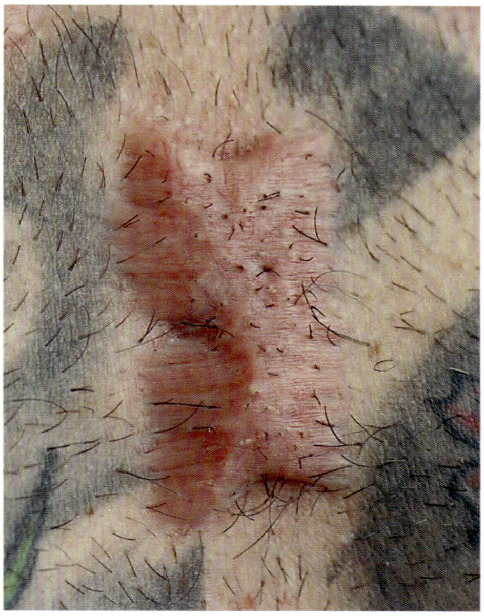

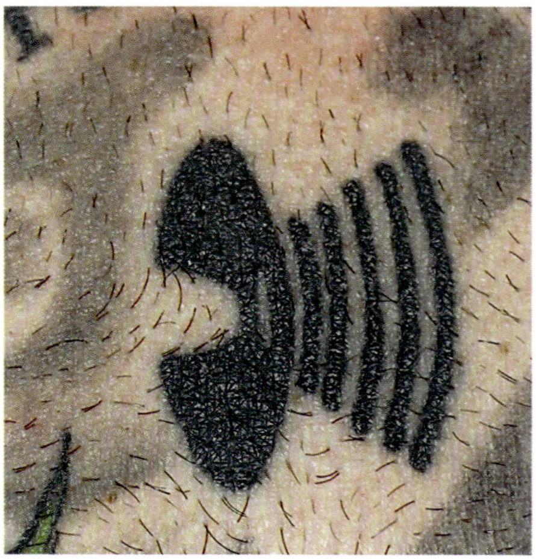

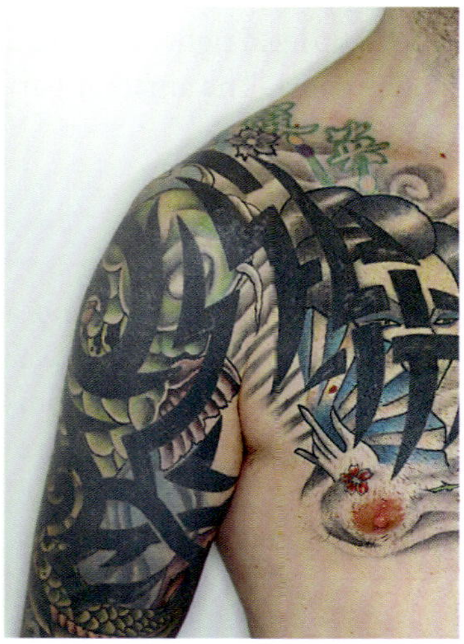

Laser Removal of a Tattoo Followed by Scarring and Chronic Itch and Pain

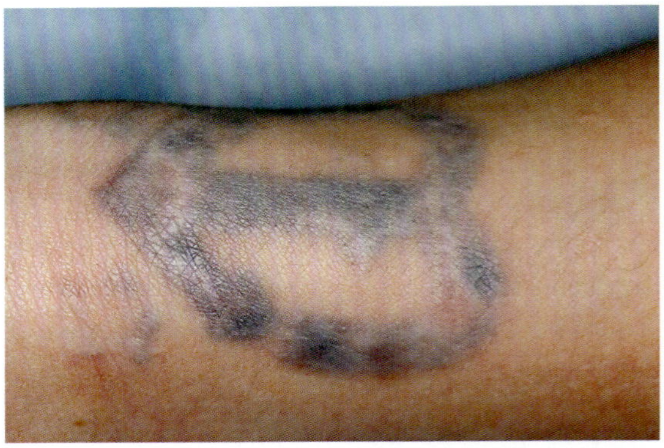

History
Shortly after having gotten a black tattoo on the hand, the patient regretted the tattoo. She received 5 laser treatments in an amateur laser removal parlor, which all caused burn and hemorrhagic bulla formation in the treated fields. She was told that this was normal and to expect. Scarring occurred, and the tattoo was not cleared. Subsequently, she received 14 successive laser treatments in a qualified parlor using a Q-switched YAG laser, with minimal burn after treatments but also without a bleaching effect on the tattoo. The outcome was unsatisfactory, and she suffered constant itching and pain when the skin was touched.

Comment
Amateur laser removal with inferior equipment and a too high dose of light poses a burn hazard to the skin, with hemorrhagic bullae followed by scarring. It has the added negative effect that subsequent, qualified treatment with Q-switched laser becomes ineffective due to skin damage from the initial amateur treatment, which was malpractice. The patient had no legal rights and could not bring her case to the court. The amateur parlor continued business as usual.

Treatment
Treatment options were surgical excision and a free transplant; however, dermatome shaving was given a try, followed by potent corticoid and compression bandage for months. Symptoms were relieved and the tattoo flattened, but some sites of pigment deep in the dermis remained. The cosmetic outcome was not satisfactory.

Laser Removal of a Tattoo in an Amateur Setting Causing Laser Burn and a Chronic Papulonodular Reaction

History

The patient wished to remove a black and green tattoo on the arm and received one treatment in a shop not considered professional, offering laser removal for a discount price. The laser instrument was very unlikely to be proper for the purpose. After one treatment she had developed bullous reaction, swelling of the arm, and pain. She was treated in the hospital casualty unit with local treatments. After 10 days, she was still burdened by pain and the remaining local reaction, which had developed into a papulonodular pattern.

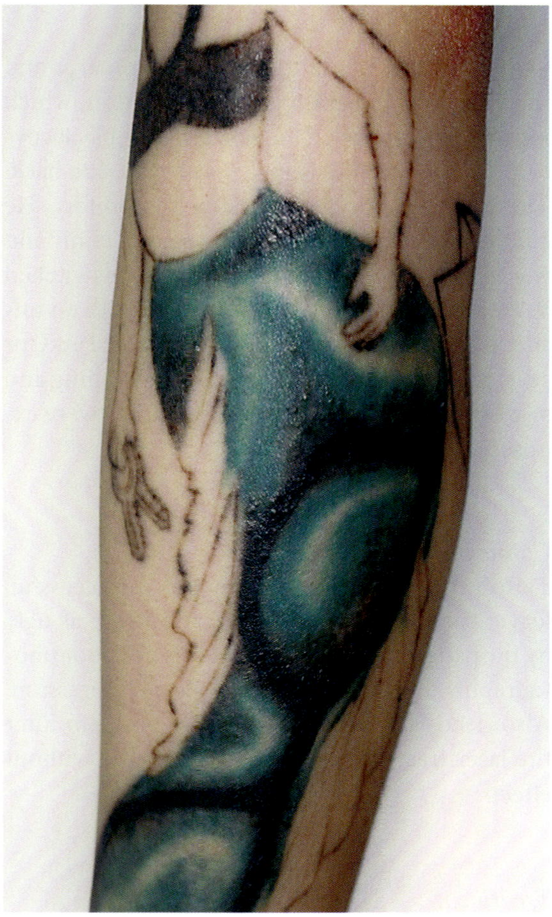

Comment

The subsequent papulonodular reaction following laser burn was prominent in the black-tattooed skin with higher pigment absorbance of light. The reaction in the black color continued and was present after 1 year. The skin subjected to laser burn, fortunately, recovered with only minute local sites with scarring. Black pigment has a special tendency to aggregate in the skin and induce chronic local reaction of the papulonodular type, in this case provoked by laser treatment.

Treatment

Treatment was a local corticoid and observation. A professional laser surgeon who was contacted after the episode found that laser removal with a good outcome could not be predicted. Thus, the patient could not be offered a proper method of removal, taking the size of the tattoo and the color green into consideration.

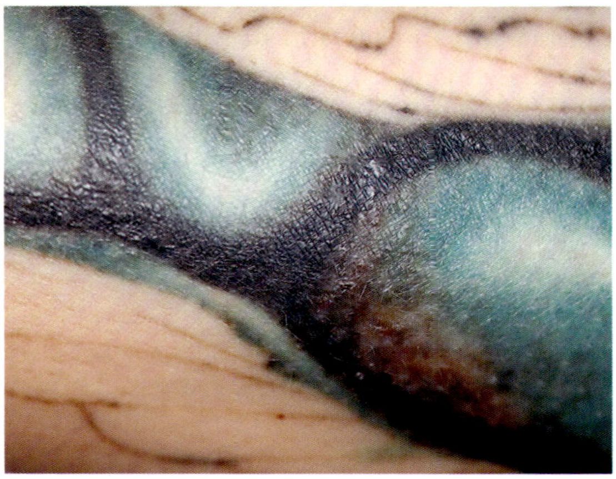

Laser Removal of a Tattoo with Poor Outcome and Followed by Scarring and Urticaria Factitia in the Treated Field

History

Shortly after being tattooed on the forearm and the hand, the patient regretted his tattoo, which illustrated a bird up in the sky. He got a black cover-up tattoo but still wanted his normal skin back. There was no kind of physical discomfort. He contacted a professional tattoo removal clinic and was treated in both tattoos with 9 Q-switched YAG laser treatments, unfortunately with an unsuccessful outcome. During laser removal and for several months after treatment, he felt itching and swelling of the treated tattoos when they were exposed to various physical contacts.

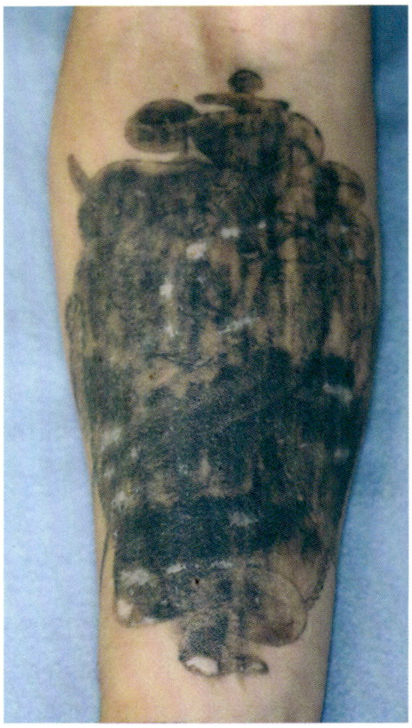

Comment

Tattoo removal by YAG laser was unsuccessful, leaving scars and a disfigured tattoo seen as ugly by the patient. Blurring of photos is not poor photographic focusing but the real visual impression. Also, factitial urticarial became a problem after the laser treatment. Local corticoid was without effect.

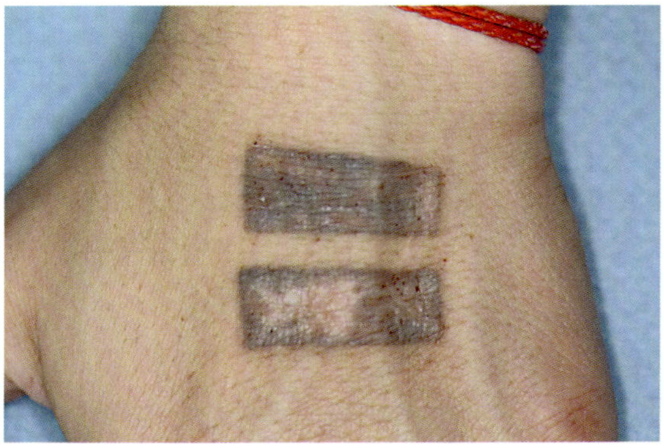

Treatment

Treatment was primarily observation without active therapy. Laser treatment with a fraxel CO_2 laser or dermatome shaving might be considered at a later stage. Excision surgery covered with a transplant was not considered realistic. The patient was warned about future cover-up of the problematic areas.

Tattoo Removal by Laser with Yellow, Green, and Blue Pigment Resistance to Treatment

History

Ten years ago, the patient had acquired a colorful tattoo on his arm. Shortly after the tattoo had been made, he developed severe photosensitivity with major swelling and pain in parts of the tattoo directly exposed to the sun. Sunscreen could not prevent sensitivity reactions. He had a special photoprotective sleeve designed, which he wore in the summertime. A specialist laser surgeon had treated the sun-sensitive sites a number of times and with different lasers, which lessened the patient's intolerance to sun significantly. However, he wanted the pigment remnants to be completely removed.

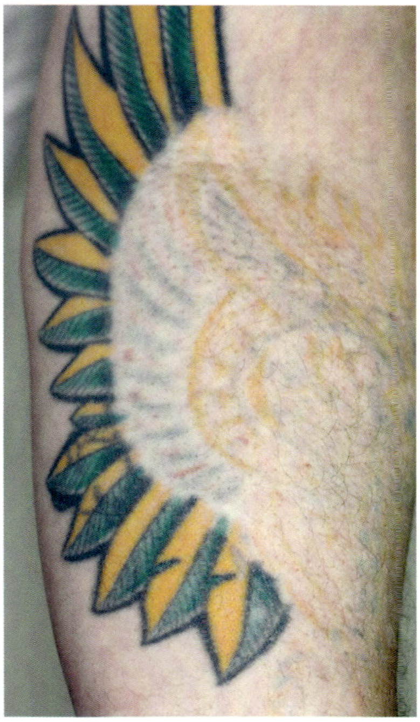

Comment

The colors yellow, green, and blue are difficult if not impossible to remove to perfection with any nonablative laser. The many laser treatments given by the laser specialist had caused remarkably little scarring or dyspigmentation, and hair and skin markings appeared to be untouched. The patient's medical problem, i.e. photosensitivity, had been cured.

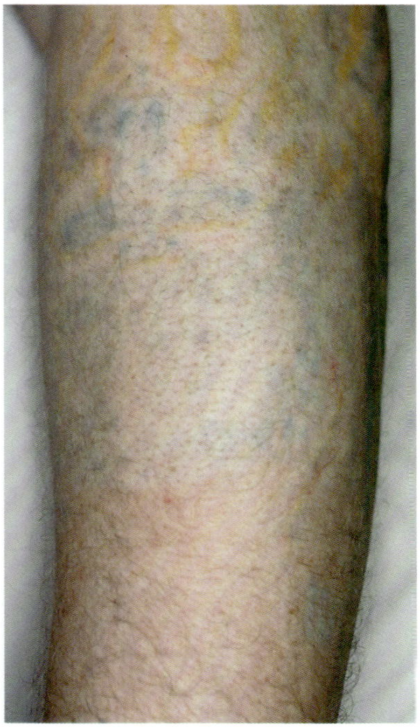

Treatment

Treatment with laser removal had been an efficient cure of photosensitivity. However, the yellow, green, and blue pigments were recalcitrant and beyond eradication by laser.

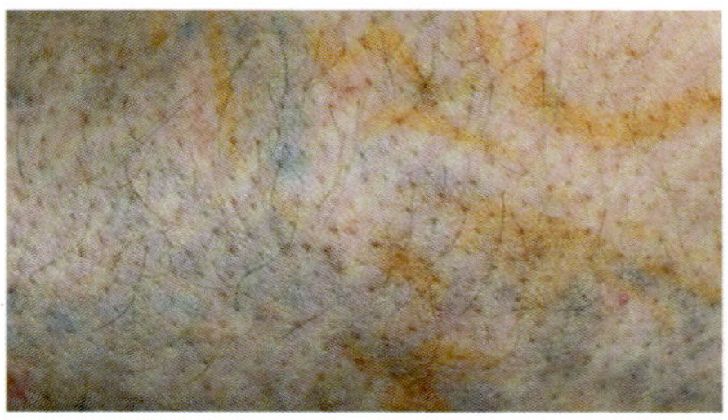

Tattoo Removal by a Caustic Product Causing a Scar

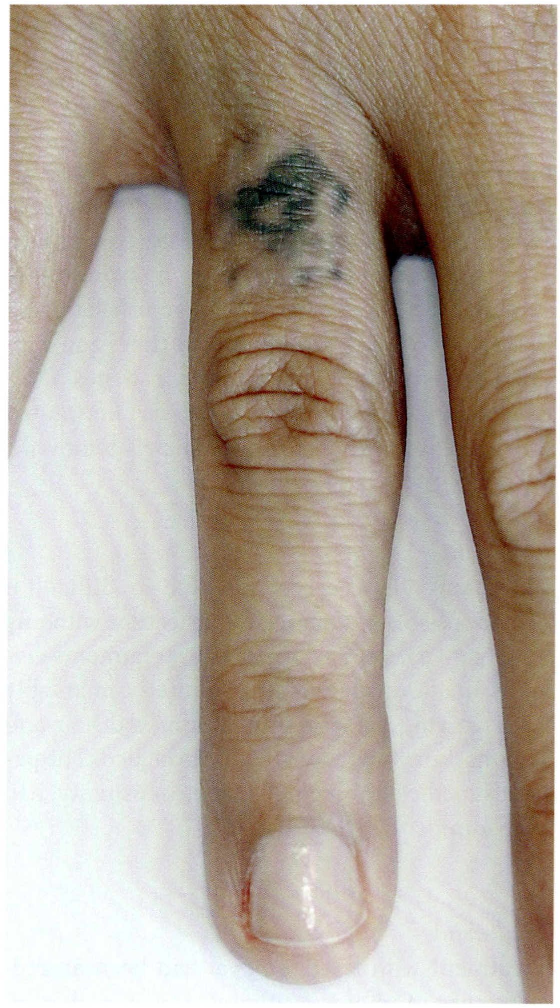

History
The patient had acquired a black tattoo on the ring finger with her boyfriend's initials, which she soon regretted. She received 2 treatments with a caustic product ('Rejuvi'), which is not based on lactic acid. The product is hyperosmolar and contains metal oxides. It is tattooed into the skin in small circles with a tattoo machine. Treatment was followed by caustic wounds and swelling of the entire finger. The tattoo was not removed. The caustic wounds healed but left major scarring. The cosmetic result was unsatisfactory.

Comment
Tattoos were removed with caustics a long time ago. This treatment is nonselective and inevitably and as a mode of action causes necrosis and scarring. General experience over decades shows that strong caustics are very difficult to dose since the response is dependent on the chemical, dosing, anatomical site, individual factors, etc. The dose-effect curve is nonlinear and the therapeutic index narrow or negative. Thus, disfiguring scarring is the typical result. Providers of such treatment are often amateurs and unauthorized. The legal situation of sufferers of malpractice from caustic tattoo removal is very weak.

Treatment
Treatment was surgical excision and plastic operation.

Caustic Tattoo Removal with Lactic Acid Causing a Scar and Psychological Complications

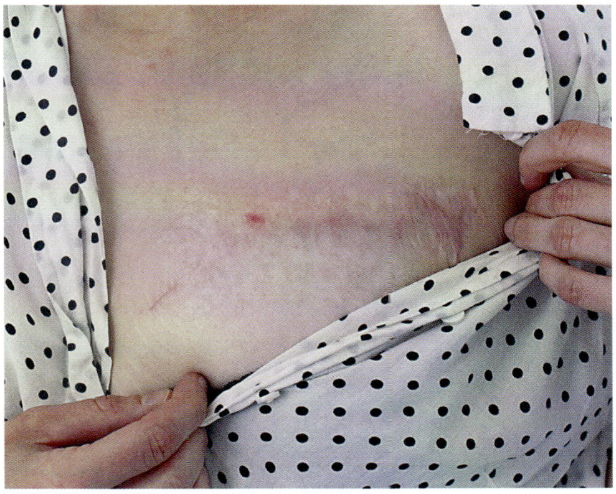

History
The patient had 2 multicolored tattoos, hand sized and symmetrical in the pectoral regions. She regretted the tattoos shortly after they had been acquired. The tattooist had made them much bigger than she had wished. Laser surgeons anticipated complications and did not dare to treat the tattoos. She had 8 treatments with lactic acid ('Tat-2-away') installed by tattoo needle injections in small circular fields scattered in the tattooed skin. The outcome was a caustic wound that healed with major scarring. The patient developed depression and required medication as well as support of a psychologist.

Comment
The scar was a psychological ruin for the patient, who felt that her breasts were destroyed and her self-esteem and sexuality invalidated. She engaged in a long series of treatments as described below, however, with only limited esthetic improvement. Her breasts ended up disfigured and asymmetrical, with an abnormal upwards position of the areola on one side as well as scars. The patient was unhappy with the outcome.

Treatment
Treatments were sequential surgical excisions by plastic surgeons, intralesional corticoid, YAG laser removal of the remnant pigment, and fractional CO_2 laser to modify the scar.

Caustic Tattoo Removal with Lactic Acid Followed by a Disfiguring Scar

History
The patient regretted a tattoo in the pectoral region. The tattoo was uncomplicated except for the regret. Removal with Q-switched laser had been attempted and was given as a treatment course of 7 treatments, which was unsuccessful but not with any clinically significant scarring. The patient tried another advertised method promising good results. He received 1 treatment with lactic acid 40% removal by tattoo needle injections in 5- to 7-mm circular treatment fields scattered in the tattoo field ('Tat-2-Away'). The treatment caused a caustic wound, which healed over about 2 months, leaving the patient with major scarring.

Comment
Injection of lactic acid 40% with a pH of about 3 by tattoo needle injection in the outer dermis is a caustic method that is very difficult to dose and individualize. The treatment principle is caustic burn of dermal tissue and the tattoo pigment, with a dermal wound leaving a scar in every case. The epidermis and the melanocytes are gone, too. Sequential treatment of scattered small circular application fields is the treatment strategy thought to help cosmetically acceptable healing. However, the method is unpredictable and unreliable in preventing disfiguring post-treatment scarring. The treatment is *high risk* with an unsatisfactory therapeutic index.

Treatment
Treatment could not be offered. Intralesional corticoid was attempted but caused telangiectasia. Plastic surgeons denied excisional surgery and correction, and tissue expansion was not an option. Fractional CO_2 laser was not considered applicable. A negative initial experience with Q-switched laser indicated that the tattoo pigment was located too deep in the dermis and out of reach of the laser.

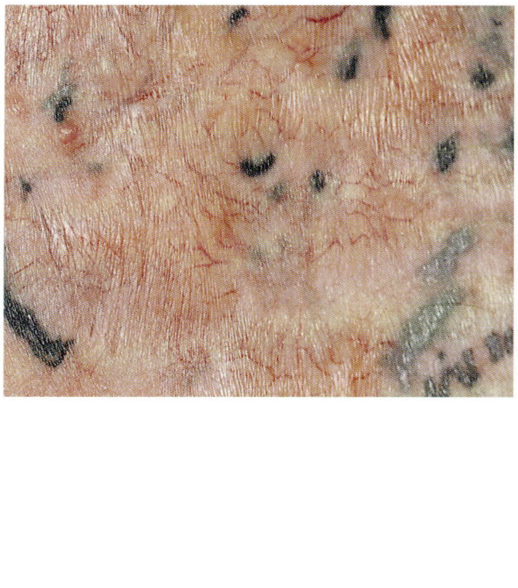

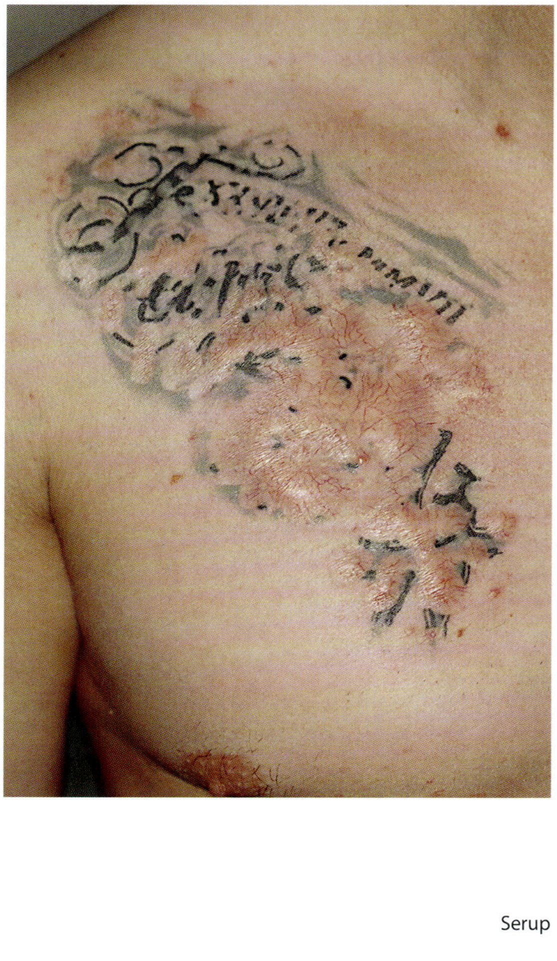

Caustic Tattoo Removal with Lactic Acid in a Person Predisposed to Abnormal Scarring

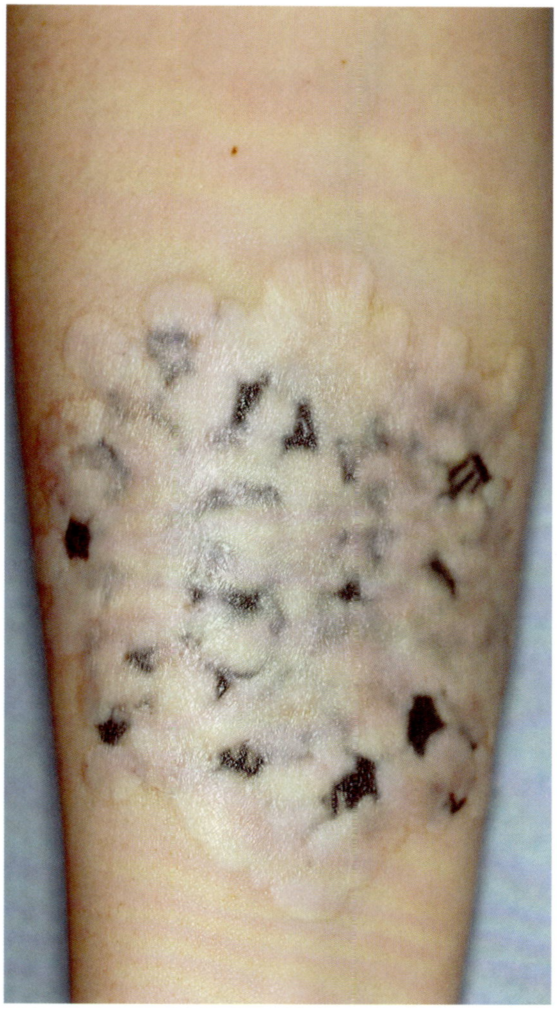

History
Four years ago, the patient regretted a multicolor tattoo on the arm and got a black cover-up tattoo. The result was unsatisfactory, and the patient wished her normal skin back. Over a period of 1 year, she received treatments with lactic acid applied in small circles and injected in the skin with a tattoo needle device ('Tat-2-Away'), made by a nurse and owner of a parlor claiming to be specialized in this treatment. The patient informed the provider that she was prone to abnormal scarring and demonstrated an abdominal scar, which had been corrected by a plastic surgeon. During the course of lactic acid treatments, the patient was told that scarring in the treatment field was 'simply normal'.

Comment
The outcome of tattoo removal with lactic acid, obviously, was highly unsatisfactory. Treatment should never have been instituted. The treatment is allowed in most countries and can be legally practiced by anyone. The patient could not go to the court with her case. Authorities are unable to close the parlor.

Treatment
Treatment could not be offered. The mix of various tattoo pigments deep in the dermis and scarring after caustic burn makes laser removal not applicable in this case. Surgical excision covered with a free transplant is considered despite the patient's predisposition to abnormal scarring.

Author Index

Subject Index